THE TEXTBOOK OF

HEALTH AND SOCIAL CARE

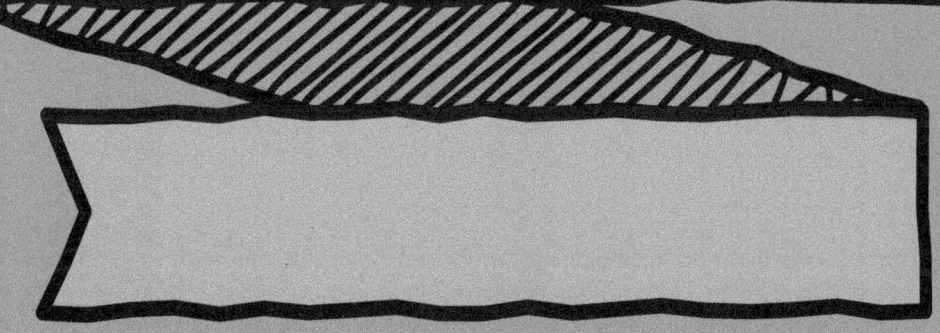

Sara Miller McCune founded SAGE Publishing in 1965 to support the dissemination of usable knowledge and educate a global community. SAGE publishes more than 1000 journals and over 800 new books each year, spanning a wide range of subject areas. Our growing selection of library products includes archives, data, case studies and video. SAGE remains majority owned by our founder and after her lifetime will become owned by a charitable trust that secures the company's continued independence.

Los Angeles | London | New Delhi | Singapore | Washington DC | Melbourne

THE TEXTBOOK of
HEALTH AND
SOCIAL CARE

EDITED BY
DARREN J. EDWARDS
STEPHANIE BEST

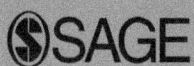

Los Angeles | London | New Delhi
Singapore | Washington DC | Melbourne

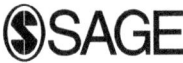

Los Angeles | London | New Delhi
Singapore | Washington DC | Melbourne

SAGE Publications Ltd
1 Oliver's Yard
55 City Road
London EC1Y 1SP

SAGE Publications Inc.
2455 Teller Road
Thousand Oaks, California 91320

SAGE Publications India Pvt Ltd
B 1/I 1 Mohan Cooperative Industrial Area
Mathura Road
New Delhi 110 044

SAGE Publications Asia-Pacific Pte Ltd
3 Church Street
#10-04 Samsung Hub
Singapore 049483

Editor: Alex Clabburn
Assistant editor: Jade Grogan
Production editor: Tanya Szwarnowska
Copyeditor: Neil Dowden
Indexer: Melanie Gee
Marketing manager: George Kimble
Cover design: Wendy Scott
Typeset by: C&M Digitals (P) Ltd, Chennai, India
Printed in the UK

Library of Congress Control Number: 2019949442

British Library Cataloguing in Publication data

A catalogue record for this book is available from the British Library

ISBN 978-1-5264-5909-1
ISBN 978-1-5264-5910-7 (pbk)

At SAGE we take sustainability seriously. Most of our products are printed in the UK using responsibly sourced papers and boards. When we print overseas we ensure sustainable papers are used as measured by the PREPS grading system. We undertake an annual audit to monitor our sustainability.

CONTENTS

ABOUT THE EDITORS

Darren J. Edwards has a PhD in health psychology and is Senior Lecturer in Psychology and Social Policy at Swansea University. He is also a registered Chartered Health Psychologist with the British Psychological Society (BPS). For the last five years he has taught and module led on the Psychology of Health and Illness course as part of the BSc Health & Social Care degree at Swansea, as well as various research methodology courses at MSc level. His research focuses largely on the development of psychological complex interventions such as acceptance and commitment therapy (ACT) for treating anxiety and depression in a variety of populations such as for those living with chronic pain.

Stephanie Best is a health services researcher from the UK now based in Melbourne. She is a Chartered Physiotherapist by background with many years of international clinical and managerial experience. Her PhD undertaken at University of Wales Institute, Cardiff, centred on innovating in health and social care. In 2013 she moved to Swansea University and took up the role of Programme Director for the Masters in Health Care Management. She is a Senior Fellow of the Higher Education Academy. She moved to Australia in 2017 and is now a Senior Research Fellow with Macquarie University and the Murdoch Children's Research Institute. Based with the Australian Genomics Health Alliance, where her focus is implementation of genomic medicine into the Australian health care system, she is engaged with a wide array of implementation projects from community engagement to health systems barriers and enablers to implementation. Other international research activities include ongoing studies focused on integrated teamworking and professional identity in health and social care, with a particular interest in working across professional and organisational boundaries.

ABOUT THE CONTRIBUTORS

Michelle Anderson is a Senior Lecturer working in the College of Human and Health Science. She holds an MSc in Health Promotion (Distinction) from Swansea University, and is a Senior Fellow of the HEA and a qualified nurse. Her research interests include health promotion, public health, health behaviours, health psychology, men's health and occupational stress reduction. Her teaching areas include public health, health promotion and health behaviours.

Sue Bond-Taylor is Senior Lecturer in the School of Social and Political Sciences at the University of Lincoln, where she contributes to the Criminology, Social Policy and Sociology degree programmes. Her research explores the connections between social care provision, crime prevention and youth justice. In particular, her PhD in Social Policy evaluated the use of family intervention services in supporting families with complex needs, in the context of the UK's controversial Troubled Families Programme. Since then, she has developed an interest in how early help approaches can be used to support young people in conflict with the criminal justice system, as well as exploring the potential of community-based strategies for improving the opportunities, well-being and outcomes for vulnerable children and young people. Her research is underpinned by feminist theory, with an emphasis on intersectionality and the ethics of care.

Keith Bradley-Adams (RMN, RNT, MSc, MHSM, PGCE, Cert HMS) graduated as a mental health nurse in Cardiff in 1986. He worked for a year at the University Hospital of Wales as a Staff Nurse before becoming a Charge Nurse in 1987. In 1991 he became a hospital manager within Older Persons Services and enrolled on a management degree with the Institute of Health Service Managers. On completion of this programme he undertook an MSc in Interprofessional Studies at Cardiff University followed (because of a life-long interest in education and continuous professional development) by a PGCE. Although remaining in clinical practice, he utilised this knowledge through teaching within both the health board and Swansea University where he was employed as a visiting lecturer. He moved away from clinical practice into a role within the education department of the local health board in 2007 before becoming a full-time Senior Lecturer at Swansea University in 2009. On joining the university, he became module lead for the Return to Practice module, which enables former NMC registrants to return to nursing. This award-winning course has helped over 300 nurses to return to their vocation during this period. Since 2016 he has been the lead nurse for mental health in Swansea University, managing a team of 11 lecturers. He has written a number of journal articles focusing on mentorship, preceptorship and the transition from student to newly qualified nurse, as well as authoring a chapter on mental health nursing for the world's highest-selling nursing textbook.

Gideon Calder, PhD, is Associate Professor in Sociology at Swansea University, where he directs the Social Policy programme and the Research Institute of Ethics and Law. His current research and teaching interests include co-production, the relationship between care and inequality, and how social justice issues apply to children, and he has written widely on these and other issues. He co-edits the journal *Ethics and Social Welfare*, and is author or editor of ten books, most recently the *Routledge Handbook of the Philosophy of Childhood and Children* (2018).

Hazel M. Chapman is Postgraduate Tutor at the University of Chester, Faculty of Health and Social Care. She is a Registered General and Learning Disabilities Nurse who gained her PhD in the health consultation experience for people with learning disabilities. She has also studied nurses' attitudes of respect in interactions with service users, developing a teaching tool to help student nurses manage challenging situations. She uses her degree in psychology and her research experience to teach across undergraduate nursing first-year psychology and biology, second-year evidence-based practice, and master's and doctoral level research methods in health and social care, as well as supervising postgraduate student research. She is currently engaged in exploring the service-user experience of acute psychiatric care interventions and developing an inclusive training programme for people with learning disabilities who wish to study, facilitate learning and co-research at the University.

Charlotte Chisnell is a Senior Lecturer in Social Work at the Eastern Institute of Technology, New Zealand. She has been involved in social work education for the past 15 years. She previously worked as a social worker with children and families and youth justice. Her research interests include safeguarding, promoting rights and social justice.

Ceryl Davies is a qualified solicitor and social worker, with a PhD in Social Policy. She has extensive practice-based experience across social care, criminal justice and learning disability services, including work on a multi-agency basis to support children, young people and vulnerable adults at practitioner, middle- and senior-management level. She has taught at undergraduate and postgraduate level across several disciplines, including education, law, criminology and social work degrees. Her research interests are focused on exploring the nature of young people's intimate relationships, domestic abuse, child to parent/carer violence and abuse, healthy relationships and youth justice matters. Her research is underpinned by feminist theory and Goffman's ideas on the presentation of self, shame and stigma.

Andrew Dunning (MA, BA Hons, CQSW, PGCHE, FHEA) is a Senior Lecturer in Social Policy at Swansea University. He previously worked as a social worker, advocacy scheme co-ordinator, policy researcher, deputy director of a national voluntary organisation and associate director of the Better Government for Older People programme. He is founder of the Older People's Advocacy Alliance (OPAAL) UK and is a current member of the Disability Wales Disability Research on Independent Living and Learning (DRILL) advisory group and the Welsh Assembly Cross-Party Groups on Older People and Ageing and the Human Rights Stakeholder Group. He is a member of the editorial board of *The Journal of Adult Protection*. He has published widely on advocacy, disability and ageing issues. His undergraduate teaching currently includes disability policy, advocacy, rights and representation, and the principles of social policy. He also undertakes postgraduate gerontological teaching on citizenship, participation and older people. His current research interests include power and participation, human rights and advocacy, disability and dementia, and critical social gerontology. He has lived experience of mental distress and services.

Ashley Frawley is a sociologist and Senior Lecturer in Sociology and Social Policy at Swansea University. She teaches modules in the Sociology of Health and Illness on the BSc Health and Social Care degree at Swansea. Her research focuses on the construction of social problems and in particular their growing medicalisation and emotionalisation. She is the author of *Semiotics of Happiness: Rhetorical Beginnings of a Public Problem*.

Benny Goodman is an independent scholar with an MSc in Nursing. He was formerly a lecturer and Registered Nurse with the School of Nursing and Midwifery at the University of Plymouth. He has written and co-written a number of articles and textbooks focusing on the social sciences and sustainability in health. The politics and the sociology of health are core interests rooted in critical social theory.

Pete Hanratty is a study skills lecturer at Swansea University with ten years' experience in writing and delivering sessions for students from a range of academic disciplines. He works mainly with Health and Social Care students across the range of levels in higher education. His research interests include communication and rhetoric, and he is currently pursuing a PhD in these areas.

Caroline Kelly is a Senior Lecturer in Social Work and Course Leader for the MA Social Work at Teesside University. She qualified as a social worker at the University of Edinburgh, achieving an MA in Social Work and a CQSW. Her social work background spans across adults and children, but particularly people with learning disabilities, people with mental health problems and older people. Interests include achieving service improvements in safeguarding adults, anti-discriminatory practice and inclusion.

Pete King has a PhD in Childhood Studies and is currently the Programme Director for the MA Developmental and Therapeutic Play and MA Childhood Studies courses at Swansea University. He has been published in journals both nationally and internationally on children's play, and has co-edited and co-authored books on research and play theory. His most recent publication is *Researching Play from a Playwork Perspective* and *The Play Cycle: Theory, Research and Application.* His professional background is in playwork and childcare where as a practitioner, trainer and development officer/manager he has been involved in children's play within the statutory and third (voluntary) sector in both England and Wales. He has contributed to the development of playwork and childcare strategy, education and training. He is also an advocate for children's rights, in particular Article 31 of the United National Convention on the Rights of the Child (UNCRC), children's right to play. His current research includes playworkers' and childcare workers' understanding of the play cycle.

John Knight is Associate Professor in Biomedical Science within the College of Human and Health Sciences at Swansea University. For the last 20 years he has taught anatomy, physiology and pathophysiology on a wide variety of professional degree and diploma programmes including health and social care, paramedic science, nursing and midwifery. His first degree is in microbiology; additionally, he holds a PhD in immunology and has over 50 published articles in peer-reviewed journals. His teaching at Swansea University has recently been recognised by the presentation of a Distinguished Teaching Award. He has a variety of research interests including the use of maggots and their secretions to promote wound healing, the physiological effects of ageing and the use of virtual reality simulations in the teaching of anatomy and physiology.

Tracey Maegusuku-Hewett has worked in health and social care since leaving school. Initially she was a support worker and state registered nurse with people with learning disabilities. She later trained as a professional social worker, practising primarily within the voluntary sector with children, young people and families. She has worked in social work education since 2007. She completed her PhD on the subject of UK Immigration Policy and the Welfare of Children Seeking Asylum in Wales. Her research interests include the welfare and rights of children and young people.

Ben Martin is a freelance writer and study skills lecturer at Swansea University, where he has spent more than seven years developing courses and materials to help students become better writers. He is a Fellow of the Higher Education Academy and has an MA in Creative Writing. His research interests include creativity and learning.

Llewellyn Morgan is a Nursing & Midwifery Council registered children's nurse and school nurse. He is employed as a lecturer in children's nursing at Swansea University. His professional expertise relates to safeguarding children, public health nursing and health promotion practice, and he lectures in these areas amongst other children's nursing specific subjects. He has particular research interests related to safeguarding children, including father's perspectives and experiences within this. He holds a Master's Degree in Advanced Practice (Child Health) awarded by Cardiff University. Prior to becoming a lecturer in 2017, he was employed as a Specialist Community Public Health Nurse in School Nursing in South East Wales. During this period, he worked across health, education and social care boundaries, and in partnership with all professionals in these areas, thus developing a keen insight into the challenges and priorities of the health and social care fields, through the lens of a public health professional.

Julia Parkhouse (LLB (Hons), PgDip LP, PGCert Ed for Health Professionals, RMN, EN(M), FHEA) is a Senior Lecturer at Swansea University. She initially trained as an Enrolled Nurse (Mental Health) prior to being one of the first enrolled nurses to undertake a conversion course, qualifying as a Registered Mental Health Nurse (RMN) in 1989. With steady career progression, she became ward manager at a local psychiatric hospital working in adult acute care. Caring for patients subject to the provisions of the Mental Health Act 1983 led to her developing an interest in the law. She undertook further education where she gained a first class honours degree in Law (LLB (Hons)) and a Postgraduate Diploma in Legal Practice at Cardiff University. She secured a training contract and qualified as a solicitor in 2006 specialising in private practice in mental health law (becoming a member of the Law Society Mental Health Law Panel) and child care law going on to join the local authority where she worked as a senior child care lawyer. She maintained her nursing registration throughout her career and was able to draw on all her nursing and legal professional experience when she joined Swansea University in 2015. She teaches health care law across a number of modules to both undergraduate and postgraduate students on professional and non-professional programmes (including health and social care, midwifery, nursing, paramedic science, physician associate studies, graduate entry medicine and osteopathy). As part of her role at Swansea University, she also teaches professionals at local health boards on a range of legal topics (including documentation, the Mental Capacity Act and deprivation of liberty safeguards). In terms of research, her interests include mental health law, mental capacity law and child protection law.

Sally Riggall is a Senior Lecturer at the University of Lincoln in the School of Health and Social Care (since 2005) where she teaches communication skills, counselling, and professional skills to undergraduate and postgraduate students. She gained an MSc in Counselling from the University of Hull in 1996. Her professional background is in counselling and for many years she trained professional counsellors in further education colleges. She is an experienced counsellor and previously worked in the public sector with doctors' patients and local authority employees. She teaches reflective practice to students across a range of programmes, including counselling, health and social care, and social work. Her research interest is in how the Egan Skilled Helper model can assist social workers and other professionals in placing service users at the centre of decision-making.

Angela Smith (LLB (Hons), LLM, FHEA) is a Senior Lecturer within the College of Human and Health Sciences at Swansea University. Having initially worked in the banking industry, she later achieved a 1st Class Honours in Law in 2003 before completing her PGCE (FE) (Distinction) at Cardiff University. She obtained a master's degree (LLM) at Bristol University and is currently in the final year of her master's degree in Ethics and Social Policy at Cardiff University. Prior to joining Swansea University, she taught in further education through the medium of video conferencing. Currently she teaches on a variety of modules, including teaching undergraduate and postgraduate students on professional and non-professional programmes including Health and Social Care, Nursing, Paramedic Science, Osteopathy, Physician Associate Studies and Graduate Entry Medicine on a range of legal and ethical topics (e.g. law on consent, equality, principles of medical ethics). She also teaches professionals at local health boards on a range of topics (including documentation, the Mental Capacity Act and deprivation of liberty safeguards). She is Chair of the Research Ethics Committee within the College of Human and Health Sciences. Her research interests include law and reproduction, do not resuscitate orders and mental capacity.

Hugh Upton studied philosophy at University College London and lectured in London and St Andrews before moving to Swansea University. His doctoral thesis was on moral theory and applied philosophy, and he lectures on philosophy as well as on applied ethics in the context of medicine, nursing and social care. His research interests are mainly in ethics, currently in the areas of truth-telling and lying.

EDITORS' ACKNOWLEDGEMENTS

The authors would like to thank Ms Julie Burton, University of Lincoln and Dr Jan Lewis, Swansea University, for their help in developing the book.

This textbook originated in Swansea University and Stephanie Best moved to Australia as the book was developing. Stephanie would like to thank the Australian Institute of Health Innovation, Macquarie University in Sydney and the Murdoch Children's Research Institute, Melbourne, for their support while completing this book.

PUBLISHER'S ACKNOWLEDGEMENTS

On behalf of the editors and contributors, the publisher would like to thank the academic reviewers whose comments and insight helped to shape the book into the comprehensive resource it is now.

Many thanks to:

Claire Bellamy, Manchester Metropolitan University

Sarah Burch, Anglia Ruskin University

Julie Burton, University of Lincoln

Yolanda Eraso, London Metropolitan University

Ceri Anwen Jones, Liverpool John Moores University

Joanne Smith, University of Bolton

INTRODUCTION

Darren J. Edwards and Stephanie Best

Health and social care refers to the services which are available from health and social care providers in the UK, and includes the whole of health care and social care provision and infrastructure, public and private. People involved in the delivery of health and social care include doctors, nurses, social workers, physiotherapists, counsellors, carers, play workers, psychotherapists and paramedics, to name just a few.

Topics covered within the study of health and social care typically include illness and treatment, nutrition, childcare, study of public health, campaigns, policy, effects of smoking, poor diet, lack of exercise and poor mental health. Given this is the fundamental study of the entire national health and social care provision, studying health and social care today is extremely important. The subject area is diverse and multidisciplinary, incorporating, for example, sociology, psychology, policy-making and health care professions, as well as law and ethics. The potential career options for those studying health and social care are broad and you may find your ideas on your future career direction changing as you gain more knowledge in different areas as your course progresses.

This textbook on health and social care offers a broad overview of the central topics within the discipline and has been developed primarily for university students studying a BSc in Health and Social Care. However, the chapters here are likely to be useful for a range of other programmes such as sociology, psychology, social policy, medical and social science courses, and other health care practitioner degree subjects. The book may also serve as an introduction for many postgraduate-level students.

This textbook has been designed to be interactive and each chapter has a series of participatory activities to help you apply the reading. These include (but vary for each chapter):

- **Pause for Thought**, where you will be encouraged to stop and think about how you could use the information provided in the chapter;
- **Case Studies**, which will include a real life example related to the chapter content (you will be able to look up further information about the case study if it is an area of particular interest to you);
- **Activities**, where you will be invited to complete a task to cement your learning;
- **Go Further Activities**, where the author will make some suggestions as to how you can deepen your learning and understanding; and
- **Further Reading and Useful Websites**, which include the author's own reflections on key sites and readings for the chapter subject.

Answers to some of the activities are highlighted in the activity boxes themselves, and can be found at the end of each chapter. You will find a different selection of activities in each of the chapters; some chapters are very activity heavy such as Chapter 3 on 'Academic Skills and Practice', while others may encourage you to reflect more. All of the chapters will have at least four or five opportunities for you to undertake one or other of the activities.

The textbook is broken down into three sections: (1) 'Underpinning Knowledge'; (2) 'Health and Social Care in Action'; and (3) 'Contemporary Topics'. The first section, 'Underpinning Knowledge', introduces you to some of the essential areas you will need to understand as you start your health and social care studies. There are a wide range of topics in this section with the first chapter, 'Sociology of Health and Illness', covering health and illness from a sociological perspective. Key concepts from the sociology of health and illness are introduced, beginning with an exploration of the 'sociological imagination' and the importance of 'context' to understanding human social life. The second chapter, 'Psychology of Health and Illness', relates to the psychology of health and illness, and introduces the principal topics of health psychology, illness representation and the limitations of the biomedical model in dealing with psychological disorders. The third chapter, 'Academic Skills and Practice', will explain some of the essential skills (through five core principles) you will need to succeed in the academic element of your Health and Social Care degree. The fourth chapter, 'The Research Process in Health and Social Care', is an introduction to research, which gives insight into the research process within a health and social care context, and explains how research is important for all types of professional practice to support both policy and practice. The next two chapters, 'The Law Relating to Health and Social Care: Introduction to Key Principles' and 'The Law Relating to Health and Social Care: Further Key Principles', provide some discussion of some key legal and ethical issues that occur in the area of health and social care in modern society, including some controversial areas such as abortion, in vitro fertilisation (IVF), surrogacy, dementia care and end of life issues. The seventh chapter, 'Reflective Practice and Critical Thinking', focuses on reflective practice and explores some of the core attributes that are necessary to a health and social care professional on their journey to becoming a skilled, intuitive, reflective practitioner; for example how well we understand how our upbringing, background and unconscious processes have shaped our views. The last chapter in this section, 'Physiological Effects of Ageing in the Older Adult', relates to the normal physiological effects of ageing in older adults, exploring the current knowledge of how ageing affects the anatomy and physiology of the human body, examining how ageing can predispose older people to a variety of age-related diseases.

The second section, 'Health and Social Care in Action', highlights a variety of different aspects of health and social care in practice. There are six chapters and the first, 'Safeguarding Children and Adults', aims to provide students of health and social care and related studies with a foundational knowledge of safeguarding children and adults in the United Kingdom (UK). The second chapter, 'Childcare in the UK', centres on childcare provision and considers the role of childcare within a health and social care context. The chapter explores how childcare practice has had to change in relation to the introduction of statutory legislation reflecting changes in the societal role of children. The next chapter, 'Health Promotion and Health Psychology', explores various psychological theories, models and approaches to behavioural ideation, intention and change, through the context of promoting healthy behaviour and positive behaviour change. Chapter 12, 'Children's Rights and Participation', relates to working with children and young people, and will provide insight into factors that hinder or promote children's participation, for example in the decision-making process. Chapters 13 and 14, 'Working with People Experiencing Mental Health Disorder: Mental Health Conditions' and 'Determinants of Poor Mental Health and the Road to Recovery', relate to working with people with mental illness, addressing mental health conditions and determinants respectively. These chapters cover mental illness as a societal problem, and the difficulty many who have not experienced mental ill-health or do not know someone with mental ill-health have in differentiating between the terms mental illness and mental health.

In the final section, 'Contemporary Topics', eight chapters consider some of the challenges faced in present-day health and social care. The first, 'Using and Developing Evidence in Health and Social Care Practice', relates to current perspectives on evidence-based practice and making sense of the evidence which will outline the processes of developing evidence-based practice and carrying out research. It will also highlight the similarities and differences between the two. Chapter 16, 'Leadership and Management', will open by considering what is leadership and management and what their relevance is in contemporary health and social care. The debate around leadership and management will be explored and, in the age of populist leaders, the need to consider theory will be discussed. Chapter 17, 'Legal and Ethical Considerations in Health and Social Care', will focus on providing discussion of some key legal and ethical issues that occur in the area of health and social care in modern society. Chapter 18, 'Equity, Intersectionality and Anti-Oppressive Practice', will provide the reader with an introduction to the key issues relating to equity, intersectionality and anti-oppressive practice as a starting point for their professional development. Chapter 19, 'Social Justice Issues in Health and Social Care', relates to care and social justice and considers questions that apply to issues in health and social care, such as: What should citizens be entitled to? What do they owe each other? How should they expect to be treated? Chapter 20, 'Disability Policy and Provision in Health and Social Care', relates to disability policy and provision in health and social care and explores key concepts, including policy and provision in health and social care with regard to disabled people in the UK. It begins by scoping out disability followed by a discussion of historical responses of the state towards people with impairments and a brief outline of the policy across the four nations of the UK. The final chapter of this section, 'Health Inequalities', relates to inequalities, and outlines the influence of the wider determinants of health on life expectancy and years of good health such as social, economic, policy, housing, education, employment and access to health services.

Of course, we are not able to cover each and every area in health and social care as the area is vast, and a SAGE textbook could be devoted to each chapter in order to do this subject area justice. However, we hope this textbook provides you with a useful resource and introductory overview of the fascinating area of health and social care. You will have ample opportunity to explore areas of particular interest to you using the activities in the book and through discussion with your colleagues and lecturers. We trust this textbook will help you all the way through your Health and Social Care BSc course and into your future career.

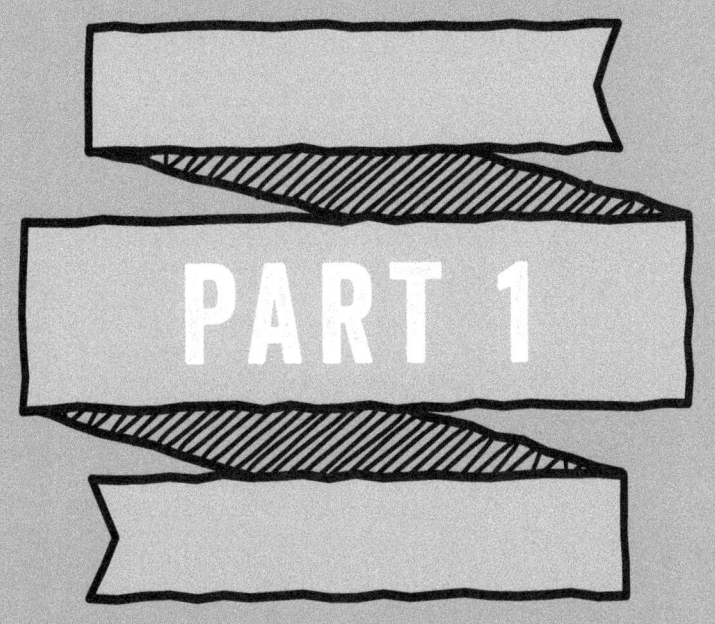

PART 1

UNDERPINNING KNOWLEDGE

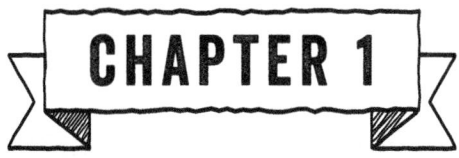

SOCIOLOGY OF HEALTH AND ILLNESS

Ashley Frawley

OVERVIEW

This chapter introduces the sociology of health and illness, first by considering the meaning of the 'sociological imagination' and associated importance of the concept of *context* to understanding human social life. It then discusses three contexts of health: socio-economic, institutional/professional and cultural. Within these contexts a number of key issues in the sociology of health and illness are considered: the social determinants of health, health inequalities, challenges to medical authority, social construction and health panics, medicalisation and growing cultural preoccupations with health risks.

LEARNING OUTCOMES

By the end of this chapter you will be able to:

- Define the 'sociological imagination' and its relationship to the concept of context
- Discuss the relationship between socio-economic context and health inequalities
- Critically examine different explanations of health inequalities
- Discuss several developments argued to indicate the decline of medical authority
- Explain and apply theories of social construction and medicalisation to think critically about health risks and panics

INTRODUCTION

Health and illness may seem solely individual matters. However, sociologists draw attention to social patterns in health and illness, seeking to situate our experiences and beliefs within broader social, historical and cultural contexts. This chapter introduces key concepts from the sociology of health and illness, beginning with an exploration of the 'sociological imagination' and importance of 'context' to understanding human social life. First, we examine socio-economic contexts of health in relation to social determinants and health inequalities. The context of health care professions is then considered with attention to changing professional relationships as well as challenges to medical authority. Introducing social constructionism, the cultural context of health is explored with reference to medicalisation, moral panics and risk.

THE SOCIOLOGICAL IMAGINATION

A wide-ranging discipline, sociological studies span examinations of everyday social interactions through to global social processes (Giddens and Sutton, 2017). American sociologist C. Wright Mills famously described the ideal mindset of the social scientist as the 'sociological imagination' or the ability to grasp 'history and biography and the relations between the two' (Mills, 2000, p. 6). This outlook connects personal troubles to public issues, seeing individual problems as intimately tied to broader social structures like institutions, social divisions (e.g. class), and the economic system as a whole. Sociology is thus about delineating the social forces that affect ordinary lives (Dunn, 2018, p. 38).

For the sociological imagination, context is key to understanding human social life. Among animals, human beings are relatively unique in being born with comparatively little instinct. What it means to be human is fundamentally different depending on how our societies are organised at particular places and times. Even the most intimate aspects of personal experience like fear, hatred, love and rage can only be fully understood within the 'social context in which they are experienced and expressed' (Mills, 2000, pp. 161–162). Thus, the sociological imagination is above all an injunction to appreciate the deeply contextual nature of human experience.

But what is context? Erving Goffman described context as a 'frame' surrounding social phenomena that allows something to be understood (Goodwin and Duranti, 1992, p. 4). Context may be the immediate facts necessary to understand 'what is going on', for instance a doctor–patient consultation versus a conversation between two strangers on the street. Another level may be institutional context, such as the organisation of the National Health Service (NHS) or a private health care system. Intelligibility may also depend on cultural context. Culture refers to prevailing norms and values, where norms are expected and accepted ways of behaving and values more abstract beliefs about what is worthwhile. As Giddens et al. (2017, p. 3) summarise:

> Sociology teaches us that what we regard as natural, inevitable, good, or true may not be such and that the 'givens' of our life—including things we assume to be genetic or biological—are strongly influenced by historical, cultural, social, and even technological forces. Understanding the subtle yet complex and profound ways in which our individual lives reflect the contexts of our social experience is central to the sociological outlook.

In other words, thinking like a sociologist involves critically examining taken for granted assumptions about the world, adopting a range of historical, structural and cross-cultural approaches to do so.

THE SOCIO-ECONOMIC CONTEXT OF HEALTH

One of medical sociology's key contributions is the situation of health outcomes within a broader socio-economic context. This perspective, known as the social determinants of health, draws attention to the 'conditions in which people are born, grow, live, work and age' which are 'shaped by the distribution of money, power and resources at global, national and local levels' (WHO, 2019). These might include (but are not limited to):

- Education
- Housing
- Employment status
- Income
- Social class
- Gender
- Ethnicity

Inequalities in these areas can lead to health inequalities, or disparities in health between advantaged and disadvantaged groups.

Growing attention to social determinants of health and health inequalities arose from criticisms of health policy dating at least to the 1970s. Critics argued that too much research and expenditure had focused on individuals and illnesses and not enough on the broader social context producing ill-health, nor the factors involved in keeping people well. For instance, McKeown (1976a, 1976b) studied centuries of mortality records in England and Wales, arguing socio-economic improvements and public health measures had done more to improve population health than technological advancement. Thus, critics argued greater attention be paid to social policy and the effects of social factors like poverty rather than treatment of disease solely within health care settings.

Since the 1970s, systematic research and review have tended to reproduce the finding that while the overall health of people living in developed countries has improved, there remain strong and persistent inequalities in morbidity and mortality both within and between countries (Acheson, 1998; Marmot, 2015; Marmot et al., 2010; Pickett and Wilkinson, 2015; Townsend and Davidson, 1982; Whitehead, 1987). The World Health Organization (2017) collects facts on global health *inequities*, or unjust differences in health status or access to services:

- 16,000 children die every day before their fifth birthday, with those in the poorest 20 per cent of households nearly twice as likely to die than those in the richest 20 per cent.
- 99 per cent of maternal deaths around the world occur in developing countries. The lifetime risk of maternal death in Chad is 1 in 16; in Sweden it is less than 1 in 10,000.
- Wide gaps in life expectancy exist between countries. Life expectancy in Sierra Leone is 50 years; in Japan it is 84.
- Within countries and even cities large disparities exist. Travelling east from Westminster, each London tube stop represents nearly a year in lost life expectancy.

Growing recognition of health inequalities in the UK is frequently traced to the Report of the Working Group on Inequalities in Health, widely known as the Black Report (Townsend and Davidson, 1982). Commissioned in 1977, it confirmed growing suspicions that while there had been substantial improvements in health overall, there remained substantial disparities in morbidity and mortality between the richest and poorest groups in society. While the NHS was free at the point of use, it had not reduced health inequalities. Indeed, in some key areas, like infant mortality, gaps had widened. The authors made a series of recommendations including better health monitoring, setting national health goals, expanded services, taxation and benefits changes, and restrictions on advertising and sale of tobacco.

The report was not received well. While commissioned by a Labour government, the committee reported in 1980 to a recently elected Conservative government. In a dismissive foreword, Patrick Jenkin, then Social Services Secretary, wrote that altering such 'deep rooted' health inequalities would require spending on a scale 'quite unrealistic in present or any foreseeable economic circumstances' (Jenkin, 1982, p. 16). In an apparent suppression, the report was issued as 250 photocopies on a Bank Holiday Monday. Regardless, interest was piqued and subsequent reports, notably the Acheson Report (Acheson, 1998) and Marmot Review (Marmot et al., 2010) have continued to highlight significant health gaps between rich and poor in the UK. Attention has also been drawn to factors like ethnicity, gender, housing and geography which bear strong relationships to morbidity and mortality (Bartley, 2017). While Margaret Thatcher's Conservatives seemed reluctant to embrace the notion of health inequalities, subsequent governments have affirmed their importance and attention to social determinants of health has been a key aspect of the public health agenda in ensuing decades. Still, government policies, most notably the imposition of austerity measures after the 2008 financial crisis, may have exacerbated health inequalities. Some researchers argue that we are seeing the return in Western countries of 'absolute poverty', or the inability to meet basic needs such as clothing, food and decent housing (Davis and Geiger, 2017; Riches and Silvasti, 2014). Food insecurity and associated health implications, exemplified by growing use of food banks offering mainly processed foods, is a key case in point (Garthwaite et al., 2015).

ACTIVITY 1.1

Read the following article which appeared in the UK newspaper *The Independent* in 2016: www.independent.co.uk/life-style/health-and-families/healthy-living/the-real- state-of-living-below-the-poverty-line-in-britain-a7484621.html and answer the following questions:

1   What is 'relative income poverty' and how is it calculated? How is this different from absolute poverty?
2   What is 'social exclusion'?
3   Are all of those living on the poverty line unemployed?
4   What factors have increased the threat of poverty since 2010?
5   What is the average household income of those helped by charitable organisations mentioned in the article? Think about your average monthly costs and/or that of your family. What difficulties would a family of four face on this income?

Check the end of the chapter for an answer to this activity.

CAUSES OF HEALTH INEQUALITIES

Considerable debate has focused on causes of health inequalities. Following the Black Report's publication, critics questioned whether the apparent health gradient was simply an artefact of the measurements and definitions of class utilised in the report (e.g. Illsley, 1986). However, subsequent research employing a variety of definitions and measures reproduced its essential findings. Early debate also questioned the direction of causation. That is, while poorer health outcomes may correlate with social class, this does not necessarily mean social class causes ill health. Unhealthy people may experience downward mobility while healthy people move up, leaving those suffering poorer health accumulated in lower classes. Longitudinal studies have attempted to parse out causation revealing complex relationships between health, social mobility and social class (Bartley, 2017; Bartley and Plewis, 2002; Goldblatt, 1989). However, health-related social mobility does not fully account for health disparities across social classes and longer-term debate has centred on the relative importance of material inequalities, lifestyle and psychosocial factors.

MATERIAL EXPLANATIONS

Material or structural explanations of health inequalities point to the significance of the social, political and economic context for people's health. Factors emphasised include poor housing, unemployment, living and working conditions, transport, nutrition, and environmental and occupational hazards. This explanation was favoured in the Black Report which suggested, 'much [...] can only be understood in terms of the more diffuse consequences of class structure: poverty, work conditions [...] and deprivation in its various forms' (Townsend and Davidson, 1982, p. 207). While any one factor like education or poor housing may contribute modestly to health outcomes, a lifetime accumulation of disadvantage can produce significant health disparities (Smith et al., 2016). From this perspective, material improvements in people's lives will have the most impact on health.

LIFESTYLE EXPLANATIONS

Lifestyle or 'behavioural' explanations recognise the social gradient in morbidity and mortality but explain these as the result of 'lifestyle choices'. There is considerable evidence that poor diet, lack of exercise and risky behaviours such as smoking tend to be more prevalent amongst socio-economically disadvantaged groups. In its 'stronger' orientation, this perspective explains health inequalities entirely individualistically, resulting from ignorance, recklessness or fatalism (Asthana and Halliday, 2006, p. 26). From this perspective, improvements will come from encouraging people to adopt healthier lifestyles. It is worth noting the Black Report explicitly referenced such explanations but dismissed them as incapable of fully explaining health inequalities. Nonetheless, policy-makers have been receptive to variations of this explanation for a variety of reasons. With material inequalities stubbornly resistant to change and costly hi-tech treatments making little headway against some diseases, health promotion and prevention offer apparently simple and cost-effective solutions (Wainwright, 2008).

Nonetheless, this perspective has been subject to criticism. Studies linking lifestyle risks and ill health often lack scientific rigour, with correlations treated causally and confounding variables (factors that might better explain a relationship) not accounted for. Critics claimed people are not simply morally feckless or irresponsible. For instance, Graham (1987) studied smoking among low-income mothers who used it as a coping mechanism as they struggled to care for children and make ends meet. Choices are often constrained by financial and geographical barriers to accessing healthy food (see, e.g., Caraher et al., 2010; Morris et al., 2014). Recognition of peer pressure and difficulties associated with overcoming addiction have led to approaches aiming to encourage healthier choices, for instance through raising self-esteem or providing nicotine patches (Wainwright, 2008). However, less research focuses on cultural factors involved in lifestyle choices, the role of free will, the comparative value attributed to health between different groups, and the potential for rational trade-offs between short-term pleasure and long-term health.

PSYCHOSOCIAL EXPLANATIONS

Clearly, serious poverty is detrimental to health. However, as living standards have improved across all social classes, inequalities have remained. The psychosocial explanation makes sense of this by considering the psychological impacts of social inequality. A key moment for this explanation was publication of the Whitehall Studies of British civil servants (Marmot et al., 1978; Marmot et al.,

1991) which found strong associations between employment grade and morbidity and mortality. Since the groups being studied were not suffering absolute poverty, it followed hierarchical position must determine health outcomes. The stress of subordinate status and low job control were posited as potential explanations (Marmot et al., 1991). The thesis that stress, status hierarchies and health are intimately linked is closely associated with social epidemiologist Richard Wilkinson. In an impactful book published in 2009, Wilkinson and Pickett argued more egalitarian nations produced healthier populations and fewer social problems generally (Wilkinson and Pickett, 2010). Advocating this explanation, the Equality Trust (2012) summarises:

> Researchers sometimes disagree about the pathways leading from inequality to worse population health. The most consistent interpretation of all the evidence is that the main route hinges on the way inequality makes life more stressful. Chronic stress is known to affect the cardiovascular and immune systems and to lead to more rapid aging. Inequality makes social relations more stressful by increasing status differences and status competition. These effects are important: Americans living in more equal states live around 4 years longer than those living in more unequal states.

However, this explanation has been controversial. For instance, Wilkinson and Pickett (2010) highlight countries supporting their thesis, downplaying contrary evidence (Nettleton, 2013). Critics accuse opponents of singling out primate species showing increased stress among lower-ranking animals while ignoring primates for whom the opposite is true (Lynch et al., 2004). In an influential criticism, Lynch et al. (2000) draw an analogy with airline travel in which first-class passengers arrive refreshed and rested while economy passengers 'arrive feeling a bit rough' (p. 1202). They conclude that economy passengers felt worse because they had worse food, less comfortable seats and were not able to sleep. 'The fact that they can see the bigger seats as they walk off the plane is not the cause of their poorer health' (p. 1203).

To summarise, the social determinants of health extends aetiology to include social and economic factors. There is a strong socio-economic gradient for most diseases, but there remains considerable disagreement between whether material inequalities, unhealthy lifestyles or psychosocial factors are most responsible. Recognising the broader socio-economic context of health reminds practitioners to take into account persistent inequalities when treating people and realise the 'bigger picture' represented by individual lives.

THE PROFESSIONAL CONTEXT OF HEALTH CARE

Sociologists have devoted considerable attention to the professional context of health care and to the concept of a 'profession' in general. Consideration of what makes a profession is tied to basic sociological questions of social cohesion, or what keeps society together. In an early functionalist interpretation, Emile Durkheim situated professions at the heart of maintaining social order. For Durkheim, modern society is sustained by people playing roles that, while different, ultimately depend on each other. From this perspective, key attributes of professions account for their cohesive role. They possess *specialised knowledge* not available to laypeople, acquired through lengthy training. Because others depend on this knowledge, they must be *altruistic* and act in others' best interests. They have *monopoly* over practice (only professionals can carry out certain tasks) and a high degree of *autonomy* since only members are able to assess competency (Nettleton, 2013, pp. 183–184).

For functionalist sociologist Talcott Parsons (1951), illness represents a potential threat to social order because the sick are unable to perform expected duties. Society deals with this by entrusting medical professionals with power to sort legitimate from illegitimate claims. The doctor verifies illness by giving a diagnosis, allowing entry to the 'sick role' which entails certain rights and responsibilities including exemption from normal duties (e.g. education, work) in return for a quick and concerted effort to get better. In many ways, this view represents common beliefs at the mid-point of the twentieth century, often seen as the 'golden age' of medicine. Medical advances inspired growing trust in medical professionals and a sense that medicine would eventually solve most medical and even social problems. However, this would not last. The latter half of the twentieth century saw the rise of criticism of the medical profession and the view that functionalist interpretations of its power and authority had represented things too smoothly.

CHALLENGES TO PROFESSIONAL DOMINANCE

Critics argued functionalists assumed the profession's power and authority straightforwardly resulted from societal recognition of their attributes. However, assuming altruism ignores that becoming a doctor often entails financial reward. Indeed, Ehrenreich and Ehrenreich (1975) pointed out that the nineteenth-century poor were largely left untreated by the medical profession since prior to the welfare state their treatment provided little financial or status gains. Similarly, Freidson (1970) argued doctors are frequently self-interested and politically rather than altruistically motivated. Assuming power is a corollary of specialised knowledge also ignores power struggles and processes of 'occupational closure' through which existing forms of knowledge were devalued. Feminists in particular argued a male-dominated medical profession belittled and accorded lower status to activities typically associated with women like nursing, health visiting and midwifery (Gabe and Monaghan, 2013, p. 16).

Marxists challenged professions for contributing to the maintenance of capitalism. Professionals may not be capitalists, but they nonetheless legitimate and perpetuate capitalist relations of production through maintaining a healthy workforce (to be exploited by capitalists), justifying inequalities (professional privileges seem to result from specialist expertise) and locating illness in the diseased body rather than broader social inequalities.

Finally, the ideal of the disinterested, objective professional, acting purely rationally and on the basis of empirical evidence, has been challenged. Jeffery (1979) observed medical staff evaluating patients on both social and medical grounds. 'Good patients' were those with conditions allowing staff to practise and develop their skills and specialities. 'Rubbish patients' were those breaking unwritten rules of appropriate patient behaviour ('trivia', drunks, regular overdoses and tramps) (Scambler, 2008, p. 79). Hughes and Griffiths (1996) studied cardiac catheterisation conferences in which cardiologists presented cases to a cardiac surgeon making decisions regarding acceptance for surgery. They found acceptance was not solely based on technical assessments but also on interpretation of social information (p. 192). Age, lifestyle (smoking, drinking, obesity) and wider social structural factors (social status, ethnicity) were utilised to decide whether a patient was given an operation or not. Thus it was argued doctors police sick role entry, making decisions about legitimate and illegitimate candidates including both biological and social judgements.

DECLINING PROFESSIONAL DOMINANCE

These and other challenges have led to the argument that, while still enjoying considerable status, the medical profession's dominance over health care provision is in decline. While medical dominance is a complex concept, it generally refers to medicine's authority over others and the treatment of disease. This is related to the concept of medical autonomy, which refers to the degree of oversight an occupation exercises over its own work (Elston, 1991). That these are in decline has been argued to be evident in a number of developments including calls for greater regulation and oversight, the rise of 'patient-centred medicine' and 'medical pluralism'.

Regarding the first, socialised systems such as the NHS had the effect of protecting the medical profession's autonomy. Errors were seen as 'internal matters' and, unlike the United States, litigation was rare (Bury, 2010, p. 417). However, rising expectations and cultural diffusion from the US saw a marked increase in clinical negligence claims in the 1990s. While litigation can make doctors more accountable, it can also decrease trust. Moreover, the expectation professionals cannot make mistakes may lead to flight from high-risk (but no less important) specialities (Bury, 2010). Since the 1990s, a series of policy reforms also strengthened managerial control and oversight, decreasing the autonomy once assumed of health care professions (Traynor, 2012).

A second challenge has been the rise of patient-centred medicine and recognition of patient expertise. A 'patient-led NHS' reconceptualises the doctor–patient relationship as partnership. As Coulter (1999, p. 719) describes:

> Partners work together to achieve common goals. Their relationship is based on mutual respect for each other's skills and competencies and recognition of the advantages of combining these resources to achieve beneficial outcomes. Successful partnerships are non-hierarchical and the partners share decision making and responsibility. The key to successful doctor patient partnerships is therefore to recognise that patients are experts too.

Patient-centred models of care and shared decision-making have replaced the older norm of knowledgeable and skilful doctors making decisions on behalf of patients (Rogers et al., 1998). According to *Creating a Patient-Led NHS* (Department of Health, 2005), 'good practice' will involve:

- Respecting people for their knowledge and understanding of their own experience, clinical condition, and how illness impacts their life
- Ensuring people always feel valued by health service, treated with respect, dignity, compassion
- Understanding that individual is best judge of own experience
- Explaining what has happened if things go wrong and why, mutually agree way forward

One example of this turn is the 'Hello, my name is' initiative, instigated in 2013 by Kate Granger, herself a medical doctor and at the time a terminally ill cancer patient. During a hospital stay following an operation, Granger had been dismayed at how few members of staff had introduced themselves before providing care. The campaign, which has since been widely adopted, reminds of the importance of communication in providing patients with dignity and respect. According to Granger, simply introducing oneself is the first step in providing compassionate care (Ford, 2015).

ACTIVITY 1.2

Why is it important to introduce oneself when you are providing care? Take one minute to jot down as many reasons as you can.

Check the end of the chapter for an answer to this activity.

Other initiatives such as the Healthcare Commission (replaced in 2009 with the Care Quality Commission) aimed to regulate the quality of health and social care services and put patient voice at the heart of clinical performance appraisal. Attention to patient satisfaction has been described as a 'patient-led revolution' (Sky News, 2013). Announcing a digital initiative in which 'every patient in England should be able to access their medical records and book an appointment with a GP via an app by the end of 2018', then Health Secretary Jeremy Hunt referred to the next ten years as 'the decade of patient power' (Hunt, 2017). These initiatives represent a departure from the period of professional dominance. Increasingly, 'doctor knows best' is seen as paternalistic and outdated. 'Patients have grown up and there's no going back' (Coulter, 1999, p. 719).

It is possible the partnership approach may fuel the decline of trust in the medical profession. For instance, conflicts can arise where there are disagreements, differing desires and goals, or where patient empowerment is perceived as an unwelcome challenge to medical authority (see, e.g., Maslen and Lupton, 2018). A case in point is the MMR vaccine in which professional opinion contradicts parental choices to forgo or stagger immunisations. Age and competency present additional conflicts. For instance, paediatric care raises questions about the relative weight given voices of parents, professionals and children which do not yet appear to be resolved (Wyatt et al., 2015). On the other hand, patients may find it difficult to weigh benefits and risks and value professional judgement. Responsibility for major decisions can lead to worry and stress, and some may prefer a more passive role (Lyttle and Ryan, 2010).

Finally, declining professional dominance may be evident in the rise of medical pluralism, or arguments that there should be greater space for complementary and alternative medicines (CAM). CAM denotes treatments falling outside mainstream health care including homeopathy, acupuncture, osteopathy, chiropractic and herbal medicines. NHS (2018) distinguishes between *complementary* treatments used alongside conventional treatment (e.g. providing pleasant experiences, aiding coping) and *alternative* treatments used in place of conventional medicine. Emphasising nature, holism and tradition, CAMs are typically based on principles and evidence not recognised by Western science. At least since the 1980s, CAM has been growing in popularity. Data shows 44 per cent of UK adults will use CAM in their lifetime (Posadzki et al., 2013).

Criticism that medical knowledge became dominant not necessarily through superior knowledge but by subordinating other knowledges makes space for CAM therapies. As Bowler (2008, p. 39) describes, 'At the same time as modern scientific medicine [...] is experiencing a drop in confidence [...] a rise in the fortunes of [CAM] is evident.' Growing suspicion of commercial interests in medicine may also lead people to seek alternative treatments (Goldacre, 2009). However, it is worth noting CAM is also 'big business', experiencing strong commercial success on the high street. For instance, Boots began selling several remedies in 1991, extending in 2000 to include consultations in osteopathy, herbalism, nutrition, aromatherapy and reflexology. In 2001 Tesco took over the complementary Hale Clinic and began selling Hale Clinic products worldwide.

CAM may also appeal to those for whom conventional treatments have failed. However, therapies do not need to promise actual cures in order to 'deliver' (Tallis, 2004, p. 131). Where conventional medicine may offer little in the way of deeper meaning to patients, CAM therapies imbue suffering with personal and sometimes spiritual significance. This not only helps patients cope, but gives a greater sense of control (Tallis, 2004).

On the one hand, CAM answers to many criticisms of the medical profession. It offers greater patient choice, autonomy and control; it is a holistic approach dealing with both mental and bodily sides of illness, aiding relaxation and increasing coping; it respects different belief systems and offers hope where hope may be lost. On the other hand, alternative medical treatments and practitioners have been accused of preying on the hopeless, giving false or overblown promises where treatments lack evidence, channelling resources away from proven treatments or discovering new ones. Moreover, it may encourage an overly rosy view of the 'natural' and 'traditional' that can lead to unhelpful rejections of warranted medical authority and proven medical interventions.

THE CULTURAL CONTEXT OF HEALTH

Sociologists are concerned with the cultural context of health and health beliefs. Social constructionism represents a key theoretical perspective within this area. Social constructionism views scientific knowledge and discourse about bodies, health and illness as socially produced, shaped by human interests and prevailing moral and cultural belief systems (Gabe and Monaghan, 2013, p. 115). Human beings are different from animals in that we categorise and label reality and give it meaning (Berger and Luckmann, 1967). However, over time social categories do not seem like human products, but rather 'just the way things are'. For example, while race is popularly considered biological, social scientists have argued race is a social construction. It has a history, emerging as a justification for colonialism and existing social hierarchies (Malik, 1996; Painter, 2010). Racial categories vary across cultures and have been argued to possess little meaningful scientific basis (Gould, 1996). However, revealing a category as socially constructed does not remove its social power. 'If men [sic] define situations as real they are real in their consequences' (Thomas and Thomas, 1928, pp. 571–572). Race is 'real' because it has real social consequences. Moreover, while people really do vary, culture ignores some characteristics while attributing others meaning and significance.

SOCIAL CONSTRUCTION OF OBESITY

There is sometimes confusion between social causation and social construction. Sociological considerations of the 'obesity problem' illustrate differences between these perspectives. Obesity can be understood as socially caused, for instance pointing to its social determinants (e.g. unavailability or expense of nutritious food) or the power of advertising to encourage unhealthy choices. However, this is quite different from saying obesity is socially *constructed*. From the social constructionist perspective, the *labelling* of certain bodies as problematic and undesirable and others as 'healthy' and desirable is of central concern.

From this perspective, societal concern about obesity can be understood through studying changing cultural norms and values. For instance, in cultures where it is easier to become fat and expensive to remain lean, thinness is preferred (Brown and Konner, 1987). Tiggemann and Zaccardo (2018) argue 'strong' or muscular physiques are currently replacing the thin ideal, particularly on social media sites like Instagram. While promoted as a healthy alternative to Internet-based pro-weight loss trends like 'thinspiration', 'fitspiration' often nonetheless emphasises very slim 'toned' figures, tends to objectify particular body parts and advocates extreme dietary restriction (ibid.). Some research has associated internalisation of these ideals with body dissatisfaction and disordered eating (Robinson, et al., 2017; Tiggemann and Zaccardo, 2015).

A social constructionist approach would understand these trends in terms of changing norms and values regarding behaviour, class and gender. For instance, maintaining this culturally valued body shape is a symbol of economic status, as it requires large amounts of time, money, education and even surgery to achieve. Similarly, 'moral panic' perspectives focus on how 'panic' can result when an issue threatens a culture's norms and values (Cohen, 1972; Young, 1971). Applying this framework, Campos et al. (2006) describe how obesity statistics are often inflated by eliding 'over-weight' and 'obese' categories when there is limited evidence that the former is bad for health and may even be protective. They suggest this disproportionate concern highlights that panic about obesity is really a panic about social change. For instance, attention to 'fast food' implies that people are no longer cooking 'nutritious meals' at home, something women are 'supposed' to do. Thus, growing societal concern about obesity is attributed to hierarchical values associated with certain body types and anxiety about, among other things, changing gender roles.

ACTIVITY 1.3

Search your favourite social media site for #fitspiration or #fitspo.

1   What are some characteristics of the bodies represented by this hashtag?
2   In what ways do the images represented accord with your own views of ideal and/or 'healthy' bodies?
3   In what ways do you think researchers are correct/incorrect that this new ideal of health is potentially damaging?
4   In what ways is the 'fit' body ideal relevant to what some researchers call a 'panic' about obesity?

Check the end of the chapter for an answer to this activity.

MEDICALISATION

Medicalisation is the process through which previously non-medical phenomena come to be defined and treated as medical problems (Gabe and Monaghan, 2013, p. 49). It usually refers to over-medicalisation, or unwarranted expansion of medical categories to encompass more and more aspects of personal and social life. Many aspects of life once considered the product of bad people (volitional deviance) are now considered illnesses, the product of sick people (unintentional deviance) (Cockerham and Ritchey, 1997). 'Right' and 'wrong' have been supplanted by 'healthy' and 'unhealthy'. Criminals are often referred to as requiring 'treatment'. Children once classed as unruly or disruptive are routinely labelled with disorders for which a variety of drug treatments are available (Bergey et al., 2018). Solutions to social problems like poverty, inequality or unemployment are increasingly sought not in deep underlying economic structures, but through, for example, the provision of therapy or close medical or other expert surveillance of families or even pregnant women.

The medicalisation of social life has a variety of consequences. It locates problems inside diseased bodies and minds rather than in society. Wide knowledge of medical categories can encourage people to think of themselves as ill rather than using other identities, frames of reference or labels to understand their experience. This can encourage dependence on professionals, disempowering and thwarting self-care (Illich, 1976; Zola, 1972). Communicated through the language of science, medical labels appear empirically verified and therefore unquestionable. Many psychiatric categories have been argued to be particular to Western cultures. Nonetheless, they are exported to other cultures, potentially undermining self-determination and existing ways of coping and making sense of life (Million, 2013; Summerfield, 2017). Ideological and moral crusades may also be obscured by medical language. For instance, in Nazi Germany, smoking was considered antithetical to the ideology of racial hygiene. It was thus banned in public places. However, this was justified on medical rather than ideological grounds. Medical knowledge about harm and risk thus masked underlying moral and ideological judgements.

RISK

A useful way of understanding cultural conceptualisations of risk is through the 'paradox of health'. People today live longer and are less likely to suffer disease their ancestors took for granted. Yet they feel increasingly unhealthy and anxious about their health. In many ways, we are doing better but feeling worse (Barsky, 1988; Buckingham, 2008; Cederström and Spicer, 2015). While health improvements have engendered rising expectations, growing risk consciousness accounts for some of this phenomenon.

Although media constantly report on putative cancer risks from aspirin to yoghurt (Battley, 2019), some features of lifestyle risk research itself compound anxieties. For instance, correlations are often treated causally, and relative rather than absolute risks are highlighted, amplifying risk perceptions. For instance, the statement that heavy smokers are '24 times' more likely to die from lung cancer sounds more probable than the absolute risk for smokers alone – 16 per cent for men and 9.4 per cent for women (Buckingham, 2008, p. 25). Moreover, many lifestyle risk studies are produced through questionable methodologies including 'data-dredging' or performing many statistical tests to find any statistically significant (though likely spurious) association (Vigen, 2015). This is exacerbated by publication bias towards positive results, so that studies failing to find significant associations will not be published nor reported.

However, even given risk amplification, whether and how we respond to risk depends on cultural context. As older structures like tradition or religion are decreasingly able to dictate what people become, the self becomes a project people construct for themselves through a variety of lifestyle choices (Giddens, 1991). Expert communication of risk becomes a resource in this 'project of the self', whose goal is not religious salvation nor political change but physical and mental well-being. Moreover, as traditional political affiliations have waned, politicians have increasingly used the language of health to connect with people. However, this can deepen medicalisation, as the perennial problems of capitalist societies are recast as health threats, remediable through medical or therapeutic intervention. The result is a society producing ever increasing health alarms and in which people are more receptive to and anxious about health risks.

CONCLUSION

Sociologists are concerned with the broader contexts of health, from socio-economic contexts to the contexts in which professionals work and interact, to the cultural context of beliefs about health and illness. Social determinants of health and health inequalities represent key contributions of medical sociology. Those with access to greater material resources tend to experience better health than those without. As Cockerham puts it, 'To be poor is by definition to have less of the good things in life, including health and longevity' (2016, p. 55). Sociologists have also studied changing contexts of health care professions, describing the relative decline of medical authority and rise of greater oversight, patient-led approaches and medical pluralism. Finally, the cultural context of health is brought into focus by constructionist approaches that consider the cultural norms and values often obscured by medical labelling and the influence of changing cultural contexts on risk perception. To have a sociological imagination is to see beyond the limited realm of individual patients and connect them to their broader contexts.

GO FURTHER ACTIVITY

The Marmot Review (Marmot et al., 2010) discussed above, which detailed the continued existence and even widening of health inequalities, was produced nearly ten years ago (at the time of writing). It is highly likely that since that time, health disparities in connection with socio-economic inequalities have not disappeared. Reflect on some of the reasons why this might be the case. Keeping in mind the broader socio-economic context of health, what can and can't health professionals contribute to narrowing these gaps?

Check the end of the chapter for an answer to this activity.

ANSWERS TO CHAPTER 1 ACTIVITIES

——— Activity 1.1: Answers

1   Relative income poverty refers to households making 60 per cent or less of the country's median household income. Median household income refers to the point that divides the country's income distribution in two, with half of the population making more and half making less. As of 2019, the median income in the UK is £29,400. By this measure, households bringing in less than £17,640 would be considered to be living in poverty.

2   The article quotes a UK Government definition: 'The lack or denial of resources, rights, goods and services, and the inability to participate in the normal relationships and activities, available to the majority of people in a society, whether in economic, social, cultural or political arenas.'

3   According to the article, many of those on the poverty line are employed and work several jobs. Much of their work is insecure and subject to low pay and/or unpredictable hours (zero-hours contracts).

4   A representative of the Joseph Rowntree Foundation interviewed for the article points to high rents, low wages and cuts to government benefits as factors increasing the threat of poverty since 2010.

5   The average household income of those helped by charitable organisations discussed in the article was £14,000 per year. There are many difficulties that a family of four might experience on this income including appropriate housing, basic necessities, and extras that many take for granted but which make life comfortable.

——— Activity 1.2: Answers

There are many answers you might offer. Humanity and compassion are a large part of health care and are practised in both large and small gestures. Simply introducing

(Continued)

yourself can indicate compassion through a sense of shared humanity. It improves communication and allows us to see others as people and as individuals first, rather than just as users of health care.

——— Activity 1.3: Answers

Your answers to these questions will vary depending on your search results and personal opinions. However, most images are of slim and 'toned' individuals. It takes large amounts of information and time to achieve and maintain this ideal. Critical obesity researchers would argue that such ideals are related to social class and valued for their connotations of intensiveness. Larger bodies are deviant from this model and are thus more likely to be singled out as problematic and unhealthy.

——— Go Further Activity: Answers

Health inequalities are likely to be difficult to tackle because of their relationships to socio-economic factors which have themselves proved resistant to change. Health professionals may be able to contribute information, support, understanding and empathy, but work at the individual level may be limited in its ability to overturn large scale social structures.

REFERENCES

Acheson, D. (1998). *Independent Inquiry into Inequalities in Health: Report*. London: HM Stationery Office.

Asthana, S. and Halliday, J. (2006). What works in tackling health inequalities? *Pathways, Policies and Practice through the Lifecourse* (1st edn). Bristol: Policy Press. https://doi.org/10.2307/j.ctt9qgq7k

Barsky, A. (1988). *Worried Sick: Our Troubled Quest for Wellness*. Boston: Little, Brown and Company.

Bartley, M. (2017). *Health Inequality: An Introduction to Concepts, Theories and Methods*. Cambridge: Polity Press.

Bartley, M. and Plewis, I. (2002). Accumulated labour market disadvantage and limiting long-term illness: data from the 1971–1991 Office for National Statistics' Longitudinal Study. *International Journal of Epidemiology* 31(2), 336–341. https://doi.org/10.1093/ije/31.2.336

Battley, P. (2019). Kill or cure? Available at: http://kill-or-cure.herokuapp.com/ (accessed 18 March 2019)

Berger, P. L. and Luckmann, T. (1967). *The Social Construction of Reality*. London: Penguin.

Bergey, M. R., Filipe, A. M., Conrad, P. and Singh, I. (eds) (2018). *Global Perspectives on ADHD: Social Dimensions of Diagnosis and Treatment in Sixteen Countries*. Baltimore: JHU Press.

Bowler, S. (2008). The object of medicine. In D. Wainwright (ed.), *A Sociology of Health*. London: Sage.

Brown, P. J. and Konner, M. (1987). An anthropological perspective on obesity. *Annals of the New York Academy of Sciences* 499(1), 29–46.

Buckingham, A. (2008). Doing better, feeling scared: health statistics and the culture of fear. In D. Wainwright (ed.), *A Sociology of Health*. London: Sage.

Bury, M. (2010). The British healthcare system. In W. C. Cockerham (ed.), *The New Blackwell Companion to Medical Sociology*. Malden: Blackwell.

Campos, P., Saguy, A., Ernsberger, P., Oliver, E. and Gaesser, G. (2006). The epidemiology of over-weight and obesity: public health crisis or moral panic? *International Journal of Epidemiology* 35(1), 55–60.

Caraher, M., Lloyd, S., Lawton, J., Singh, G., Horsley, K. and Mussa, F. (2010). A tale of two cities: a study of access to food, lessons for public health practice. *Health Education Journal* 69(2), 200–210. https://doi.org/10.1177/0017896910364834

Cederström, C. and Spicer, A. (2015). *The Wellness Syndrome*. Cambridge: Polity Press.

Cockerham, W. C. (2016). *Medical Sociology* (13th edn). Boston: Pearson.

Cockerham, W. C. and Ritchey, F. J. (1997). *Dictionary of Medical Sociology*. Westport: Greenwood Press.

Cohen, S. (1972). *Folk Devils and Moral Panics*. London: MacGibbon and Kee.

Coulter, A. (1999). Paternalism or partnership? Patients have grown up – and there's no going back. *BMJ* 319(7212), 719–720.

Davis, O. and Geiger, B. B. (2017). Did food insecurity rise across Europe after the 2008 crisis? An analysis across welfare regimes. *Social Policy and Society* 16(3), 343–360. http://dx.doi.org/10.1017/S1474746416000166

Department of Health (2005). Creating a patient-led NHS – Delivering the NHS improvement plan. Available at: http://webarchive.nationalarchives.gov.uk/20130107105354/http://www.dh.gov.uk/prod_consum_dh/groups/dh_digitalassets/@dh/@en/documents/digitalasset/dh_4106507.pdf

Dunn, R. G. (2018). *Toward a Pragmatist Sociology: John Dewey and the Legacy of C. Wright Mills*. Philadelphia: Temple University Press.

Ehrenreich, B. and Ehrenreich, J. (1975). Medicine and social control. In B. R. Mandell (ed.), *Welfare in America: Controlling the Dangerous Classes*. Englewood Cliffs: Prentice Hall.

Elston, M. (1991). The politics of professional power: medicine in a changing health service. In J. Gabe, M. Calnan and M. Bury (eds), *The Sociology of the Health Service*. London: Routledge.

Equality Trust (2012). Physical health. Available at: www.equalitytrust.org.uk/physical-health (accessed 15 March 2019)

Ford, S. (2015). 'Hello my name is' campaign adopted by 100 plus NHS trusts. *Nursing Times*, 2 February. Available at: www.nursingtimes.net/roles/nurse-managers/hello-my-name-is-campaign-adopted-by-100-plus-nhs-trusts/5081757.article (accessed 10 June 2019)

Freidson, E. (1970). *Profession of Medicine: A Study of the Sociology of Applied Knowledge*. New York: Dodd, Mead and Company.

Gabe, J. and Monaghan, L. F. (2013). *Key Concepts in Medical Sociology*. London: Sage.

Garthwaite, K. A., Collins, P. J. and Bambra, C. (2015). Food for thought: an ethnographic study of negotiating ill health and food insecurity in a UK foodbank. *Social Science & Medicine* 132, 38–44. https://doi.org/10.1016/j.socscimed.2015.03.019

Giddens, A. (1991). *Modernity and Self-Identity*. London: Polity Press.

Giddens, A., Duneier, M., Appelbaum, R. P. and Carr, D. (2017). *Essentials of Sociology* (6th edn). New York: W.W. Norton & Company.

Giddens, A. and Sutton, P. W. (2017). *Essential Concepts in Sociology*. John Wiley & Sons.

Goldacre, B. (2009). *Bad Science: Quacks, Hacks, and Big Pharma Flacks.* London: Fourth Estate.

Goldblatt, P. (1989). Mortality by social class 1971–85. *Population Trends* 56, 6–15.

Goodwin, C. and Duranti, A. (eds.) (1992). *Rethinking Context: Language as an Interactive Phenomenon*. Cambridge: Cambridge University Press.

Gould, S. J. (1996). *The Mismeasure of Man*. New York: W.W. Norton & Company.

Graham, H. (1987). Women's smoking and family health. *Social Science & Medicine* 25(1), 47–56.

Hughes, D. and Griffiths, L. (1996). 'But if you look at the coronary anatomy…': risk and rationing in cardiac surgery. *Sociology of Health & Illness* 18(2), 172–197.

Hunt, J. (2017). Health Secretary challenges NHS to deliver digital services nationwide. *Department of Health and Social Care*, 12 September. Available at: www.gov.uk/government/news/health-secre tary-challenges-nhs-to-deliver-digital-services-nationwide (accessed 18 March 2019)

Illich, I. (1976). *Medical Nemesis: The Expropriation of Health*. New York: Pantheon Books.

Illsley, R. (1986). Occupational class, selection and the production of inequalities in health. *The Quarterly Journal of Social Affairs* 2, 151–165.

Jeffery, R. (1979). Normal rubbish: deviant patients in casualty departments. *Sociology of Health & Illness* 1(1), 90–107.

Jenkin, P. (1982). Foreword by Patrick Jenkin. In *Inequalities in Health: The Black Report*. London: Penguin.

Lynch, J., Smith, G. D., Harper, S. A., Hillemeier, M., Ross, N., Kaplan, G. A. and Wolfson, M. (2004). Is income inequality a determinant of population health? Part 1. A systematic review. *The Milbank Quarterly* 82(1), 5–99.

Lynch, J., Smith, G. D., Kaplan, G. A. and House, J. S. (2000). Income inequality and mortality: impor- tance to health of individual income, psychosocial environment, or material conditions. *BMJ* 320(7243), 1200–1204.

Lyttle, D. J. and Ryan, A. (2010). Factors influencing older patients' participation in care: a review of the literature. *International Journal of Older People Nursing* 5(4), 274–282. https://doi.org/10.1111/ j.1748-3743.2010.00245.x

Malik, K. (1996). *The Meaning of Race: Race, History and Culture in Western Society*. Basingstoke: Macmillan International Higher Education.

Marmot, M. (2015). *The Health Gap: The Challenge of an Unequal World*. London: Bloomsbury.

Marmot, M., Allen, J., Goldblatt, P., Boyce, T., McNeish, D., Grady, M. and Geddes, I. (2010). *The Marmot Review: Fair Society, Healthy Lives. Strategic Review of Health Inequalities in England Post-2010*. Available at: www.parliament.uk/documents/fair-society-healthy-lives-full-report.pdf (accessed 10 September, 2019)

Marmot, M., Rose, G., Shipley, M. and Hamilton, P. J. (1978). Employment grade and coronary heart disease in British civil servants. *Journal of Epidemiology and Community Health* 32(4), 244–249.

Marmot, M., Stansfeld, S., Patel, C., North, F., Head, J., White, I., … Smith, G. D. (1991). Health inequali- ties among British civil servants: the Whitehall II study. *The Lancet* 337(8754), 1387–1393.

Maslen, S. and Lupton, D. (2018). 'You can explore it more online': a qualitative study on Australian women's use of online health and medical information. *BMC Health Services Research* 18(1), 916. https://doi.org/10.1186/s12913-018-3749-7

McKeown, T. (1976a). *The Modern Rise of Population*. New York: Academic Press.

McKeown, T. (1976b). *The Role of Medicine: Dream, Mirage, or Nemesis?* London: Nuffield PHT.

Million, D. (2013). *Therapeutic Nations: Healing in an Age of Indigenous Human Rights*. Tucson: University of Arizona Press.

Mills, C. W. (2000). *The Sociological Imagination*. Oxford: Oxford University Press.

Morris, M. A., Hulme, C., Clarke, G. P., Edwards, K. L. and Cade, J. E. (2014). What is the cost of a healthy diet? Using diet data from the UK Women's Cohort Study. *Journal of Epidemiology and Community Health* 68(11), 1043–1049. https://doi.org/10.1136/jech-2014-204039

Nettleton, S. (2013). *The Sociology of Health and Illness*. Cambridge: Polity Press.

NHS (2018). Complementary and alternative medicine. Available at: www.nhs.uk/conditions/comple mentary-and-alternative-medicine/ (accessed 18 March 2019)

Painter, N. I. (2010). *The History of White People*. W.W. Norton & Company.

Parsons, T. (1951). *The Social System*. London: Routledge & Kegan Paul.

Pickett, K. E. and Wilkinson, R. G. (2015). Income inequality and health: a causal review. *Social Science & Medicine* 128, 316–326.

Posadzki, P., Watson, L. K., Alotaibi, A. and Ernst, E. (2013). Prevalence of use of complementary and alternative medicine (CAM) by patients/consumers in the UK: systematic review of surveys. *Clinical Medicine* 13(2), 126–131. https://doi.org/10.7861/clinmedicine.13-2-126

Riches, G. and Silvasti, T. (2014). *First World Hunger Revisited*. Basingstoke: Palgrave Macmillan.

Robinson, L., Prichard, I., Nikolaidis, A., Drummond, C., Drummond, M. and Tiggemann, M. (2017). Idealised media images: the effect of fitspiration imagery on body satisfaction and exercise behaviour. *Body Image* 22, 65–71. https://doi.org/10.1016/j.bodyim.2017.06.001

Rogers, A., Entwistle, V. and Pencheon, D. (1998). A patient led NHS: managing demand at the interface between lay and primary care. *BMJ* 316(7147), 1816–1819.

Scambler, G. (2008). *Sociology as Applied to Medicine (E-Book)*. London: Elsevier Health Sciences.

Sky News (2013, 29 July). NHS ward ratings a 'patient-led revolution'. Available at: https://news.sky.com/story/nhs-ward-ratings-a-patient-led-revolution-10438835 (accessed 18 March 2019)

Smith, K. E., Bambra, C. and Hill, S. E. (eds) (2016). *Health Inequalities: Critical Perspectives*. Oxford: Oxford University Press.

Summerfield, D. A. (2017). Western depression is not a universal condition. *The British Journal of Psychiatry*, 211(1), 52–54. https://doi.org/10.1192/bjp.211.1.52

Tallis, R. (2004). *Hippocratic Oaths: Medicine and its Discontents*. London: Atlantic Books.

Thomas W, I. and Thomas, D. S. (1928). *The Child in America: Behavior Problems and Programs*. New York: A.A. Knopf.

Tiggemann, M. and Zaccardo, M. (2015). 'Exercise to be fit, not skinny': The effect of fitspiration imagery on women's body image. *Body Image* 15, 61–67. https://doi.org/10.1016/j.bodyim.2015.06.003

Tiggemann, M. and Zaccardo, M. (2018). 'Strong is the new skinny': a content analysis of# fitspiration images on Instagram. *Journal of Health Psychology* 23(8), 1003–1011.

Townsend, P. and Davidson, N. (1982). *Inequalities in Health: The Black Report*. London: Penguin.

Traynor, M. (2012). *Managerialism and Nursing: Beyond Oppression and Profession*. London: Routledge.

Vigen, T. (2015). *Spurious Correlations*. New York: Hachette books.

Wainwright, D. (2008). The changing face of medical sociology. In *A Sociology of Health* (pp. 1–18). London: Sage.

Whitehead, M. (1987). *The Health Divide: Inequalities in Health in the 1980s: a Review Commissioned by the Health Education Council, London*. London: Health Education Council.

WHO (2017). 10 facts on health inequities and their causes. Available at: www.who.int/features/factfiles/health_inequities/en/ (accessed 6 March 2019)

WHO (2019). About social determinants of health. Available at: www.who.int/social_determinants/sdh_definition/en/ (accessed 12 March 2019)

Wilkinson, R. and Pickett, K. (2010). *The Spirit Level: Why Equality is Better for Everyone* (rev. edn). London: Penguin.

Wyatt, K. D., List, B., Brinkman, W. B., Lopez, G. P., Asi, N., Erwin, P., ... LeBlanc, A. (2015). Shared decision making in pediatrics: a systematic review and meta-analysis. *Academic Pediatrics* 15(6), 573–583. https://doi.org/10.1016/j.acap.2015.03.011

Young, J. (1971). *The Drugtakers: The Social Meaning of Drug Use*. London: MacGibbon and Kee.

Zola, I. K. (1972). Medicine as an institution of social control. *The Sociological Review* 20(4), 487–504. https://doi.org/10.1111/j.1467-954X.1972.tb00220.x

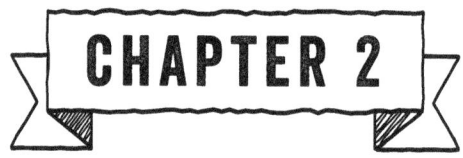

CHAPTER 2

PSYCHOLOGY OF HEALTH AND ILLNESS

Darren J. Edwards

OVERVIEW

This chapter will first introduce the key concepts of health psychology, illness representation and the limitations of the biomedical model in dealing with psychological disorders. It will explore: (1) the historical perspective of psychology, health, illness representation, and medicine; (2) the role of learning and expectation in the treatment of illnesses such as the behavioural models of stimuli–response and findings from the contextual effects literature; (3) the role of personality theories such as trait theories in illness and treatment; (4) social cognition such as schemas which are cognitive categories storing patterns about the world, implications of attribution theory such as health locus of control, self-concept and self-blame, and how these can lead to poor mental health; (5) implicit and explicit models of attitude, models of health belief such as the theory of reasoned action, and their theory of planned behaviour in explaining how individuals cope with health and illness representation; (6) some applied health psychology approaches to well-being which have shown to be effective for reducing mental health problems such as phobias, anxiety and depression.

LEARNING OUTCOMES

By the end of this chapter you will be able to:

- Describe the role of modern health psychology within the broader context of psychological history and illness representation
- Identify the different ontological approaches used and how they apply to health psychology
- Understand the role of learning and expectation in illness and treatment
- Discuss how personality trait theories play a role in illness and treatment
- Understand how social cognition can affect illness representation
- Identify how implicit and explicit attitudes, models of health belief and reasoned action predict behaviour in relation to coping with illness
- Discuss some specific psychological therapies used by health psychologists

INTRODUCTION

The World Health Organization (WHO) has defined health for over half a decade as 'a state of complete physical, mental and social well-being, and not merely the absence of disease or infirmity' (World Health Organization, 1948). This is different from the dominant view of the bio-medical model which has dominated medicine for many years and which defines health strictly as the absence of disease (Rosen, 1991). This strict definition referring to the absence of disease has been challenged in medicine more recently and these challenges have given rise to the biopsychosocial model of health where other factors of social, psychological, as well as biological components are now accepted in mainstream medicine (Engel, 1977). It has now been recognised that people's perceptions and expectations about their health, symptoms and treatment can have profound effects on their actual health and well-being (Di Blasi et al., 2001).

The relationship between health and psychology are substantial; for instance, a meta-review including over 1.7 million patients and a quarter of a million deaths found that patients with affective disorders have a reduced life expectancy equivalent to the effects of heavy smoking (Chesney et al., 2014). Unfortunately, though, the WHO definition for health has been criticised as being unachievable, contributing to the over-medicalisation of society and minimising the human capacity to cope (Huber et al., 2011). The numbers of people who need mental health treatment and do not receive it exceeds 50 per cent in all countries and reaches 90 per cent in those with less resources (Patel et al., 2010). This problem is apparent in some evidence which has highlighted a treatment gap combined with a treatment lag – the delay in receiving mental health treatment when it is required has been estimated to be as long as ten years (Wang et al., 2004), and represents a serious obstacle that remains to be overcome.

As a result of these problems health psychologists are now focusing their attention on promoting positive social ties and social connectedness (Kemp et al., 2017) as a means to increase physical and mental health more generally, with the focus on preventing mental health problems in the first place. With respects to well-being, a focus on happiness (hedonia) and realising our full potential (eudaimonia) has been criticised as a socio-cultural construction of Western individualism that neglects global (environmental) well-being (Carlisle et al., 2009). These criticisms have led to broader conceptualisations of well-being spanning seven components that include prosperity, resilience, health, equality, community, culture and global responsibility, leading to, for example, the Wellbeing of Future Generations Act 2015 in the UK.

Health psychologists today have a broad range of psychological approaches and theories which help them to understand the contemporary issues of health and illness representation today globally. These theories include behavioural, cognitive, personality and attitude theories, and have been manifested in many forms of mental health therapies such as cognitive behavioural therapy (CBT), goal-directed therapies such as motivational interviewing (MI), positive psychology, and mindfulness-based therapies such as acceptance and commitment therapy (ACT). With these psychological theories and therapies, health psychologists are in a good position to help facilitate positive change in mental health and well-being not just at an individual level but on a societal and global level as a whole.

THE DEVELOPMENT OF HEALTH PSYCHOLOGY
AND ITS HISTORICAL ORIGINS

The etymology of the word 'psychology' translates directly from Latin as 'the study of the soul', and was first referenced in 1693 by the Dutch physician Steven Blankaart, who defined the difference between the studies of anatomy and psychology as: 'Anatomy, which treats the body, and psychology which treats the soul' (Dictionary of Psychology, 2009). The historical origins of psychology can be traced back even further to ancient Greece; for example, Aristotle's *De Anima treatise*, written in 350 BC, which translates to 'On the Soul', is perhaps the first piece ever written about psychology within a biological framework (Hicks, 2015).

For many centuries, humoral theory was the dominant perspective in clinical psychology. Humoral theory, which dates back to ancient Greece and dominated European medicine up until the sixteenth century, suggested that psychological illness was the result of an imbalance in various fluids of the body, which were blood, black bile, yellow bile and phlegm. In treating this imbalance, physicians would bleed the patient (drain the patient of some blood) or place hot cups on certain areas of the body to restore the balance of fluid.

By the mid-nineteenth century, humoral theory was replaced by the biomedical approach as the dominant model in clinical psychology. This started in the form of diagnosis through phrenology, which explored the shape and bumps of the head to help understand mental traits. Though this practice is now understood today as a primitive and obsolete therapy it had been influential in shaping modern psychiatry and neuroanatomy (Fodor, 1983). This eventually brought about the modern biomedical model which focuses on the biological aspects of disease and illness and assumes that health constitutes of freedom from pain, disease and defect. It has long been considered as the dominant model of the day for reducing or removing disease and uses molecular biology as its basis for a scientific discipline. This includes the field of psychology in treating psychological disorders in the form of psychiatry (Engel, 1977; Rosen, 1991).

However, in the 1970s the field in relation to psychiatry began to consider broadening the scope of therapy outside of this strict biomolecular approach of using psychopharmacology to treat depression, anxiety and other mental-health-related disorders, to include the biopsychosocial model (Engel, 1977). This biopsychosocial model is more inclusive of psychological theories, principles and practice, in the form of therapy to reduce mental health problems and promote positive affect.

Perhaps the earliest theory of clinical psychology was psychoanalysis developed by Sigmund Freud (Freud, 1916). Freud suggested that patients could be cured from their depression and anxiety by making conscious what was stored in their unconscious. This, Freud believed, led to a process called catharsis. In doing this, Freud employed a wide range of introspective techniques to lead to a cathartic process such as dream analysis (exploring dream content), free association (exploring the patients' free speech), exploring the patients' responses to ink bolts (symbolic analysis) and finally looking out for Freudian slips (where the patient says something unintentionally).

However, the work of Freud was later suggested to be unscientific by the positivist movement of more contemporary researchers of the time who demanded a scientific approach to psychological therapy. This scientific approach came in the form of behaviourism, where John B. Watson suggested: 'Psychology as the behaviourist views it is a purely objective experimental branch of natural science. Its theoretical goal is the prediction and control of behaviour. Introspection forms no essential part of its methods, nor is the scientific value of its data dependent upon the readiness with which they lend themselves to interpretation in terms of consciousness' (Watson, 1913, p. 158).

Behaviourism developed in the early nineteenth century in the form of Ivan Pavlov's account of associations and conditioned responses (Pavlov, 1897). Pavlov had demonstrated that by pairing the association of a bell ringing with food led to, after several pairings, a conditioned response where the dog would salivate simply by the sound of the bell alone – a process which he called classical conditioning. Burrhus Frederic Skinner (Ferster and Skinner, 1957; Skinner, 1938) developed this model further by suggesting that operant conditioning behaviours which led to some form of pleasant outcome (positive reinforcement) would be likely to be repeated, whilst behaviours which led to less pleasant outcomes or painful outcomes (negative reinforcement) would be less likely to be repeated.

This operant conditioning was utilised as a means for behavioural modification, for example in the case of aversion therapy, where induced vomiting or an electric shock would be paired with an addictive impulse (such as alcoholism) to reduce this addictive behaviour (McGuire and Vallance, 1964).

However, perceptions of psychology changed when cognitive psychology developed through Noam Chomsky who criticised Skinner's explanation of operant conditioning to adequately explain the emergence of language (Chomsky, 1957, 1959). He suggested that verbal behaviour could not be explained simply by reinforcement and that this model was incomplete. Cognitive psychology has thus explored the mediating factors between stimuli and response such as memory and attention. Ulric Neisser (Neisser, 1967) used the term 'cognitive psychology' for the first time to describe a person as a dynamic information-processing system, where mental operations can be given in computational terms.

The merging of ideas from cognitive and behavioural psychology has led to one of the most successful treatments for mental health disorders such as depression and anxiety in the form of cognitive behavioural therapy (CBT). This uses a symptom reduction approach through thought reconstruction and systematic desensitisation. That is, its focus is on removing or reducing disorder symptoms (Beck, 2011).

This shift to CBT demonstrates how psychotherapy has evolved towards an evidence-based approach (Sackett, 1997). This approach explores the available evidence to identify the most effective forms of treatment, the specific needs of the patient, and the clinical expertise of the therapist delivering the treatment (American Psychological Association Presidential Task Force on Evidence Based Practice, 2006). In light of this, various agencies such as the National Registry of Evidence Based Programs and Practices (NREPP) of the US Substance Abuse and Mental Health Service Administration have compiled lists of evidence-based psychotherapy efficacy and best practices (Hofmann and Hayes, 2018).

In addition to this, Division 12 of the American Psychological Association, the Society of Clinical Psychology, created a Task Force on 'Promotion and Dissemination of Psychological Procedures' with the goal of collating a list of research supported psychological treatments for multiple domains and associated meta-analyses (Tolin et al., 2015). These included psychodynamic, interpersonal, cognitive behavioural and systemic points of view. Their finding suggested that CBT demonstrated the largest evidence base. As such, mental health today is assessed through the Diagnostic and Statistical Manual of Mental Disorders 5 (DSM 5) (American Psychiatric Association, 2000, 2013) which is the most modern collection of diagnosis classifications system available. Today, clinical psychologists can identify mental health disorders through this DSM5 classification system in order to appropriately treat a condition and with the appropriate evidence base. This usually means a course of CBT for many disorders involving depression and anxiety.

PAUSE FOR THOUGHT 2.1

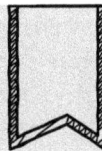

- Consider how early philosophers in ancient Greece, and those from the time of Sigmund Freud, may have considered mental health. Did they have any evidence to base or formulate their theories from? How is this different from today?
- Do you think the ideas around the humorous theory of mental health conditions were based in good scientific methodology and evidence?

(Continued)

- Consider the advantages and disadvantages of the biomedical model and biopsychosocial model. Which of these do you feel is more inclusive of a broader range of possible factors which can lead to possible mental health issues?

Check the end of the chapter for an answer to this activity.

THE ROLE OF LEARNING IN ILLNESS AND TREATMENT

The role of learning vs biological factors which determine behaviour can be centred around the nature vs nurture debate (Schaffner, 2001). On the one side, researchers have suggested that genetics and biology play a more important role in the psychology of an individual, and on the other side, arguments have been made which suggest that the environment plays a more important role.

One of the major theories which supports the environmental and learning side of that debate is behaviourism. Behaviourists attempt to explain psychological phenomenon through empirically defined objective phenomena in the form of overt stimuli – responses which can be objectively measured. In this way they focused on what people and animals do in response to different environmental situations (Klimenko and Golikov, 2003).

Albert Bandura developed the behavioural ideas even further by agreeing with the classical and operant theories but by adding two important ideas: (1) there are mediating (cognitive) processes that occur between stimuli and response; and (2) behaviour is also learned from the environment through the process of observational learning and not just the product of direct reinforcement (Bandura, 1978). This observational learning was demonstrated through the famous Bobo doll experiment where children learned (and then mimicked) aggressive behaviour by watching the behaviour of another aggressive person (e.g. hitting the Bobo doll) through varying levels of rein-forcement contingencies. So, they learned aggressive behaviour through this process of imitation (called vicarious reinforcement) (Bandura, 1965; Bandura et al., 1961).

In terms of mental illness being learned, one famous study called the Little Albert study (Watson and Raynor, 1920) demonstrated that phobias can be learned in the same way that Pavlov had demonstrated that salivation can be learned through association. In this study, Little Albert was exposed to a loud noise every time he was in the presence of a white rat. The noise would distress him, and he cried each time. Eventually, he learned to associate the distress with the presence of the white rat and became distressed at the sight of the white rat without the presence of the noise. He had learned to fear white rats, and this fear generalised to other white furry objects. Similarly, eating disorders and other unhealthy coping behaviours such as smoking and drinking heavily may also be learned in a similar way, as the individual may associate comfort when smoking, eating unhealthily, and so on.

Some therapies such as CBT utilise learning principles (i.e. behaviourism) to reduce mental health problems through systematic desensitisation (Beck, 2011). Systematic desensitisation (SD) is used to unlearn their fears through the use of classical conditioning and has been very successful for the treatment of phobia. This involves exposing the patient with phobia to the stimuli which is causing the fear (e.g. a spider) and it prevents them from avoiding it. SD is typically done progressively, starting with maybe a picture of a spider and then, as the patient becomes more relaxed, progressing to an actual spider. As the patient becomes more desensitised through exposure, the negative reinforcement of the stimuli causing distress (in this case a spider) is reduced and the phobia has been treated.

THE ROLE OF PERSONALITY TRAIT THEORIES IN ILLNESS AND TREATMENT

Personality may be defined as 'the characteristics or blend of characteristics that make a person unique' (Weinberg and Gould, 1999). Gordon Allport defined personality as 'the dynamic organisation within the individual of those psychophysical systems that determine his characteristics behaviour and thought' (Allport, 1961).

Sigmund Freud was perhaps the first psychologist to try to develop a model for personality and suggested that personality was tripartite in the sense that there was the id, ego and superego, which he referred to as the psyche (Freud, 1923). He assumed that the id was the primitive and instinctive component of personality whilst the superego represented the morality of the individual learned through society and similar to conscience. The superego, he suggested, could punish the ego through feelings of guilt, and thus moderate the behavioural impulses of the id. The ego represented the reality principle through working out realistic ways the id's and superego's demands could be met. The ego was thought to consider social norms and reality, and decided how to behave based on this (Freud, 2017).

Another theory, Allport's trait theory (Allport, 1961), emphasised the uniqueness of the individual as well as the cognitive and motivational processes that influence behaviour such as intelligence, temperament, habits, skills, attitudes and traits. Allport believed that personality is biologically determined at birth and is shaped by the environmental experience (Allport, 1937). He suggested that there are three trait levels: cardinal traits, central traits and secondary traits. Cardinal traits, he suggested, were the dominant traits of a person's life such as being assertive, Machiavellian, etc. Central traits were ones that made up your personality such as being intelligent, shy and honest. Secondary traits were harder to detect and could be situational. For example, if a person had the cardinal trait of being assertive generally they may be submissive in certain situational encounters, perhaps with parents for example.

Later, Eysenck developed his personality theory which was called the Big Two, referring to introversion and extroversion (Eysenck, 1964, 2017) and suggested that this was based on biologically inherited factors. These biological factors meant that individuals had unique nervous systems which affected the way in which they learned and adapted to the environment. He developed what he called second-order personality traits which he reduced from a much larger battery of questions he was developing for a questionnaire (first-order traits). He then applied a statistical technique called a factor analysis which reduced all these into two binary factors: Introversion/Extroversion (E); Neuroticism/Stability (N). In 1966, Eysenck then added a third trait called psychoticism, which he referred to as someone who lacked empathy, and was cruel, a loner and aggressive (Eysenck, 1966).

Raymond Cattell (Cattell, 1945; Rothe, 2017) disagreed with Eysenck's view that personality could be reduced to just two or three factors. Cattell explored a much greater range of individuals, whereas Eysenck had only explored servicemen of similar backgrounds. Cattell utilised L-data, which is the individual's life record such as grades, absence from work, and so on. He also used Q-data, which was designed to rate the individual's personality, and T-data, which was data from the objective tests designed to capture the personality construct. Using a mathematical model called factor analysis he reduced data from the T-data and Q-data and grouped the behaviour of similar people, identifying that there were 16 personality traits common to all people.

Due to such criticism from researchers such as Cattell, Eysenck's two-factor model was later expanded upon by Paul Costa and colleagues with the development of the Big Five model for personality traits. This suggested that the main components of personality were: openness vs closed; introverted vs extroverted; conscientiousness; agreeableness; and neuroticism (Costa et al., 1991). This five-factor model represents the most dominant theory on personality today.

In terms of the personality disorders which have led to mental illness, Freud had suggested that events in childhood shaped our personalities and caused many forms of mental health problems which were hidden from consciousness but then formed into neurosis in adult life (Freud, 2017). He suggested that through free association and dream analysis a state of catharsis could be reached which would reduce the effects of neurosis.

Today, the DSM 5 has recognised several problematic personality type disorders. One of these is borderline personality disorder (BPD), which is a mood-related disorder and affects how the individual relates to others. It is characterised by emotional instability, disturbed patterns of thinking, impulsive behaviour and intense unstable relationships. Similar to the theory of psychoanalysis, BPD is thought to originate through childhood trauma where there was some form of neglect, or emotional abuse. BPD is often associated with high levels of neuroticism, closed mindedness and low levels of agreeableness. Associated with BPD are other common mental health problems such as misusing alcohol, generalised anxiety, bipolar disorder, depression, misusing drugs, self-harm, and eating disorders such as bulimia and anorexia.

Another form of personality disorder is antisocial personality disorder (ASPD) which is often characterised by impulsive, reckless behaviour and lacking compassion for others. Psychopaths are considered to have a severe form of ASPD. In terms of mental health problems, ASPD can be associated with depression and substance misuse, and many social problems.

In terms of treating these personality disorders, the biomedical model suggests the use of selective serotonin reuptake inhibitors (SSRIs), which promotes an increased volume of serotonin in the synaptic gaps of the neurons. In terms of biopsychosocial models, CBT has been used to treat this disorder effectively through thought reconstruction and are supported by current NICE guidelines (NICE, 2019).

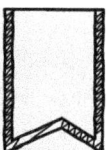

PAUSE FOR THOUGHT 2.2

- Which do you feel is the better approach, psychopharmacology or psychological therapies relating to personality disorders? Do they both have a place in treatment?
- When it comes to personality disorders is it better to develop preventative methods such as dealing with aspects of the society, or individual methods of fixing the problem when it occurs? Perhaps both?
- Where does psychology and psychopharmacology go from here for the treatment of personality disorders?

Check the end of the chapter for an answer to this activity.

COGNITION AND ILLNESS REPRESENTATION

Social cognition was perhaps first developed by Jean Piaget who developed the idea of schema in the 1930s even before cognitive psychology had been formally developed (Piaget and Cook, 1952). Piaget referred to a schema as a building block of knowledge which allows the individual to form a mental representation of the world such as objects, actions and other concepts. Schema processing specifically refer to cognitive processes of attention, encoding and the retrieval of information (Cohen, 1981), whereby the receiving of external stimuli, learning and reinforcement stored in memory are combined to form a schema which is a pattern or model of the world we live in. The function of the schema is to interpret the world information in order to help with decision-making when new stimuli or situations are presented. Illness beliefs (according to this model) are assumed to be organised in memory into schema representations in the same way. Through these schemas, illness representation can guide our reactions to symptoms, diagnosis and other types of illness related information.

Piaget referred to two processes in relation to schemas, called assimilation and accommodation, where assimilation was where the existing schemas would change new incoming information (e.g. about an object or situation) to fit into existing schemas and accommodation was where the existing knowledge contained in a schema changed to deal with the new incoming information (Piaget and Cook, 1952; Wadsworth, 1996).

Though it has been suggested that schemas are very important in day-to-day life such as facilitating decision-making and reducing the information processing cost of these mental processes (Derry, 1996), there may be many problems which can occur as a result of schemas. One of these problems is attribution bias due to the overreliance on schemas which can occur when one selectively remembers only information which is consistent with their schema representation rather than the facts (Kleider et al., 2008). In the area of self-schema, this has been found to be a determinant of several mental health problems such as depression where an individual may use new information to confirm negative representations about the self which leads to a negative downward spiral of self-beliefs (Dykman et al., 1991; Roberts and Monroe, 1994).

Self-regulation model of illness cognition and behaviour (Leventhal et al., 1992) offers another example of how schemas may affect our illness representation and coping ability. This theory suggests that people are active problem solvers, and central illness beliefs in the form of schemas guide the individual's coping in response to the illness belief. The theory suggests that self-regulation is a function of the representation of health threats and the ongoing targets for coping set by the individual's own schema representation about the procedures to regulate these targets and the appraisal of potential coping outcomes. Individuals are thought to be biased in the way they test potential coping methods based on concrete symptom-based schemata as well as abstract disease labels.

In another example of social cognition and illness representation, Fritz Heider (Heider, 1958) through attribution theory suggested that individuals try to find causal explanations for what happens to them like naïve intuitive scientists. These causal explanations can be either internal or external attributions. Errors such as the fundamental attribution error (FAE) can mean that we can overestimate how much a person's behaviour is explained by dispositional personality-based factors and underestimate (situational) factors. In terms of the development of mental illness, for example, the individual, as a result of FAE, may overemphasise personal rather than situational factors for negative events in one's life (such as failing a driving test) and as a result place blame on oneself rather than an unfortunate situation.

Self-blame is a cognitive process in which the individual attributes the stressful event to oneself (Brickman et al., 1978). Two forms of self-blame have been identified: (1) behavioural self-blame which involves attributions to a modifiable source (i.e. one's behaviour); (2) characterological self-blame which is esteem related and involves attributions to a relatively non-modifiable source (i.e. one's character) (Janoff-Bulman, 1979). This categorical self-blame relates to other theories around self-concept. Self-concept is an organisation of beliefs and perceptions about oneself, and can include present self, future self and working self-concept (Rosenberg, 1986). It has also been defined as 'The individual's belief about himself or herself, including the person's attributes and who and what the self is' (Baumeister, 1999). This can include self-esteem which is the attitude about the self (Harter, 1993). Attitudes about the self can be positive or negative depending on the representation of the self-concept. Negative beliefs about the self may lead to harmful attributions about events which lead to self-blaming.

Related to this attribution of cause is the theory of locus of control, which refers to a component in social-learning theory of personality, suggested by Julian B. Rotter (Rotter, 1954). This theory suggests that individuals have a cognitive construct for the degree to which they believe they have control over the outcomes of the events in their lives. So, the theory suggests that a high locus of control is related to a belief of high control over the environment and low locus of control is related to the belief of low control over one's life. This was then later adapted for health locus of control (Wallston et al., 1976) which consists of having internal or external locus of control over individual beliefs on health issues in a way which could affect health (Wallston, 1992; Wolinsky et al., 2009). For example, if one believes that their illness was outside of their control they may not try to take the appropriate steps in order to manage the problem. This could then lead to the mental illness (e.g. stress) to spiral out of control thus leading to further distress.

MODELS OF HEALTH BELIEF IN ILLNESS REPRESENTATION

Attitudes may also play an important part in illness representation. Attitudes are thought to be common sense representations that the individual holds in relation to objects, people and events (Eagly and Chaiken, 1993). Another definition is that they are 'a relatively enduring organization of beliefs, feelings, and behavioural tendencies towards socially significant objects, groups, events or symbols' (Hogg and Vaughan, 2005).

The principle of consistency refers to expectation that people are rational and their behaviour should be consistent with their attitudes. One such study that explored this was conducted by LaPiere (LaPiere, 1934); however, he did not always find consistency between behaviour and attitudes. Attitudes have been found to be better predictors of behaviour when they are strong and have importance, personal relevance or valued by a group the individual is a member of. Another aspect in determining attitude strength and predicting behaviour is the influence of knowledge, which is how much the individual knows about the object, situation, and so on. A third factor that may influence the strength of the attitude is whether the attitude is based on direct or indirect experience (e.g. reading, television, hearsay).

As with the debate on personality, there is some debate about whether attitudes are genetically orientated or completely learned through the environment (Tesser, 1993), and this has largely been explored through studies involving twins (Martin et al., 1986). There is likely to be a substantial learning component to attitudes. Daniel Katz (Katz, 1960) identified that attitudes can provide knowledge for life in a consistent and relatively stable world. As attitudes involve knowledge they would need to be learned through environmental factors. Katz suggested that attitudes allow us to predict what is likely to happen and give us a sense of control as they help us to organise the structure of our experience. Katz also suggested that attitudes help us be ego expressive, whereby they help us communicate who we are, assert our identity, feelings, values and beliefs, whether verbally or non-verbally. Thirdly, Katz suggested that attitudes are adaptive in the sense that when they are socially accepted they are usually expressed as they gain approval from peers and are kept hidden when this is not the case. Finally, Katz suggested that attitudes provide a mechanism for ego defence, in that they can provide the function of protecting the individual's self-esteem or justify actions that may make us feel guilty. Katz suggested that attitudes may help the individual mediate their inner needs (expression and defence) with the outside world.

It is also interesting to note that attitudes can be implicit and explicit (Greenwald and Banaji, 1995). Explicit attitudes are attitudes that exist at the conscious level; they are deliberately formed and easy to self-report. Implicit attitudes are attitudes that are at the unconscious level, which are involuntarily formed and are typically unknown to us. So, sometimes our behaviours and responses to the threat of illness or coping may be shaped by attitudes which are not readily apparent to us.

In terms of specific models of attitudes, the three-component model (Eagly and Chaiken, 1998) suggested that attitudes can be described by three processes: (1) affective component – personal emotions ('I am scared of spiders'); (2) behavioural component – the way that attitudes affect behaviour ('I will avoid spiders'); and (3) cognitive component – this involves beliefs/knowledge about the object or event ('I believe spiders are dangerous').

Another model called the health belief model (HBM) tried to explain and predict behaviour (Hochbaum et al., 1952; Rosenstock et al., 1994) and has been used to explore a variety of health behaviours. This includes several factors which influence and predict the likelihood of engaging in health-promoting behaviour such as perceived seriousness, perceived threat, benefits vs barriers and self-efficacy. However, this model was criticised as it did not consider emotions. The theory of reasoned action (TRA) (Fishbein and Ajzen, 1975) was developed in response to problems with the HBM. TRA included emotions into the model such as the role of fear as an important determinant of health behaviour (Witte, 1992). This model included attitude, subjective norm, perceived behavioural control which are all thought to lead onto intention and behaviour. This model was developed further in order to increase the predictive power and now included perceived behavioural control in the theory of planned behaviour (Ajzen, 1991).

APPLIED HEALTH PSYCHOLOGY APPROACHES TO WELL-BEING

The first and most widely utilised psychological intervention is cognitive behavioural therapy (CBT), a second-wave behavioural therapy, which uses a symptom reduction approach of thought reconstruction to reduce disorder symptoms (Beck, 2011). However, other approaches are available which include acceptance and commitment therapy (ACT) (Hayes et al., 2011; Strosahl and Wilson, 1999), positive psychology (Seligman, 2012), dialectical behavioural therapy (DBT) (Linehan, 2018), metacognitive therapy (MCT) (Wells, 2002) and mindfulness-based cognitive therapy (MBCT) (Segal et al., 2018).

ACT is different to more traditional (second wave) therapies such as CBT as it emphasises psychological flexibility, a fundamental component of individual health and well-being (Kashdan and Rottenberg, 2010). Psychological flexibility in ACT revolves around the six key properties, which are: (1) the here and now (mindfulness); (2) acceptance; (3) cognitive defusion; (4) values; (5) commitment; (6) self as context (Hayes et al., 2011; Strosahl and Wilson, 1999). Through ACT, an individual builds skills in these six key areas, which helps clients change the way they relate to negative thoughts, emotions and memories, and commit action to what they value which ultimately leads to greater quality of life (Hayes, 2005).

In terms of societal issues, ACT has been usefully applied to problems of smoking cessation (Gifford et al., 2004), burnout at work (Hayes et al., 2004), stress management (Bond and Bunce, 2000), diabetes management (Gregg et al., 2007), depression (Hayes et al., 2006), psychosis (Gaudiano and Herbert, 2006) as well as pain-related distress, anxiety and depressive symptoms (Buhrman et al., 2013), to name a few.

CONCLUSION

Broadly, health psychology and understanding of illness have been shaped through the different approaches within the development of psychology. From this, we have identified that mental illness, and our coping responses to illness, can be formed through attitudes, our personality, learning theories such as behaviourism, social schemas and our attitudes. Though some of these psychology traditions may be distinct and utilise their own ontologies, there may be overlap between these theories, particularly when it comes to treatment. This is clear with the use of CBT which combines behavioural and cognitive components to help alleviate destructive learned associations as well as maladaptive thinking. Given the broad range of effective interventions such as positive psychology, CBT and ACT, health psychologists are well placed to help people in society with many of their mental health problems as well as facilitate other health care professionals such as social and community workers.

ACTIVITY 2.1   TEST YOURSELF

Having read this chapter:

- What do you feel are the main theories in psychology which best explain health and illness from a psychology perspective?
- How can personality theories be used by health psychologists to understand illness representation?
- What are the main differences between cognitive and behavioural models in relation to illness representation?
- How can implicit and explicit attitudes play a role in mental illness?
- Please reflect for a moment on everything you have learned. Where do you feel psychology is going in the future in terms of developing better models to account for health and illness representation?

ANSWERS TO CHAPTER 2 ACTIVITIES

——— Activity 2.1: Test Yourself: Answers

- The learning (behavioural), personality, and cognitive theories listed in the chapter.
- By explaining how personality traits lead to illness representation. This informs health psychologists in terms of which psychological treatment is appropriate.

- Behavioural models focus on learning whilst cognitive models focus on processing.
- Implicit is the non-conscious attitudes whilst explicit are the conscious attitudes. Both have an effect on how we represent mental illness.
- More evidence is developing the behavioural, personality, and cognitive models. There seems to be some overlapping between models as these develop such as Bandura's model which included both cognitive and behavioural elements. There may be more overlapping of this kind in the future.

——— Pause for Thought 2.1: Answers

- Early philosophers and those from the time of Sigmund Freud had very little evidence to base their theories from.
- No, humorous theories were not grounded in good methodology and evidence.
- Biopsychosocial model is more inclusive.

——— Pause for Thought 2.2: Answers

- They both have a place in treatment.
- Both. Individual treatments and preventative methods are useful approaches.
- More evidence is needed for both of these approaches in treatment to develop treatment further. Greater communication between psychopharmacologists and psychologists may be needed.

REFERENCES

Ajzen, I. (1991) The theory of planned behavior. *Organizational Behavior and Human Decision Processes* 50(2), 179–211.

Allport, G. W. (1937) *Personality: A Psychological Interpretation*. New York: Holt.

Allport, G. W. (1961) *Pattern and Growth in Personality*. New York: Holt, Rhinehart & Wilson.

American Psychiatric Association (2000) *Diagnostic and Statistical Manual of Mental Disorders*. Washington, DC: American Psychiatric Association.

American Psychiatric Association (2013) *Diagnostic and Statistical Manual of Mental Disorders (DSM-5)*. Washington DC: American Psychiatric Publishing.

American Psychological Association Presidential Task Force on Evidence Based Practice. (2006). *APA Presidential Task Force on Evidence Based Practice*. Washington, DC: American Psychological Association.

Bandura, A. (1965) Influence of models' reinforcement contingencies on the acquisition of imitative responses. *Journal of Personality and Social Psychology* 1(6), 589–595.

Bandura, A. (1978). Social learning theory of aggression. *Journal of Communication* 28(3), 12–29.

Bandura, A., Ross, D. and Ross, S. A. (1961). Transmission of aggression through imitation of aggressive models. *The Journal of Abnormal and Social Psychology* 63(3), 575–582.

Buhrman, M., Skoglund, A., Husell, J., Bergström, K., Gordh, T., Hursti, T., et al. (2013). Guided internet-delivered acceptance and commitment therapy for chronic pain patients: a randomized controlled trial. *Behav. Res. Ther.* 51, 307–315. doi: 10.1016/j.brat.2013.02.010

Baumeister, R. F. (1999) Self-concept, self-esteem, and identity. In V. Derlega, B. Winstead, and W. Jones (eds), *Personality: Contemporary Theory and Research* (2nd ed.) (pp. 339–375). Chicago: Nelson-Hall.

Beck, J. S. (2011). *Cognitive Behavior Therapy: Basics and Beyond*. New York: Guilford Press.

Bond, F. W. and Bunce, D. (2000). Mediators of change in emotion-focused and problem-focused work-site stress management interventions. *Journal of Occupational Health Psychology* 5(1), 156 –163.

Brickman, P., Coates, D. and Janoff-Bulman, R. (1978). Lottery winners and accident victims: is happiness relative? *Journal of Personality and Social Psychology* 36(8), 917–927.

Carlisle, S., Henderson, G. and Hanlon, P. W. (2009). 'Wellbeing': a collateral casualty of modernity? *Social Science & Medicine* 69(10), 1556-1560.

Cattell, R. B. (1945). The description of personality: principles and findings in a factor analysis. *The American Journal of Psychology* 58(1), 69–90.

Chesney, E., Goodwin, G. M. and Fazel, S. (2014). Risks of all-cause and suicide mortality in mental disorders: a meta-review. *World Psychiatry* 13(2), 153–160.

Chomsky, N. (1957). *Syntactic Structures*. The Hague: Mouton.

Chomsky, N. (1959). A review of BF Skinner's verbal behavior. *Language* 35(1), 26–58.

Cohen, L. J. (1981). Can human irrationality be experimentally demonstrated? *Behavioral and Brain Sciences* 4(3), 317–331.

Costa, P., McCrae, R. R. and Dye, D. A. (1991). Facet scales for agreeableness and conscientiousness: a revision of the NEO Personality Inventory. *Personality and Individual Differences* 12(9), 887–898.

Derry, S. J. (1996). Cognitive schema theory in the constructivist debate. *Educational Psychologist* 31(3–4), 163–174.

Di Blasi, Z., Harkness. E., Ernst, E. et al. (2001). Influence of context effects on health outcomes: a systematic review. *The Lancet* 357(9258), 757–762.

Dictionary of Psychology (2009). Edited by Andrew M. Colman. Oxford University Press.

Dykman, B. M., Horowitz, L. M., Abramson, L. Y. et al. (1991). Schematic and situational determinants of depressed and nondepressed students' interpretation of feedback. *Journal of Abnormal Psychology* 100(1), 45.

Eagly, A. H. and Chaiken, S. (1993). *The Psychology of Attitudes*. Fort Worth, TX: Harcourt Brace Jovanovich.

Eagly, A. H. and Chaiken, S. (1998). Attitude structure and function. In D. T. Gilbert, S. T. Fiske and G. Lindzey (eds), *The Handbook of Social Psychology* (pp. 269–322). New York: Oxford University Press.

Engel, G. L. (1977). The need for a new medical model: a challenge for biomedicine. *Science* 196(4286), 129–136.

Eysenck, H. (1964). *The Eysenck Personality Inventory*. London: University of London Press.

Eysenck, H. (1966). Personality and experimental psychology. *Bulletin of the British Psychological Society*, 19, 1–28.

Eysenck H. (2017). *The Biological Basis of Personality*. New York: Routledge.

Ferster, C. B. and Skinner, B. F. (1957). *Schedules of Reinforcement*. New York: Appleton-CenturyCrofts.

Fishbein, M. and Ajzen, I. (1975). *Belief, Attitude, Intention and Behavior: An Introduction to Theory and Research*. Reading, MA: Addison-Wesley.

Fodor, J. (1983). *The Modularity of Mind*. Cambridge, MA: MIT Press.

Freud, S. (1916). Introductory lectures on psycho-analysis. The Standard Edition of the Complete Psychological Works of Sigmund Freud, Volume XVI (1916-1917): Introductory Lectures on Psycho-Analysis (Part III), 241–463.

Freud, S. (1923). The ego and the id. In the *Standard Edition of the Complete Psychological Works of Sigmund Freud* (trans. & ed. Strachey, J.), vol 19: 3–66. London: Hogarth Press.

Freud, S. (2017). *Jenseits des lustprinzips*. Litres.

Gaudiano, B. A. and Herbert, J. D. (2006). Believability of hallucinations as a potential mediator of their frequency and associated distress in psychotic inpatients. *Behavioural and Cognitive Psychotherapy* 34(4), 497–502.

Gifford, E. V., Kohlenberg, B. S., Hayes, S. C. et al. (2004). Acceptance-based treatment for smoking cessation. *Behavior Therapy* 35(4), 689–705.

Greenwald, A. G. and Banaji, M. R. (1995). Implicit social cognition: attitudes, self-esteem, and stereotypes. *Psychological Review* 102(1), 4–21.

Gregg, J. A., Callaghan, G. M., Hayes, S. C. et al. (2007). Improving diabetes self-management through acceptance, mindfulness, and values: a randomized controlled trial. *Journal of Consulting and Clinical Psychology* 75(2), 336–343.

Harter S. (1993). Causes and consequences of low self-esteem in children and adolescents. In R. F. Baumeister (eds), *Self-esteem* (pp. 87–116). New York: Plenum Press.

Hayes, S. C. (2005). *Get Out of Your Mind and into Your Life: The New Acceptance and Commitment Therapy*. Oakland, CA: New Harbinger Publications.

Hayes, S.C, Bissett, R., Roget, N. et al. (2004). The impact of acceptance and commitment training and multicultural training on the stigmatizing attitudes and professional burnout of substance abuse counselors. *Behavior Therapy* 35(4), 821–835.

Hayes, S. C, Luoma, J. B., Bond, F. W., Masuda, A. and Lillis, J. et al. (2006). Acceptance and commitment therapy: model, processes and outcomes. *Behaviour Research and Therapy* 44(1), 1–25.

Hayes, S.C., Strosahl, K.D. and Wilson, K.G. (2011). *Acceptance and Commitment Therapy: The Process and Practice of Mindful Change*. New York: Guilford Press.

Heider, F. (1958). The psychology of interpersonal relations. *The Journal of Marketing* 56, 322.

Hicks, R. D. (2015). *Aristotle De Anima*. Cambridge: Cambridge University Press.

Hochbaum, G., Rosenstock, I. and Kegels, S. (1952). Health belief model. United States Public Health Service.

Hofmann, S. G. and Hayes, S. C. (2018). The history and current status of CBT as an evidence-based therapy. In S. G. Hofmann and S. C. Hayes (eds), *Process-Based CBT: The Science and Core Clinical Competencies of Cognitive Behavioral Therapy*. Oakland. CA: New Harbinger Publications.

Hogg, M. A and Vaughan G. M. (2005). *Social Psychology* (4th ed). London: Prentice Hall.

Huber, M., Knottnerus, J. A., Green, L., van der Horst, H., Jadad, A. R., Kromhout, D., ... and Schnabel, P. (2011). How should we define health? *BMJ*, 343, d4163.

Janoff-Bulman, R. (1979). Characterological versus behavioral self-blame: inquiries into depression and rape. *Journal of Personality and Social Psychology* 37(10), 1798–1809.

Kashdan, T. B. and Rottenberg, J. (2010). Psychological flexibility as a fundamental aspect of health. *Clinical Psychology Review* 30(7), 865–878.

Katz, D. (1960) The functional approach to the study of attitudes. *Public Opinion Quarterly* 24(2), 163–204.

Kemp, A. H., Arias, J. A. and Fisher, Z. (2017). Social ties, health and wellbeing: a literature review and model. In *Neuroscience and Social Science* (pp. 397–427). Springer, Cham.

Kleider, H. M., Pezdek, K., Goldinger, S. D. et al. (2008). Schema-driven source misattribution errors: remembering the expected from a witnessed event. *Applied Cognitive Psychology: The Official Journal of the Society for Applied Research in Memory and Cognition* 22(1), 1–20.

Klimenko, V. M. and Golikov, J. P. (2003). The Pavlov department of physiology: a scientific history. *The Spanish Journal of Psychology*, 6(2), 112–120.

LaPiere, R. T. (1934). Attitudes vs. actions. *Social Forces* 13(2), 230–237.

Leventhal, H., Diefenbach, M. and Leventhal, E. A. (1992). Illness cognition: using common sense to understand treatment adherence and affect cognition interactions. *Cognitive Therapy and Research* 16(2), 143–163.

Linehan, M. M. (2018). *Cognitive-Behavioral Treatment of Borderline Personality Disorder*. New York: Guilford Publications.

Martin, N. G., Eaves, L. J., Heath, A. C. et al. (1986). Transmission of social attitudes. *Proceedings of the National Academy of Sciences* 83(12), 4364–4368.

McGuire, R. J. and Vallance, M. (1964). Aversion therapy by electric shock: a simple technique. *British Medical Journal*, 151–153.

Neisser, U. (1967). *Cognitive Psychology*. New York: Appleton-Century-Crofts.

NICE (2019). Antisocial behaviour and conduct disorders in children and young people: recognition and management. NICE Clinical Guidelines, No. 158. National Collaborating Centre for Mental Health (UK); Social Care Institute for Excellence (UK).Leicester (UK): British Psychological Society; 2013.

Patel, V. and Prince, M. (2010). Global mental health: a new global health field comes of age. *Jama*, 303(19), 1976-1977.

Pavlov, I. (1897). *The Work of the Digestive Glands* (trans. W. H. Thompson). London: Griffin. (Original work published in 1897)

Piaget, J. and Cook, M. (1952) *The Origins of Intelligence in Children*. New York: International Universities Press.

Roberts, J. E. and Monroe, S. M. (1994). A multidimensional model of self-esteem in depression. *Clinical Psychology Review* 14, 161–181.

Rosen, R. (1991). Some systems theoretical problems in biology. *Facets of Systems Science* (pp. 607–619). Springer.

Rosenberg, M. (1986). *Conceiving the Self*. New York: Basic Books.

Rosenstock, I. M., Strecher, V. J. and Becker, M. H. (1994). The health belief model and HIV risk behavior change. *Preventing AIDS*. (pp. 5–24). Boston, MA: Springer.

Rothe, J. P. (2017). *The Scientific Analysis of Personality*. Abingdon: Routledge.

Rotter, J. B. (1954). *Social Learning and Clinical Psychology*. Englewood Cliffs, NJ: Prentice Hall.

Sackett, D. L. (1997). *Evidence-Based Medicine How to Practice and Teach EBM*. New York: W.B. Saunders Company.

Schaffner, K. F. (2001). Nature and nurture. *Current Opinion in Psychiatry* 14(5), 485–490.

Segal, Z. V., Williams, M. and Teasdale, J. (2018). *Mindfulness-Based Cognitive Therapy for Depression*. New York: Guilford Publications.

Seligman, M. E. (2012). *Positive Psychology in Practice*. New York: John Wiley & Sons.

Skinner, B. (1938). *The Behavior of Organisms: An Experimental Analysis*. New York: Appleton-Century.

Strosahl, K. and Wilson, K. (1999). *Acceptance and Commitment Therapy: An Experiential Approach to Behavior Change*. New York: Guilford Press.

Tesser, A. (1993). The importance of heritability in psychological research: the case of attitudes. *Psychological Review* 100(1), 129–142.

Tolin, D. F., McKay, D., Forman, E. M et al. (2015). Empirically supported treatment: Recommendations for a new model. *Clinical Psychology: Science and Practice* 22(4), 317–338.

Wadsworth, B. J. (1996). *Piaget's Theory of Cognitive and Affective Development: Foundations of Constructivism*. New York: Longman Publishing.

Wallston, B. S., Wallston, K. A., Kaplan, G. D. et al. (1976). Development and validation of the health locus of control (HLC) scale. *Journal of Consulting and Clinical Psychology* 44(4), 580.

Wallston, K. A. (1992). Hocus-pocus, the focus isn't strictly on locus: Rotter's social learning theory modified for health. *Cognitive Therapy and Research* 16(2), 183–199.

Wang, P. S., Berglund, P. A., Olfson, M. and Kessler R. C. (2004) 'Delays in initial treatment contact after first onset of a medical disorder' *Health Services Research*, 39(2), 393–415.

Watson, J. and Raynor, R. (1920). Emotional reactions. *Journal of Experimental Psychology* 3, 1–14.

Watson, J. B. (1913). Psychology as the behaviorist views it. *Psychological Review* 20(2), 158–177.

Weinberg, R. and Gould, D. (1999). Personality and sport. *Foundations of Sport and Exercise Psychology*, 25–46.

Wells, A. (2002). *Emotional Disorders and Metacognition: Innovative Cognitive Therapy*. Chichester: John Wiley & Sons.

Witte, K. (1992). Putting the fear back into fear appeals: the extended parallel process model. *Communications Monographs* 59(4), 329–349.

Wolinsky, F. D., Vander Weg, M. W., Martin, R. et al. (2009). Does cognitive training improve internal locus of control among older adults? *Journals of Gerontology Series B: Psychological Sciences and Social Sciences* 65(5), 591–598.

World Health Organization (1948) Manual of the International Statistical Classification of Diseases, Injuries, and Causes of Death. Sixth Revision of the International Lists of Diseases and Causes of Death Adopted 1948. Bulletin of the World Health Organization 1(1).

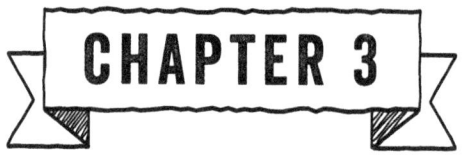

CHAPTER 3

ACADEMIC SKILLS AND PRACTICE

Pete Hanratty and Ben Martin

OVERVIEW

This chapter will take you through some of the essential skills you will need to succeed in the academic element of your Health and Social Care degree. On the following pages, you will find five core principles that will help you understand what your lecturers are looking for from your academic work and how you can achieve it.

The chapter is by no means exhaustive – there are many other skills you will develop over the course of your studies – nor does it go into detail as to how to research and write specific types of assignments such as reflective work. However, the principles do provide an introduction to the academic context in which you will be writing.

LEARNING OUTCOMES

By the end of this chapter you will be able to:

- Identify and improve instances of poor academic writing style
- Develop strategies to read more effectively
- Develop strategies to improve your paraphrasing
- Understand how to logically structure your written work
- Develop strategies to be more critical in your work

PRINCIPLE 1: ACADEMIC STYLE

Students can find it difficult to express themselves in an appropriate academic style, which can result in feedback from lecturers stating the work is 'unclear', has 'incorrect expression', is 'too informal' or 'wordy'. These kinds of problems can impact on students' marks.

Expressing yourself academically is something that requires practice, and this section will detail some common issues before suggesting solutions to these problems and providing an opportunity for you to practise identifying and editing instances of poor academic style. The most effective way for you to improve the style of your academic writing is to identify how you can be clearer in your expression. Consider the example below from a student's reflective assignment.

ACTIVITY 3.1 REFLECTIVE ASSIGNMENT

Initially, when I first went in to the communal room, I noticed that poor Mr Jones was sitting all by himself at the window, staring into space. I walked up towards him so that I could ask him whether he was ready to have his check-up, and as I approached him he jumped out of his skin and looked absolutely petrified and at sixes and sevens. The colour had gone from his face and he was now as pale as a ghost. I remember thinking that I had to be careful of how I communicated with him in his fragile state and looked him straight in the eyes and spoke out to him to let him know who I was. His face changed and he looked a bit more chilled out. Still looking at him, I decided to pull up the chair next to him so that I could keep chatting and try my best to get him to relax more. After a little while, I asked him about his last check-up and whether he was ready for another check-up. His face now lit up and he said that he was ready.

On first read, you may find a few examples in which the student could have expressed themselves in a more appropriate way. Consider Table 3.1, which illustrates some of the points that the student should address and suggests solutions.

Table 3.1 Problems with sample text and suggested solutions

Text	Problem & *Solution*	Text	Problem & *Solution*
Initially, when I first…	Repetition of idea. *This could be replaced by deleting 'Initially'/'first'*	as pale as a ghost	Idiom which could be misunderstood. *Replace with 'pale'/'visibly pale'*
went in	Two-part verb using unnecessary words. *Replace with one word alternative 'entered'*	looked him straight in the eyes	Too many words resulting in a clumsy expression. *Replace with 'made eye contact'*
poor Mr Jones sitting all by himself	Too many words resulting in a clumsy expression. No need to write 'poor' as it's too emotive. *Replace with 'Mr Jones was sitting alone'*	spoke out to him to let him know who I was	Too many words resulting in a clumsy expression. *Replace with 'introduced myself'*
staring into space	Unclear: was he **really** staring into 'space'? *Consider deleting*	His face changed	Unclear: how did his face change? *Replace with 'his expression changed'*
I walked up	Two-part verb using unnecessary word. *Replace with 'walked'/'approached'/ delete 'up'*	he looked a bit more chilled out	Idiom which could be misunderstood, and too many words used. *Replace with 'he appeared more relaxed/comfortable'*

(Continued)

Table 3.1   (Continued)

Text	Problem & *Solution*	Text	Problem & *Solution*
he jumped out of his skin	Idiom which could be misunderstood. *Replace with 'jolted'/'was surprised'*	and try my best to get him to relax more	Too many words resulting in a clumsy expression. *Replace with 'attempted to comfort him'*
absolutely petrified	Idiom which could be misunderstood: this means 'turned to stone'. *Replace with 'scared'*	After a little while	Unclear expression. *Replace with 'approximately two/ three/five minutes'*
at sixes and sevens	Idiom which could be misunderstood. *Replace with 'confused'*	His face now lit up	Idiom which could be misunderstood. *Replace with 'he smiled'/'he appeared more relaxed'*

Now consider the revised version below:

Initially, when I entered the communal room, I noticed that Mr Jones was sitting alone, staring out of the window. I walked towards him so that I could ask him whether he was ready to have his check-up, and as I approached him he jolted with surprise and appeared scared and confused. The colour had gone from his face and he was now visibly pale. I remember thinking that I had to be careful of how I communicated with him in his fragile state and made eye contact and introduced myself. His expression changed and he appeared more comfortable. Still looking at him, I decided to pull up the chair next to him and attempted to comfort him. After approximately five minutes, I asked him about his last check-up and whether he was ready for another check-up. He smiled and he said that he was ready.

Now we have identified some common issues in student work, and suggested some solutions, it is important to practise this skill – as only practice will help you to spot these problems in your own work.

ACTIVITY 3.2

Consider the exercise below from a student's assignment on methods to engage hard-to-reach groups. Can you identify the areas for improvement?

There are a lot of ways to engage with hard-to-reach groups. One of the main, most effective ways could be cognitive behavioural programmes which can be tailored to specific groups and individuals. As well as this, another way can be practitioners' advice and feedback given during the time of visits to homes and places of residence. There is, sadly, not too much evidence which has been collected on the nature of the feedback and advice given, nor how effective such interventions are. The level of engagement which can be got with hard-to-reach groups can also vary depending on the barriers to engagement which can possibly be present: each and every single one of us is different and, at the end of the day, interventions should be designed with specific groups in mind.

Check the end of the chapter for an answer to this activity.

PRINCIPLE 2: READING

For any essay or assignment in higher education, you will be required to back up the claims or ideas you include with the ideas of other academics or professionals in your field. This means reading – and a lot of it – will soon become a staple in your Health and Social Care Studies diet. Problems students usually find with reading include:

- There is too much to read and so little time.
- Knowing which texts are reliable.

We'll cover how to incorporate the ideas of others into your work in the next two sections of this chapter. But first, it's worth spending a little time learning some techniques that can help you become a more efficient academic reader.

WHEN DOES READING BEGIN?

Your lecturer hands you your first assignment title along with a recommended reading list. What's the first thing you do?

If you're like many students, you'll head straight to the library and take out all the books on the list, then start to plough through them. A* for effort – but in your diligence you've missed an important stage called 'pre-reading'.

PRE-READING

With so much to read, the sheer volume of texts, ideas and authors can soon become overwhelming. How do you know if what you are reading is even relevant to the question?

Try this. Before you even begin reading, write out a very basic plan for your answer to the question. Of course, at this stage your plan will have some gaps as there are lots of elements you don't know. But you'll also be surprised at how much you do know and the general direction that you think your assignment will take.

BOX 3.1 EXAMPLE ASSIGNMENT PLAN

Consider the question:

'Smoking is the most preventable cause of ill health in Britain today' (NHS 2016). With reference to specific smoking-related illnesses and ethical issues, discuss whether smokers should have the same access to the limited resources of the National Health Service.

Possible initial response:

- Smokers should have the same rights – despite the element of personal choice it's too hard to say other factors contributed to illness.

Situation:

- Statistics on smoking – difference between socio-demographic areas.
- List of main smoking-related diseases.

Arguments why smokers should have limited access to NHS.

- They make a choice that damages their health.

Ways to counter this:

- Human rights angle.
- Other factors that may contribute to illness.
- Other diseases where choice matters, e.g. obesity.
- Pregnant women – actually need more support.

As you can see, you don't need to have a lot of detail, but even by quickly jotting down your initial response you can start to get an idea of the direction your answer may take. This will naturally change as you read and learn more, but you have a starting point! You can use this plan as a way to guide your reading, as now you can see where the gaps are. The next step is to write a series of questions that will help you fill these gaps.

Continuing with the same example, these questions might look like this:

Situation:

- Facts and statistics on smoking – difference between socio-demographic areas.
- What are the latest figures on smoking-related diseases?
- What are smoking rates in the UK?

List of main smoking related diseases:

- What are the main smoking-related diseases?
- What qualifies as a smoking-related disease?
- What are current guidelines with regards treatment? Is there any distinction?

Arguments why smokers should have limited access:

- Who makes this argument?
- What are their reasons? Money? Choice?
- What do smoking-related illnesses cost the NHS?

Ways to counter this:

- Human rights angle.
- What do human rights bodies say about right to free choice?
- What does UK government policy say about right to free health care?

Other factors that may contribute to illness:

- What are other factors related to smoking – e.g. do smokers tend to be from lower socio-demographic backgrounds? If so what are the comparative rates of disease?
- How easy is it to definitively say that smoking causes an illness?
- Other diseases where choice matters, e.g. obesity.
- What are the obesity rates in the UK? Is it a more serious problem? To what extent is obesity a choice of diet?
- What other diseases can be caused by risky lifestyle choices? Extreme sports injuries?
- Pregnant women – do they actually have more support?

The student in the example above now has a long list of questions that need answering and can approach the texts with these at the forefront of their mind.

Important note: Your assignment plan (and perhaps your ideas) will almost certainly change as you read. The first set of questions will lead to more questions, and you may well go through this process several times as you explore your subject.

TARGETED READING: HONING IN

Armed with your list of questions, you return to your reading list. Now you can tackle your reading not one book at a time, but one question at a time.

This is a very different approach from simply reading texts in the hope that quotes or ideas jump out at you. You have a purpose for reading and you can seek out the answers to your questions. This is the difference between being an *active* or *passive* reader. We'll return to this idea later, but for now let's consider how asking questions before we read can help us be more efficient in our reading.

The first question to ask is whether a particular book or journal will be helpful in answering our particular question. You should look broadly at the title or abstract to see if you will be likely to find the answer you are looking for.

Remember also that you very rarely have to read all of a book. You can use other 'honing-in' techniques to help find the information you want.

ACTIVITY 3.3

Take a couple of minutes and jot down as many different ways of 'honing in' as you can think of.

Check the end of the chapter for an answer to this activity.

Honing in can help you out as a reader by giving you a sense of what is to come next. This can help you a lot when you're looking to answer the questions you have laid out in your plan. You can (and should) use all the techniques given in the answer to this exercise to help you read faster and pinpoint the exact answers to your questions, before you move onto the next stage.

READING FOR DETAIL

At some point the honing-in process ends and the serious business of reading begins. Problems students often face at this stage include:

- Not fully understanding information.
- Not remembering who said what when they come to write their assignments.

The ideas we'll look at next will help you do both more effectively and become a more efficient academic reader.

ACTIVITY 3.4

Can you put the following activities into order of how useful you find them when reading?

- Highlighting
- Making notes in the margin
- Paraphrasing key ideas
- Writing summaries at the end of key paragraphs
- Underlining
- Copying out good quotes

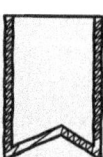

PAUSE FOR THOUGHT 3.1

How many of these techniques do you currently use when you read?

There's no one right answer here, and if you are using any of these techniques you are doing something right – much better than simply reading and putting the book to one side without picking up a pen. However, we would probably put the techniques into the following order – from least to most useful:

Copying quotes

Highlighting

Underlining

Making notes

Paraphrasing

Writing summaries at the end of chapters

We might further separate them like this:

Passive	**Active**
Copying quotes	Making notes in the margin
Highlighting	Paraphrasing key ideas
Underlining	Writing summaries of chapters

Take a moment to think about the difference between these two categories. In the first column, passive reading, none of the activities take too much extra thought. You highlight or underline a key word, or copy a quote verbatim, but you are not necessarily engaging with the material on a higher level.

In the second category, the actions all require effort on your part. To put an idea into your own words you have to understand it; to summarise the key ideas in a chapter you have to think about what the key elements are and how they link together. And your notes in the margin might be questions, comments, reminders on how this might link to other literature elsewhere, and so on.

When you are an *active reader* you are engaging with the text in a different way. You've come in with questions and you're making a concerted attempt to find the answers. You're *analysing and critiquing* the ideas expressed and thinking about how they link to those of other authors you have read.

BECOMING A CRITICAL READER

One of the most common pieces of feedback received by students in the early stages of their higher education is that their writing is not critical or analytical enough. Of course, the first step to being a critical writer is to become a critical reader. As you read any text, it can be useful to consider the following questions:

- What are the main ideas expressed?
- How does the author back up these ideas? Have they left any key points out and why?
- How do these ideas relate to what other authors have said on the same topic?
- What evidence have they used to back up their points?
- If they cite studies, are there any notable limitations to this study (size, time period, was it privately funded by an organisation with a vested interest, etc.)?

Note that it might take more than one reading of a text to answer all these questions and really engage with it on the required critical level.

TAKING NOTES

There are many different ways to take notes, and you should cultivate a range of techniques as all have their different uses.

LISTING

List should be used for taking down the main ideas and sub-points in a text quickly, and beginning to organise your ideas. Your lists can become a starting point for your paragraphs, e.g.:

DIFFICULTIES IN ADDRESSING OBESITY

- Care not to offend patients
- Often an issue in areas of lower socio-economic demographic – harder to reach
- Media arguments as to causes are confusing
- 'Nanny state' argument

MATRICES

Matrices are useful for comparing the ideas of different authors. Compiling even a basic matrix like Table 3.2 can save you a lot of time when you come to write as you won't have to go back to the book to keep looking for who said those important quotes.

Table 3.2   Basic reading matrix

Author & Date	Main point	Comments
Johnson & Bukowski (2013)	Health care practitioners should aim to maximise contact with patients	Good idea and the reasons why are valid but they fail to go into detail as to how could be achieved in practice
Powell (2017)	Increased contact increases patients' well-being	Link to Johnson & Bukowski (2013)
Jameson (2016)	A report into the trial by NHS Wales where admin duties were reduced – showed improvement in patient satisfaction	Small study – not conclusive. But seems to back up Johnson's claim. Key point = reducing admin is possible

SPIDER DIAGRAMS

Spider diagrams are great for getting all your ideas down, without necessarily putting them into order. This form of note-taking can help you see connections between ideas. Using the question

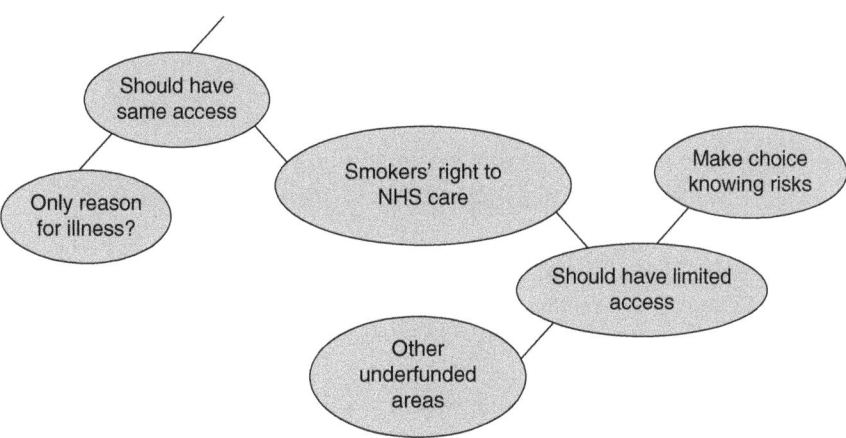

Figure 3.1 An example spider diagram

on smokers' rights as an example, see Figure 3.1. Each of the ideas in Figure 3.1 could be expanded upon with further points spanning from each of the circles.

TOP TIP: SPEED READING

Try this. Instead of focusing your eyes on every word as you read, try to take in three or four words at once. Focus just above the middle of the three or four words that you want to read and allow your eyes to 'absorb' them all at once. Then bounce your focus to a central spot above the next cluster of three or four words. You move your eye like a ball bouncing across the page. It takes some practice, but after a while you will be reading much quicker.

PRINCIPLE 3: PARAPHRASING

Sometimes it can seem as though the conventions of academic writing are asking you to do two, contradictory activities:

- Back up any point you make with evidence from another author.
- Make your work original, without plagiarising from other sources.

This conflict is something that presents students with a dilemma – 'How am I supposed to be original if all my work needs to be based on other people's ideas?'

To understand the answer, we must understand what our lecturers are looking for in our Health and Social Care assignments. At undergraduate level (and very often postgraduate level too) they do not expect you to come up with original ideas and solutions to problems. What they *do* want to see is that you have a clear understanding of the field and the current academic 'conversation' around key ideas. In Health and Social Care this means having an in-depth knowledge of everything from government policy to World Health Organization (WHO) guidelines, to a knowledge of the latest research.

But how do you prove that you really understand all the key issues and arguments in the area that you are writing about?

The answer is to employ one of the core skills of academic writing: paraphrasing.

WHY IS PARAPHRASING SO IMPORTANT?

Paraphrasing is such an important skill because it allows you to demonstrate clearly that you have grasped the point the author is trying to make. Also, it helps you to back up the points you make with reputable sources, synthesise the ideas of others and avoid penalties for plagiarism while writing with your own voice and style.

QUOTING?

Some quotes are acceptable, and in a few cases necessary. For example, if you need to mention a particular NHS guideline or WHO definition, you may be better off using the exact wording from the policy document. However, you should avoid using large chunks of quotes or quoting too often, as it is harder for a lecturer to ascertain your understanding and engagement with the topic. Anybody can copy and paste quotes that look like they might be relevant!

As a rough guide, no more than 20 per cent of the evidence you use to back up your argument should be direct quotes; that's a minimum of 80 per cent of the evidence you cite that should be paraphrased!

PARAPHRASING: A FIVE-STEP PROCESS

Let's say that you have found the following quote in a text that you are reading on barriers facing social care workers when dealing with hard to reach groups. You decide that the idea is an important one, but you don't need to quote it word for word to express it in your assignment.

Staff may have poor awareness of differing cultures or people with disabilities and could easily offend without any intention. (Reid, 2002)

STEP 1: IDENTIFY THE WORDS YOU CAN'T CHANGE

In many of the ideas you wish to paraphrase, you will find words that you can't change. This might be for the following reasons:

- The word is a key subject word relating to the issue you are talking about.
- The word is a proper noun, for example the name of a person, town or country.
- A direct synonym does not exist and explaining it would seem awkward and unnecessary in the context of the writing. 'Economy' is one such example; 'health care' might be another.

In this sentence there are no proper nouns. However, the word 'cultures' stands out as one that is very hard to accurately replace with just one word. Likewise, the word 'disabilities' has a very specific meaning that is hard to accurately replace. So in this sentence we will not try to change the words 'culture' and 'disabilities'.

STEP 2: THE WORDS YOU CAN CHANGE

Now it's time to identify the words you *can* change.

The most important thing with any paraphrase is *accuracy*. Sometimes this will be possible with a single word – sometimes it will require you to substitute a word for a phrase or vice versa to remain true to the meaning of the original.

A word of warning here: don't be tempted to use the right-click button and replace every word with the synonym you find – it can make for a very confusing sentence indeed!

Looking at our original sentence, which words or phrases do you think could be changed?

Staff may have poor awareness of differing cultures or people with disabilities and could easily offend without any intention. (Reid, 2002)

ACTIVITY 3.5

For each replaceable word in our source sentence, there are three possible synonyms below. Which one do you think is most accurate and relevant in the context of the original?

Staff – workers – employees – practitioners

Poor awareness – ignorant – oblivious – not know enough

Differing – varied – alternative – unfamiliar

Offend – upset – insult – hurt their feelings

Without any intention – unintentionally – accidentally – inadvertently

To see how far a sentence can stray from its original meaning with poor paraphrasing, consider the example below!

Employees may be oblivious to those from alternative cultures or people with disabilities and may insult them accidentally.

Check the end of the chapter for an answer to this activity.

STEPS 3 AND 4

Although our paraphrase is now noticeably different from the original, there is more that we could (and should) do to change it and make it 'our own'. At present, the sentence structure is still very similar to the original. If all our paraphrases only followed the sentence structures of the original, our writing would seem disjointed.

Therefore, two further steps can be taken to make our paraphrase more distinct from the original. These are:

- Changing the sentence structure.
- Changing the grammatical structure.

These two will often happen concurrently or even necessitate each other, so here we have presented the two stages together.

CHANGING THE SENTENCE STRUCTURE

One of the great things about English is that in most sentences with more than one clause (identifiable 'parts') the order can be changed without changing the meaning.

Taking the example that we have already worked through:

Practitioners may not know enough about unfamiliar cultural practices or people with disabilities and could easily hurt their feelings unintentionally. (Reid, 2002)

This could be altered to:

Practitioners could easily hurt patients' feelings without meaning to, as they may not know enough about unfamiliar cultural practices or people with disabilities. (Reid, 2002)

(Note that it was necessary to add the object of the sentence – 'patients' here; while it was obvious in the first example that the sentence meant patients, after switching the order it became necessary to direct the reader a little more.)

CHANGING THE GRAMMAR

One of the easiest grammatical switches to employ is going from the active voice to the passive voice, or vice versa: The nurse cared for the patient (active). The patient was cared for by the nurse (passive). When we do this we change the emphasis from who is doing the action, to who or what the action is done to (or vice versa).

In this example:

Patients' feelings could easily be hurt by practitioners who do not know enough about unfamiliar cultural practices or people with disabilities. (Reid, 2002)

You could also choose to make one sentence into two. For example:

Practitioners could easily hurt patients' feelings without meaning to. This is because they may not know enough about unfamiliar cultural practices or people with disabilities. (Reid, 2002)

The structure and grammar of the sentence can also be changed by incorporating the source in a different way:

Reid (2002) observes that practitioners could easily hurt patients' feelings without meaning to. This is because they may not know enough about unfamiliar cultural practices or people with disabilities.

Note that for this you need to add a 'reporting verb' ('observes' in this instance). You should have a good list of these to avoid using the same two or three throughout your text.

STEP 5: CHECK

Once you have written your paraphrase, it's essential that you check it again for accuracy. Is what you have written true to the original meaning?

Check it for grammatical accuracy too – have you written a correct sentence?

And finally acknowledge the source. Even if you have changed every word, you need to say where the idea came from.

PRINCIPLE 4: STRUCTURE

Once you have done all your reading and have a clear picture of the ideas you plan to include in your assignment, the next stage is to put it all together.

Remember – just because you have done all the reading and have a good understanding of the key areas of your topic, your lecturer *won't know that until you present it in your assignment.* We need to do this in a way that shows we have understood all the key points. The best way to do this effectively is to structure our work in a clear and logical fashion.

Throughout your degree you will work on a number of different projects, all of which will require a different structure. Reflective essays, for example, have a very different structure from research-based dissertations or argument-based essays. This section is not the space to go into detail about each of the various projects you will work on. However, we can outline some general structural principles which can help you write anything – from a reflective essay to a dissertation, or even an email!

THE POWER OF PREDICTION

When you are writing, it can be useful to remember one simple rule: in any situation we feel more comfortable and are more likely to enjoy ourselves if we have a reasonable idea of what to expect. We live our lives making predictions about the future – even if we do something intentionally surprising like watching a horror film, we predict that we are going to be surprised in a certain way (which allows us to enjoy it when the ghost appears in the mirror!).

Reading is no different from any other activity. It is easier and more enjoyable when you can make accurate predictions about the content. Therefore, our job as writers is to make it as easy as possible for our readers to predict what is coming. In the context of a written assignment, we can do this through three 'structural aids'.

STRUCTURAL AID #1: INTRODUCTIONS

The purpose of an introduction is to lay out clearly for the reader everything that they can expect in your assignment – even down to the conclusion that you will come to. In academic writing, unlike horror movies, there should be no surprises.

Most introductions have three distinct sections. It is often said that these sections move from the general to the specific, following a kind of 'funnel' shape.

Figure 3.2 is a very general description of the role of introductions. Some assignments, such as reflective pieces of work, may require specific elements from an introduction, and you should always be sure to follow the given guidelines. However, in any example the purpose of an introduction is the same: to prepare your reader for the journey ahead.

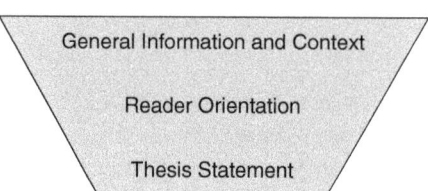

Figure 3.2   'Funnel-shaped' introduction

GENERAL INFORMATION AND CONTEXT

This is where you give some broad background information regarding the subject. You might choose to present some facts or statistics around the subject or perhaps even a relevant quote. You might also define some key terms that you will use throughout your essay.

READER ORIENTATION

Now you begin to discuss the way your answer will relate to the general issue you have described. Which of the main sub-points will you tackle? In what order will you tackle them? Which sources will you use? It is important to signpost this information to your reader here.

THESIS STATEMENT

Your thesis statement is where you outline the conclusion that you have come to over the course of your research, or your 'argument'. (For more on argument see the next Principle.)

ACTIVITY 3.6

Read the following introduction to a Health and Social Care essay and try to identify each of the three 'sections' of the introduction.

How does each section help prepare the reader for what is to come throughout the essay?

Recent statistics published by the Welsh Health Board confirm that 54 per cent of Welsh adults and 42 per cent of Welsh children can be categorised as obese (with a BMI in excess of $30kg/M^2$). The figures have remained constant since 1998, despite a number of programmes such as 'Active Wales' and 'Fit for Life Wales' being implemented by the Welsh government. Findings from two studies, 'Obesity in Wales' by the Welsh government (2012) and 'Fighting the Fat' by Active Wales (2013), agree that the central cause for this problem is a poor diet and a 'culture of inactivity' (Wilde, 2013). This essay will examine both these causes using recent case studies as examples, and will suggest that while identifying these causes is an important step, it is not enough to simply 'fire-fight'.

> Using evidence from other countries such as the United States and Mexico, this essay will argue that the most effective way to combat obesity is to educate children at a young age.
>
> Check the end of the chapter for an answer to this activity.

STRUCTURAL AID #2: PARAGRAPH HEADERS

We know that a typical assignment has an introduction, a main body and a conclusion. We understand that the purpose of the introduction is to signpost everything that a reader can expect from the assignment. The main body is where this will be delivered, and the conclusion provides a summary of the main points, perhaps guiding us to further reading or investigation.

Interestingly, the structure of a paragraph can be seen as a mini-version of the structure of an assignment. Consider Figure 3.3.

The most important feature for us to note here is that just as a good assignment begins by outlining what a reader can expect, so too a good paragraph should provide its own introduction. We often hear these called *topic sentences* or '*paragraph heads*'. These constitute simple sentences that prepare your reader for what to expect in the forthcoming paragraph.

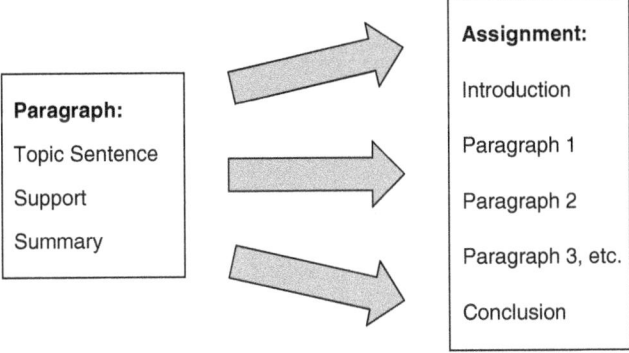

Figure 3.3   Structuring paragraphs

ACTIVITY 3.7

Consider the following example sentences. What would you expect to find in the paragraphs that follow each of these:

- The WHO (2017) outline three main benefits of giving up smoking.
- To combat the problem of disparity in care across providers, Johnson (2012) developed a framework for health care managers.

(Continued)

> - However, Graham (2018) sees the issues differently, arguing that many services fail to accurately report critical incidents in order to avoid the time-consuming administration process they entail.
>
> Check the end of the chapter for an answer to this activity.

Top Tip: Writing a list of your topic sentences can help you plan a coherent answer that covers all the points you want to make. It can also help you avoid the common problem of 'rambling' – going off on a tangent and changing topic mid-paragraph. Remember – one paragraph = one idea. Everything in your paragraph should relate to the topic sentence. When you begin to change subject, it's time for a new paragraph.

ACTIVITY 3.8

Try This – pick a magazine or newspaper article and try reading just the first sentence of every paragraph. Chances are you should be able to follow the story or catch the gist of the argument.

Your writing should be the same – can a reader pick up your assignment and skim it, but still follow the flow?

WHAT GOES INTO A PARAGRAPH?

Topic sentences outline the direction of a paragraph, perhaps presenting a stance or point of view at the same time.

The rest of the paragraph is your chance to expand upon this, developing the idea or backing up your point with the literature you have read.

Students often ask what length their paragraphs should be, but there is no fixed or 'ideal' length for a paragraph. Some points can be dealt with in just a few words – others will require a lot more explanation or discussion. In many cases three or four sources to back up your idea is enough, but don't take this as a rule. A paragraph is over when you have finished developing your point and you are ready to move on to the next one.

STRUCTURAL AID #3: TRANSITIONS AND COHESIVE DEVICES

You can help your reader find their way through your assignment by writing a clear introduction and by outlining the direction of every paragraph with a clear topic sentence. But there is one more step you can take to make sure your writing flows.

Consider the following two sentences:

Health and Social Care is a fascinating subject. It is very difficult to write about.

Now consider how the meaning changes if you add each of the following words in between the two sentences.

- However
- Therefore
- Because

These are *transition words*, and each one of them affects how we interpret the information. Correct use of these transition words has two main benefits for your writing:

- It allows you to show your understanding of the relationship between the ideas you are discussing.
- It helps your writing flow, as your reader is guided between points rather than having to make the links themselves.

The following is a list of some common transition words found within academic writing and their purposes:

Contradiction	Continuation	Meaning	Summarising
However	Furthermore	Therefore	Overall
Although	In addition	Thus	In conclusion
While	A further example	This means	In summary
... but ...			

ACTIVITY 3.9

Read the following paragraph from a Health and Social Care studies essay. All transition words have been removed. Which words might you use to help the ideas flow more clearly?

> It is clear that healthcare visitors need more support following cases of encountering traumatic incidents on their rounds. More funding was announced for counselling support in 2017. A small number of areas in England have implemented the scheme (Jones, 2017). Since the budget was announced, cases of healthcare visitors taking time off for stress has risen by more than 7 per cent (RCN, 2017). Even more strain is placed on workers, which in turn increases the chances of stress – a vicious cycle that could easily be prevented by local healthcare authorities adequately utilising their healthcare budgets.

Check the end of the chapter for an answer to this activity.

COHESIVE DEVICES

As well as transition words, good writers use a number of other cohesive devices to help their work flow.

These include:

- Use of pronouns, such as this, these, he, she, they, to avoid repeating the subject.
- Use of umbrella terms – words that capture a number of points: 'All these arguments ...'
- Use of synonyms to refer to the key words.

ACTIVITY 3.10

Identify the use of the cohesive devices outlined above in the following paragraph:

The aim of the Wanless report (2003) was to ensure patients were educated and encouraged to take care of people with long term conditions (LTC) in a community setting. It claims that doing this will reduce the pressure on the acute care wards in hospitals. The document sets out ways to continue working in tackling the changes to the way care was delivered to patients with LTC. This approach began in the hospital setting and was extended to primary care in the community. The idea was reinforced with 'Together for Health' by the Welsh government (2011), a plan for primary and community care, where professionals within diverse specialities were caring for individuals with LTC and available to give the care continuously.

Check the end of the chapter for an answer to this activity.

RECAP

Good structure is essential to help your reader understand the points you are making. You can employ structural devices at different levels throughout your writing:

- By writing a clear introduction, outlining what the reader can expect.
- By including a clear topic sentence at the start of each paragraph and making sure the points you include all relate to this.
- By using transition words and other cohesive devices to help the reader move easily between sentences.

In the next Principle, we will look at how to make sure you are using this structure to help build sound and coherent arguments.

PRINCIPLE 5: ARGUMENT

Argument is perhaps the most important element of academic writing, and this is no different for students of Health and Social Care programmes. A student who receives feedback from their markers stating that their work is 'descriptive', 'not critical enough' or has a 'weak argument' often see this reflected in their marks.

Developing an argument requires practice, and this section will provide some examples and techniques you can use to help identify your arguments and to think and write in a more critical way. A key point to remember is that being 'critical' or 'argumentative' in your writing does not necessarily mean being negative, or simply looking for fault.

Creating an argument can be best simplified by a two-stage process:

1   Understanding how your ideas connect.
2   Asking yourself the three questions of argument building.

STAGE 1: UNDERSTANDING HOW YOUR IDEAS CONNECT

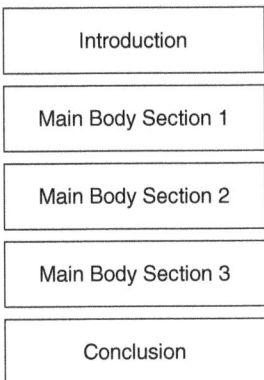

Figure 3.4   Understanding an assignment

Figure 3.4 shows the different sections of a student assignment, each represented by an orange box. In this example, all the boxes are arranged vertically; this represents a progression of ideas (i.e. from the introduction, through the various numbered main body sections and finishing with a conclusion). However, sometimes this representation doesn't translate directly into student work and this can result in a disorganised piece of writing, with no clear progression of argument.

Figure 3.4 above illustrates the reality of some student assignments. The sections seem to come as a surprise (could you guess where the next box would go?) and there seems to be no relation between sections of the assignment. For this reason, it is important that you try to avoid

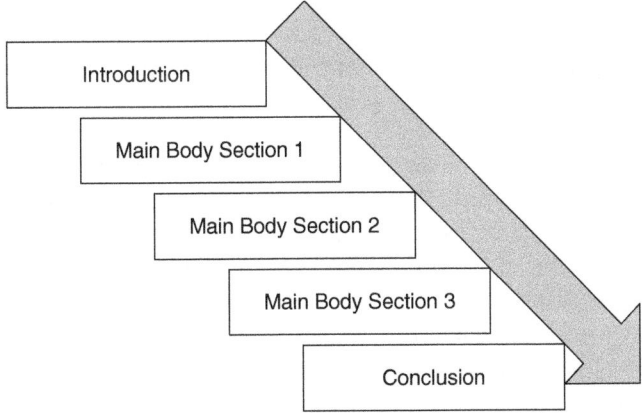

Figure 3.5   A strong assignment

this kind of disorganisation in your own work and consider how each point logically relates to the last. A good way to remind yourself of this is to consider your essay as being held together by something – represented in Figure 3.5 by the strong arrow.

Figure 3.5 represents a student assignment which has been *carefully* and *thoughtfully* constructed. Each part is a necessary point to develop in order to reach the conclusion, and each part logically flows from the last – this means that the student has considered which part of the answer should come first, and why. Next, they would have considered the following section, how it develops from the previous, and how it contributes to their conclusions. The strong arrow can be thought of as stage 1 of constructing an argument.

STAGE 2: THE THREE QUESTIONS OF ARGUMENT BUILDING

Once you have considered how your ideas connect, it is important to understand the process of developing the kind of critical thought which can help you to build a convincing, and critical, argument. The simplest way to do this is to consider the following three questions:

- What do I think?
- Why do I think that?
- What does this mean?

Of course, there is more to argument than just writing your answers to these questions, but they provide a really useful starting point for you to engage with your work in a critical way. Next, each of these questions is outlined in more detail so that you can see how they are presented in student work.

1. WHAT DO I THINK?

This is a fundamental question for you to ask yourself in your reading and your writing. Descriptive writing is often descriptive because the student hasn't asked themselves this question while reading, and this can lead to the student producing something like the below in an assignment.

Consider the example text from a student assignment below:

Smith (2014) suggests that there is a strong link between obesity and socio-economic status. Jones (2015) also indicates that low socio-economic status is linked with obesity. However, a study by Evans (2017) did not find that individuals with low socio-economic statuses had higher levels of obesity.

In the above example, the student has used different source material to construct a paragraph on the links between obesity and socio-economic status. However, all the student has done is describe the findings of the different studies which they have presented; they haven't asked themselves, 'What do I think?' The starting point for answering this question in your writing is to consider your answer to this question, and start the paragraph in a different way. You should first try to make a statement which broadly addresses your answer to this question.

There appears to be a link between obesity and socio-economic status. For example, both Smith (2014) and Jones (2015) found that individuals of low socio-economic status suffered with higher levels of obesity. However, a study by Evans (2017) did not find a clear link between socio-economic status and obesity.

Now, the student has attempted to answer the first question. The first sentence (like the arrow) indicates what the student thinks and introduces the studies to provide examples. However, it is not yet a convincing argument as the student hasn't considered the second question of argument construction.

2. WHY DO I THINK THAT?

This is the next question to consider when developing your argument. In the above examples, the student has included citations to provide examples, but hasn't really engaged with the source materials. When asking yourself this question, it is important to keep in mind that you can only *rationally* and *logically* justify your answer to the first question by engaging with the source material and *evaluating* the evidence it uses to build its own argument.

There appears to be a link between obesity and socio-economic status amongst the population of the UK. For example, both Smith (2014) and Jones (2015) found that individuals of low socio-economic status suffered with higher levels of obesity. Smith's (2014) study drew 1,000 participants from three urban areas of the UK and tracked them over a ten-year period through their interactions with their doctors. He found that over 70 per cent of participants from low socio-economic backgrounds were classed as overweight or obese. In addition, Jones's (2015) study comprised 500 participants from a low socio-economic area of Wales and compared their levels of obesity against a more affluent area of Wales. She found that those individuals from lower socio-economic areas were 68 per cent more likely to be classed as obese than their more affluent counterparts. However, a study by Evans (2017) did not find a clear link between socio-economic status and obesity. In his study, Evans asked 100 participants to fill in an online questionnaire during the summer of 2016. From his initial request, 57 participants responded, and 43 per cent of those did not indicate that they were obese. The self-reporting of obesity has been shown to provide inaccurate results in the past (see Martins, 2007, 2008) and this, together with the low participant numbers, would suggest that the findings of Evans's study would not be generalisable to the UK population.

It's clear from the above example that the excerpt is longer – and it needs to be because it provides evidence to explore and support the claim made in the first sentence.

3. WHAT DOES THIS MEAN?

The final sentence in the above excerpt starts to make sense of the evidence presented in the context of the question. Some writers may use a linking word (such as 'therefore') to link the ideas developed to the context of the question.

CONCLUSION

The five principles we have covered in this chapter demonstrate the key requirements of the kind of academic skills you will be asked to employ in your Health and Social Care studies programme. Of course, there is more to good academic writing than the principles covered here, but if (like so many students) the writing element of your programme is making you most worried, these rules are a great place to start.

ANSWERS TO CHAPTER 3 ACTIVITIES

———— Activity 3.2: Answers

- **'There are a lot of ways'** – 'a lot of' needs to be more specific.
- **'One of the main, most effective ways'** – Repetition of ideas (main/most effective). The student should choose just one.
- **'There is, sadly'** – Two problems here. Firstly, the use of 'sadly' – an emotive adverb. But secondly, the student starts the sentence with 'There is', which echoes the beginning of the previous sentence. Try to avoid this kind of repetition.
- **'not too much evidence'** – 'not too much' is too colloquial a term. The student should find a more academic way to express the idea.
- **'feedback and advice'** – again, one of these words will do.
- **'The level of engagement which can be got'** – the student should find a more specific word than 'got'.
- **'each and every single one of us is different'** – this is a colloquial phrase that contains redundancy. The student should find a more appropriate way to express the idea.
- **'at the end of the day'** – clichés such as this should be avoided and replaced with more specific language.

———— Activity 3.3: Answers

Did you think of all of these?

- Looking at chapter headings within the book
- Looking at indexes for key words
- Looking at subheadings within chapters
- Reading introduction paragraphs to chapters or sections
- Reading the topic sentences of paragraphs (usually the first one or two sentences)
- Skimming for gist
- Scanning for key words

———— Activity 3.5: Answer

In the context of the source sentence, these would be the most accurate synonyms:

Staff – workers – employees – practitioners

Poor awareness – ignorant – oblivious – not know enough

Differing – varied – alternative – unfamiliar

Offend – upset – insult – hurt their feelings

Without any intention – unintentionally – accidentally – inadvertently

Therefore our paraphrase would now look like this:

Practitioners may not know enough about unfamiliar cultural practices or people with disabilities and could easily hurt their feelings unintentionally. (Reid, 2002)

———— Activity 3.6: Answer

Background, Context and Definition of Terms

Recent statistics published by the Welsh Health Board confirm that 54 per cent of Welsh adults and 42 per cent of Welsh children can be categorised as obese (with a BMI in excess of 30kg/M^2). The figures have remained constant since 1998, despite a number of programmes such as 'Active Wales' and 'Fit for Life Wales' being implemented by the Welsh government. Findings from two studies, 'Obesity in Wales' by the Welsh government (2012) and 'Fighting the Fat' by Active Wales (2013), agree that the central cause of this problem is a poor diet and a 'culture of inactivity' (Wilde 2013).

Reader Orientation

This essay will examine both these causes via recent case studies, firstly by Proctor (2013) and secondly by the Worldwide Obesity Forum (2016), and will suggest that while identifying these causes is an important step, it is not enough to simply 'fire-fight'. Using further evidence from other countries such as the United States and Mexico …

Thesis Statement

This essay will suggest that while identifying these causes is an important step, it is not enough to simply 'fire-fight'. Using further evidence from other countries such as the United States and Mexico, this essay will argue that the most effective way to combat obesity is to educate children at a young age.

> Notice the slight overlap between the orientation and the thesis statement in the above example. Your introductions will not always be divided into three perfect sections, nor do they necessarily have to be in the order outlined above. As long as all are present, and all are helping to prepare your reader, then your introduction is doing its job.

———— Activity 3.7: Answer

The WHO (2017) outline three main benefits of giving up smoking.

We would expect the three benefits to be defined and perhaps expanded upon.

To combat the problem of disparity in care across providers, Johnson (2012) developed a framework for health care managers.

(Continued)

We would expect more information about the framework – perhaps the key features of how it works and/or how it helps managers.

However, Graham (2018) sees the issues differently, arguing that many services fail to accurately report critical incidents in order to avoid the time-consuming administration process they entail.

We would expect the writer to expand upon this point, perhaps explaining what the dangers of this might be, or suggesting ways to make sure that more services do report critical incidents.

The above topic sentences are all different, but each gives an indication of what is to come.

Check the end of the chapter for an answer to this activity.

────── Activity 3.9: Answer

As you will have noticed, while the ideas are logical in the example paragraph, the reader still has to do too much work to understand how they relate to each other. The following, in contrast, uses transition words to clearly guide the reader through the ideas.

> It is clear that healthcare visitors need more support following cases of encountering traumatic incidents on their rounds. **Although** more funding was announced for counselling support in 2017, only a small number of areas in England have implemented the scheme (Jones, 2017). **Furthermore,** since the budget was announced, cases of healthcare visitors taking time off for stress has risen by more than 7 per cent (RCN, 2017). **This means** that even more strain is placed on workers, which in turn increases the chances of stress – a vicious cycle that could easily be prevented by local healthcare authorities adequately utilising their healthcare budgets.

Check the end of the chapter for an answer to this activity.

────── Activity 3.10: Answer

It – Use of pronoun, referring to the report

Doing this – use of pronoun, referring to the action of educating and encouraging patients

The document – use of synonym to avoid repetition

This approach – referring to the 'ways to tackle change' mentioned previously

These ideas – umbrella term referring to all the previously mentioned initiatives

In the above example the writer has helped their writing flow and avoided repetition by using a variety of cohesive devices. Note that in all cases, the cohesive device is positioned towards the beginning of the sentence, helping us move easily from one idea into the next.

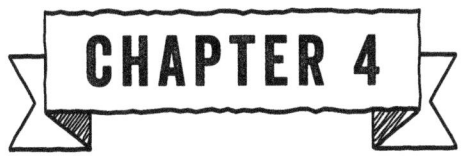

CHAPTER 4

THE RESEARCH PROCESS IN HEALTH AND SOCIAL CARE

Pete King

OVERVIEW

This chapter considers the research process within a health and social care context. The chapter starts with a brief consideration of how research is important for all types of professional practice to support both policy and practice. The chapter then explains how research is undertaken using a step-by-step cyclical process, the research process. The research process is influenced by two aspects, epistemology and ontology, which are discussed in relation to quantitative and qualitative approaches to research. These two different approaches to research will determine aspects of the research design data collection and data analysis. The chapter concludes where the chapter began, the role of research in relation to health and social care professional practice, and considers the importance of both evidence-based research and ethics for anybody involved in engaging in research.

LEARNING OUTCOMES

By the end of this chapter you will be able to:

Recall the purpose of research may be descriptive, exploratory, explanatory or correlation

Recall the research process as a six-step process

Differentiate the main differences between qualitative and quantitative research studies with respect to epistemology and ontology

Explain why research is important for evidence-based practice and the need to have an ethical approach

INTRODUCTION

This chapter will introduce the concept of the research process. The research process is used in all types of research. This could be a third-year undergraduate dissertation, a PhD postgraduate thesis or a funded research project. Through completing the various tasks within this chapter, you will start to become familiar with the basic concepts that make up the research process and the different epistemological and ontological perspectives of research. Before we start discussing research, complete Activity 4.1.

ACTIVITY 4.1

Using the two headings 'Health' and 'Social Care' write down a list of jobs and occupations that would fall under each heading.

For 'Health', you may have come up with health visitor, nurse, physiotherapist, occupational therapist or midwife. For 'Social Care' your list may have included social worker, adult care worker, childcare worker or work within the realms of disability. Whatever your chosen profession, there is a growing need for sound research to support professional practice in both health and social care.

THE RESEARCH PROCESS

Before discussing the research process, consider the problem in Activity 4.2.

ACTIVITY 4.2

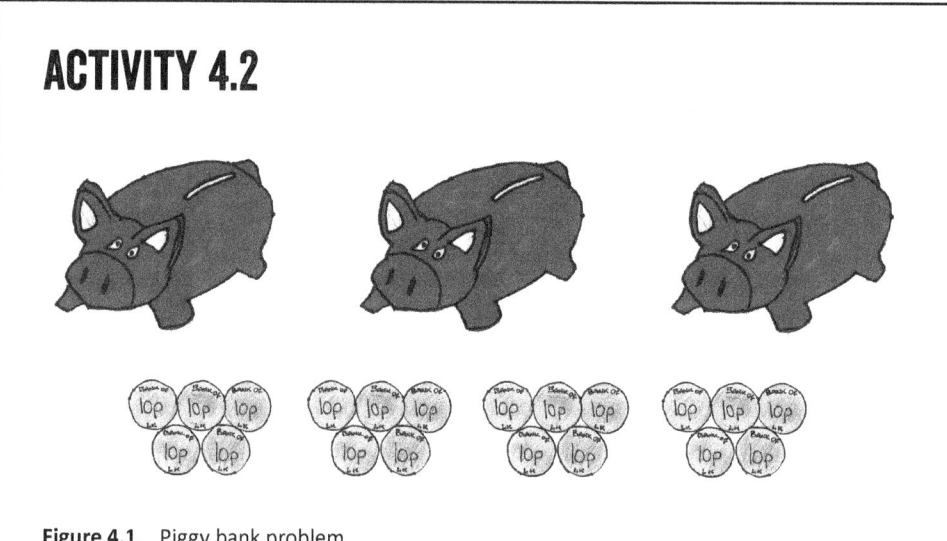

Figure 4.1   Piggy bank problem

I have 20 coins (each coin is worth 10p). I have three piggy banks, one for each of my children. I want to divide the 20 coins up so that each piggy bank has an even number of coins placed in it.

How many coins would be in each piggy bank?

Clue: there does not have to be an equal number of coins between piggy banks, but each must have an even number in each piggy bank.

How did you do? You may have come up with an answer of 8 coins in the first, 6 coins in the second and 6 coins in the third (which are all even numbers and totals 20 coins). Or you may have 6 coins in the first, 6 coins in the second and 8 coins in the third. You could also have 2 coins in the first, 4 coins in the second and 14 coins in the third. There are several different combinations to resolve this task. So, what does this have to do with research?

Research is not necessarily solving problems, but as with the activity above there are many ways to approach a given problem, or an issue within health and social care. Irrespective of how you undertake research, whether it is a third-year dissertation, a postgraduate PhD or a postdoctoral funded research project, the basic research process must be adhered to. What is the research process?

A clear definition of the research process has been defined by Gelling (2015) as 'a series of steps or stages that the researcher should progress through when planning and conducting research' (p. 44). The steps within the research process can vary depending on what research text you read (for example compare Meadows, 2003 with Gelling, 2015) and it's not to say one way is more correct than another. For this chapter, a six-step process will be discussed, where one step links into the next and the process is considered as a cycle.

THE PURPOSE OF RESEARCH

The purpose of research can be considered in relation to Kumar's (2011) outline of four types of research study:

- Descriptive: Is the research study to provide detail about something?
- Exploratory: Is the research study to investigate something new?
- Explanatory: Is the research study to clarify something?
- Correlation: Is the research study to find out a relationship?

The purpose of research study will be determined by many factors, for example personal interest, a particular need or funding by an agency or organisation. Often a descriptive-type research is undertaken as there may be some knowledge about the subject area and there may be a more specific aim or objectives to describe more fully the aspects addressed in the research study. For an exploratory-type research, there will be very little research knowledge about the phenomenon. An explanatory-type research often (but not always) involves a prediction (or hypothesis) to explain a phenomenon. A correlation looks for relationships, which again may include a prediction.

A research paper will often state if it's an exploratory, explanatory, descriptive or correlation study as it may use one of these words or within the title or the research question of the research paper. This is not always the case and you may have to read through the background or introduction section and look for the key phrases which may be 'This study aims to describe ...' or 'This exploratory study aims to ...' or 'This research aims to provide an explanation for ...' or 'the correlation between ...'. Sometimes the research purpose may not be clear and it is left to the reader to guess if the research paper has a descriptive, exploratory, explanatory or correlation purpose. Irrespective of the type of research purpose, all research studies go through a process, the research process.

STAGES IN THE RESEARCH PROCESS

The steps within the research process can vary depending on what research text you read, for example the research process is a seven-step process (Polgar and Thomas, 2008), an eight-step process (Hek et al., 2003; Polgar and Thomas, 2013) a ten-step process (Lynch, 2013; Moule, 2018) or an 11-step process (Lacey, 2015).

None of these approaches are wrong, they all cover the same aspects. The research process used for this chapter is a six-step process (which covers all the aspects in the difference research processes outlined above) to use in producing a research proposal:

1   The research question or hypothesis
2   The research design
3   Collecting the data
4   Processing and analysing the data
5   Implementation of the results
6   Dissemination of the results

This six-step approach must be considered as a cycle (see Figure 4.2).

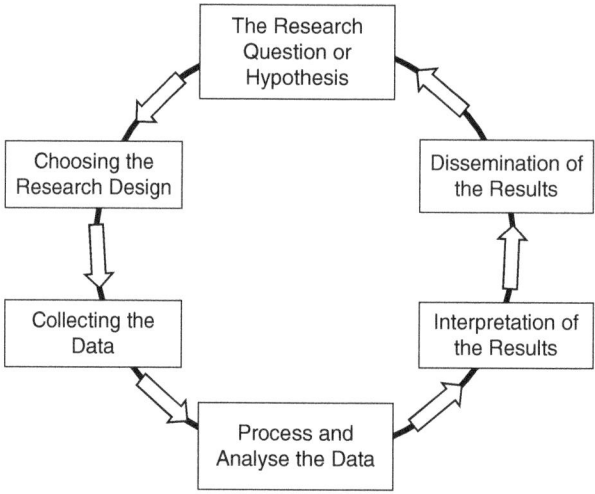

Figure 4.2   Six-step research process

The first stage of the research process is to generate the research question or hypothesis. The difference between a research question and hypothesis is that for the latter the researcher is making a prediction on what they are anticipating the results of the study will find. The research question or hypothesis should reflect the research purpose (descriptive, exploratory, explanatory or correlation) and is developed by the researchers undertaking a literature review. A literature review is where the researchers find other research studies that have already been undertaken in the same or similar area of study. Once the research question or hypothesis has been generated, the research design is chosen.

The research design is like the 'blueprint' or plan for the research study. The research design will include a consideration of the number of participants that will take part and this can range from less than ten to thousands of people. The research design will determine the type of data that will be collected and which method will be used. Following on from the data collection, the data will need to be analysed. Once the data has been collected and analysed the results are implemented. The implementation discusses the results back to the research question or hypothesis and the research purpose and could contribute professional practice or policy. The final stage of the research process is dissemination, this is where the findings from the research is circulated to relevant individuals, organisations or even governments. Using the six-step process above, have a go at Activity 4.3 below. This task requires you to use a search engine to locate a research paper.

Common search engines include Google, Yahoo! and Bing; however, for Activity 4.3 use a more research-focused search engine, such as Google Scholar, or research databases can be used. Research databases can be general and interdisciplinary, for example Web of Science, ScienceDirect and JSTOR, or more specific, such as PubMed/Medline (health), Psycinfo (psychology) and ERIC (education). What you need to do is come up with some key words in an area you are interested in within health and social care. For example, you may want to find a paper on how adults with dementia are cared for in residential care homes. Your key words may be: dementia, residential care and older people. If you use too many words, you could end up with too many 'hits' from a range of different sources; too few words and you may not end up with anything. You must 'play' around with the search engine with the choice and number of words. One useful method is using the concept of Boolean Operators (Evans et al., 2009).

Boolean Operators use the simple words of 'AND', 'OR' and 'NOT' between your key words you put in a search engine. The way Boolean Operators work Boolean logic is a bit more confusing than it seems. Search results get smaller the more 'AND' or 'NOT' is used between your key words, and larger the more 'OR' is used.

A research paper will have a basic structure of:

Abstract: this provides an overview of the research paper

Introduction: this section provides background information to the study

Methods: this section explains how the data is collected and analysed

Results: this section explains the results obtained from the research

Discussion: this section describes the significance of the research findings

ACTIVITY 4.3

Find a research paper on a particular subject area you are interested in (for example, within health or social care) from a published journal (a paper of six to eight pages would suffice). Read the paper and see if you can identify the different elements of the research process outlined above in the paper.

Research papers will differ in length, quality and clarity. Some research papers will have a clear aim, justify the research design (often including ethical issues addressed), state what and how the data is collected and analysed, discuss the results (and consider the strengths and weaknesses of the research design) and make suggestions on how the research can contribute to particular groups or policy. Other research papers may not be as clear, there is no clear research question (or aim) or the results are not clear. Whether you consider a paper to be of good quality or not, a sound piece of research would have engaged in the research process in a sequential order from research question to dissemination.

When considering types of research, there is a hierarchy of research which indicates some research is 'better' than others. Some care must be made with this statement. Whilst there is a case for stating one type of research is possibly 'more robust' than others, the key is the best research design is chosen to meet the focus of the research question. This will be discussed next with respect to the purpose of research and the hierarchy of research.

HIERARCHY OF RESEARCH

The hierarchy of research evidence consists of five aspects: systematic reviews and meta-analysis; randomised-controlled trials; quasi-experiments; non-experimental studies; and expert opinion. Ingham-Broomfield (2016) and Evans (2003) provide two detailed accounts of the hierarchy of research evidence. This hierarchy, as described by Ingham-Broomfield (2016), is shaped as a pyramid. At the base of the hierarchy is the 'expert opinion', which although may be an accurate opinion, lacks any or has poor methodology quality (Evans, 2003). At the top is the systematic reviews and meta-analysis, where several robust research studies undertaken on the same topic are analysed (Ingham-Broomfield, 2016). In between these two extremes is the focus for this chapter, the various studies which involve research that undertakes data collection and data analysis (randomised control trials, quasi-experiments and non-experimental studies). The evidence that will be generated will be determined by the type of research study undertaken, and the philosophical approach that underpins where different research theories exist (Babbie, 2013). Now do Activity 4.4.

ACTIVITY 4.4

Below is a drawing of the Earth. Get a piece of paper, something to write with and a timer of some sort.

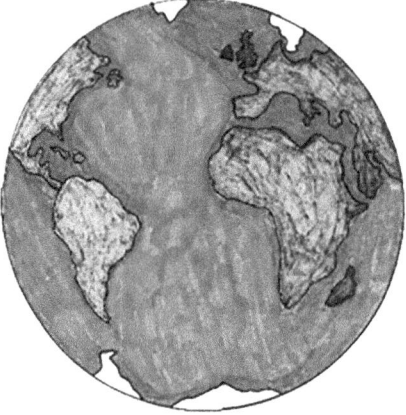

Figure 4.3   The earth

Set the timer for 100 seconds. The task is to write down everything you know about the world we live in.

Once you have created your list, group your answers into each of the three categories below:

Human

Non-human (living)

Non-human (non-living)

From your list in Activity 4.4 which category had the most? The chances are that non-human (non-living) was high which may have included the world is round (more accurately it is an ellipse), or the world is four-fifths made up of water, or if we jump up in the air gravity will pull us down. You may have come up with non-human (living) that we share the world with other animals or that plants produce oxygen by the chemical process of photosynthesis. For the category of human, we have 206 bones in our skeletal body or there are different cultures and races of people that inhabit the planet. These are all facts and wherever we are in the world, these facts would apply. For example, if you jump up and down where you are now, the effect of gravity will also apply if you flew to another country and did the same action.

However, there are aspects of the world we live in that may not apply to everyone. For example, we all have different likes and dislikes of music or the type of film we watch. We all have different feelings and thoughts about topics such as poverty, crime or even euthanasia. Not everything can be reduced to a fact that applies to everyone everywhere. This leads into the concepts in research of epistemology and ontology.

EPISTEMOLOGY AND ONTOLOGY

Epistemology is the study of knowledge and the assumptions we make about knowledge (Richards, 2003). We can consider research from 'two contrasting epistemological positions of positivism and interpretivism' (Grix, 2001, p. 27). The epistemological approach of the researcher (using positivism or interpretivism) will have a major influence on the research design. Ontology is how we view social reality (Crotty, 1998) and two different approaches to ontology are 'objectivism and constructivism' (Grix, 2001, p. 27). Objectivism holds that social reality is separate from human consciousness, whilst constructivism claims that social reality is constructed by people through their interaction in the world (Gray, 2013). The ontological approach of the researcher will influence the type of data being collected and analysed.

Rather than go into the deep and philosophical debates and arguments of what counts as knowledge and what constitutes social reality, the aspects of epistemology and ontology combined will influence the research design, data collection and analysis of the research process. Two distinct research paradigms reflect both epistemology and ontology.

A paradigm can be defined as an overarching philosophical stance, a system of beliefs about the nature of the world and, ultimately, when applied in the research setting, the assumptive base from which knowledge is produced. Kuhn (1970) defined paradigms as:

Some accepted examples of actual scientific practice – examples which include law, theory, application, and instrumentation together – provided models from which spring particular coherent traditions of scientific research. (p. 10).

The two broad paradigmatic types of research are qualitative and quantitative. Quantitative and qualitative research differ, but can also complement each other because they generate different kinds of knowledge that are useful in the context of interpreting social reality.

QUANTITATIVE RESEARCH

Quantitative research is also written as positivism derived from the French philosopher Comte (1798–1857) and developed from the nineteenth century onwards (Ryan, 2018). Detailed definitions and explanations of quantitative research can be found in many published research textbooks (see further reading list at the end of the chapter); however, the key factors of quantitative research are:

- An approach to science based on objectivity and the belief in universal laws (e.g. gravity applies to anywhere in the world we live in)
- The researcher as the scientist underpinned by an objectivist ontology (facts are facts)
- Based on testing theories and hypothesis (deductive) with a distance between the researcher and what is being studied
- Large sample size (number of people participating in the research) which could be over 1,000 people
- Universal laws can be generalised to similar situations and settings and behaviour can be predicted on the basis of these laws
- Data is collected as numbers and statistical tests are undertaken on the numerical data
- Heart of research lies with cause and effect and relationships through numerical measurability

QUALITATIVE RESEARCH

Qualitative research is also known as interpretivism whereas the origins of qualitative research are derived from sociology and developed from the 1960s (Ryan, 2018). Again, many published textbooks will provide details of what makes up qualitative research (see further reading section at the end of this chapter). However, the key factors of qualitative research are:

- The approach is subjective by interpreting and making sense of the meanings and experiences of individual humans
- Underpinned by a subjectivity, finding out what people think or feel where reality is socially constructed
- The researcher is more of a detective looking for themes of commonalities and differences
- May generate theories from the data (inductive)
- Smaller sample sizes are used (often under ten people may be involved)
- Universal laws are not generated but multiple perspectives are considered
- Heart of the research lies in understanding different perspectives where data is collected through words (narratives) and identifying for themes to look for meaning and understanding

So, to recap: Quantitative research is objective, collects numerical data from a large sample population which is often statistically analysed and the results are generalised to similar situations. Qualitative research is subjective, collects data in the form of words (narratives) from smaller sample populations and analyses it to look for meanings that are often context-based, which often are not generalised to other similar situations.

ACTIVITY 4.5

Draw out and complete Table 4.1.

Table 4.1   Quantitative or qualitative research study

	Objectivity or Subjectivity?	Researcher as Scientist or Detective?	Numbers or Words Collected?	Data Analysis Looking for Themes or Statistical Tests?	Universal Laws or Multiple Meanings?
Quantitative					
Qualitative					

Check the end of the chapter for an answer to this activity.

These are the basic factors which define whether a research study will be either a quantitative study or a qualitative study. With regards to the four types of research purpose (Kumar, 2011), a general rule of thumb is that a descriptive and exploratory study are often qualitative in nature, whereas an explanatory and correlation study is quantitative. Whatever paradigm a researcher bases their research on, this will determine the research design. However, the research design will be influenced by the researcher's epistemological and ontological standpoint; that is how they view knowledge and reality. In recent years, a third paradigm has emerged and is referred to as 'mixed-methods' (Burke Johnson and Onwuegbuzie, 2004) where a combination of both quantitative and qualitative research designs is used. Here both numerical and narrative data are collected to address the research question. Whether a quantitative, qualitative or a mixed-methods approach is taken, all researchers go through the six stages of the research process and these should be reflected in any research paper.

DIFFERENT TYPES OF RESEARCH DESIGN, DATA COLLECTION AND ANALYSIS

Quantitative research designs aim to collect and analyse numbers and common designs include randomised control trials (sometimes referred to as 'true' experiments), quasi-experiments, questionnaires and surveys. The number of people (or participants) in the study is often stated as the sample size, and for quantitative research are often large numbers. The numerical data is often (but not always) analysed using a statistical test. The statistical test does not 'prove' the results are right or wrong, but considers whether the results produced are down to the research design (randomised control trial, quasi-experiment or correlation) and not by chance.

Qualitative research does not focus on collecting numbers but is more interested in what people say, feel, perceive or think. The focus is on collecting words, or narratives or undertaking observations. The most common method of collecting data are interviews and focus groups (although surveys are often also used). Interviewing involves one-to-one interaction (although small groups of two or three are not uncommon, particularly when interviewing children) whilst focus groups can have up to eight or ten people. Qualitative research will involve a smaller sample size (fewer participants) compared with a quantitative research design. Qualitative analysis often looks for common words or themes, often termed thematic analysis (for example the framework developed by Braun and Clarke, 2006).

To sum up, quantitative research designs involve collecting and analysing numerical data from large samples to test hypotheses or look for relationships. Qualitative research designs are more concerned with narratives (words) which are analysed to look for themes (often the phrase thematic analysis is used) and may generate a hypothesis.

INTERPRETATION AND DISSEMINATION

Once the research data has been collected and analysed, the research will be interpreted and this is often in the 'discussion' section of the research paper. The discussion should link the results back to the research question and the background section of the research paper and identify the main findings from the research. This section will often consider the strengths and limitations of the research, and often identify areas for further research. The research findings may also give an indication on how far the results can be generalised to a wider population. For a quantitative study, there may be enough in the results to do this, but this will not be the case for a qualitative study.

ACTIVITY 4.6

We have now looked at the different parts of the research process of: research question; research design; data collection; data assimilation; data analysis; interpretation; and dissemination. This activity involves going back to the research paper you found (you may want to find a different one) and go through it to consider the research process in more depth using the prompt questions below:

- Is the research descriptive, exploratory, explanatory or a correlation?
- Does it have a broad theme, a more specific research question (aim or objective) or a hypothesis?
- Does the introduction/background/literature review identify any other research studies?
- What is the epistemology of the research paper (is it qualitative or quantitative?)
- What is the ontology of the research paper (what is the research design?)

- What is the sample size?
- How is the data collected?
- How is the data analysed?
- How do the results relate to the wider population?
- What were the strengths and limitations of using the research design?
- Could the study be undertaken using a different research design?

Depending on how the research paper is written, some of the questions can be answered quickly whilst other questions you have to search for the answers, or even have to make a judgement. What is important is that you should now be able to start reading research papers thinking about the research process and identify the key points if it's a qualitative and quantitative research. So why is research important in health and social care? This can be answered in relation to evidence-based practice.

EVIDENCE-BASED PRACTICE

At the start of this chapter you were asked to come up with different professions that fall under health, social care, education or law. How can we ensure professional practice reflects current research? Often professional practice is undertaken because 'This is the way we have always done it', or 'If it's not broken don't fix it', or 'We don't like change here'. All these examples may relate to professional opinion (which is at the 'lowest' point of the hierarchy of evidence). However, more and more professions are now engaging in evidence-based research to support evidence-based practice (e.g. conservation, criminology, design, government and public policies, librarianship, nursing, medicine, health care management, social work and software engineering). This is the aspect of evidence-based research which supports evidence-based practice.

Originating in health, evidence-based practice has been defined as 'the conscientious, explicit, and judicious use of current best evidence in making decisions about the care of individual patients' (Sackett et al., 1996, p. 71). Evidence-based practice is further defined by Steglitz et al. (2015) as 'an approach that aims to improve the process through which high-quality scientific research evidence can be obtained and translated into the best practical decisions to improve health' (p. 332). The aspect of using research evidence to support decisions can relate to not just individual patients or health, but children in educational and childcare contexts (childcare workers and teachers), adults in residential care (care workers) and both children and adults who require social care support from social workers. The key aspect is that evidence-based practice is not just about identifying the relevant research to support your practice, but also being the professional who undertakes research, to support both your own and others' practice.

The research design needs to fit in with the research question (not the other way around), and although the hierarchy of research evidence indicates that randomised control trial research is 'better' than research involving undertaking interviews, this may not obtain the best evidence to support practice. For example, if a new intervention programme was being introduced to lower cholesterol, then a randomised control trial may be the best design as it will provide a measure of effectiveness (whether positive or negative). However, if during the intervention, 50 per cent of the participants drop out, it might be useful for the researcher to find out why. This may involve speaking to those participants that drop out. Although interviewing is perceived to be 'lower' in the hierarchy of research evidence, a randomised control trial would not be an appropriate research design. Evidence-based research to support evidence-based practice needs to consider the relevant research to support professional practice, and again this will start from the initial research question.

Whether research is a quantitative randomised control trial reflecting a positivist perspective, or qualitative interviews underpinned by interpretivism, all research must be ethically sound and justified. Within the United Kingdom (UK), health and social care research has a set of principles and regulations set out within the 'UK policy framework for health and social care research' (Health Research Authority (HRA), 2017) as devised by the HRA and the four UK Health Departments (Department of Health in England, Department of Health in Northern Ireland, Scottish Government Health and Social Care Directorates and the Department for Health and Social Services in Wales). The framework consists of 19 principles that protect both the participants involved in the research, the researcher or researchers carrying out the study and the organisations responsible for the research (this could be a public body funding it). For any research to take place, ethical approval must be obtained through a recognised ethics research committee, and for any research within the National Health Service (NHS) this involves approval as set out by their Research Governance (Department of Health (DoH), 2005).

Ethical research must ensure all participants who take part in any research study know what the study is about and what their participation in the research will involve. Any participation must be voluntary and participants must expect anonymity, confidentiality and the right to withdraw from the study. This relates to the aspect of informed consent; that is participants voluntarily agree to take part in any research study. In addition, any data collected within the UK, must be collected and stored to meet the General Data Protection Regulations (GDPR) 2018. When planning any research, an ethical consideration needs to be considered throughout the six stages of the research process, from the initial research idea of ensuring it would be ethical to undertake the research.

ACTIVITY 4.7   TEST YOURSELF

1   What are the six stages in the research process?
2   What is epistemology and what is ontology?
3   What are the four types of research purpose?
4   How does qualitative research differ from quantitative research?
5   Give an example of a qualitative research design and a quantitative research design.
6   Why is evidence-based practice important?
7   What are the key aspects of informed consent to be considered when undertaking research?

Check the end of the chapter for an answer to this activity.

CONCLUSION

This chapter has considered the purpose of research in relation to a study being descriptive, exploratory, explanatory or a correlation (Kumar, 2011). The process of research is a six-step cyclical process starting with a research question or hypothesis, research design, data collection, data analysis, implementation and dissemination. The research design will be determined by the researchers' epistemological and ontological position on knowledge and viewing reality. Two broad paradigms exist, qualitative and quantitative, and these paradigms are compared with respect to the research design, participants, data collection, data analysis and how far results from any study can be generalised to a bigger population. The chapter concludes with a consideration of evidence-based research and the importance of addressing ethics throughout the research process.

GO FURTHER ACTIVITY

In Activity 4.6, you would have found either a qualitative or a quantitative paper. If your research paper was a quantitative paper, do the same exercise but this time for a qualitative paper (or vice versa – if your paper was qualitative, find a quantitative paper). Compare how the researchers use these two different research methods thinking about the sample size, how the data is collected and analysed, and how far the results can be generalised to a wider population.

ANSWERS TO CHAPTER 4 ACTIVITIES

───── Activity 4.5: Answers

	Objectivity or Subjectivity?	Researcher as Scientist or Detective?	Numbers or Words Collected?	Data Analysis Looking for Themes or Statistical Tests?	Universal Laws or Multiple Meanings?
Quantitative	Objectivity	Scientist	Numbers	Statistical Tests	Universal Laws
Qualitative	Subjectivity	Detective	Words	Themes	Multiple Meanings

───── Activity 4.7: Test Yourself: Answers

1   What are the six stages in the research process? Generate the Research Question or Hypothesis, research design, data collection, data analysis, implementation of results and dissemination of results.
2   What is epistemology and what is ontology? Epistemology is the study of knowledge, ontology is how we view social reality

(Continued)

3   What are the four types of research purpose? Descriptive, Exploratory, Explanatory and Correlation

4   How does qualitative research differ from quantitative research? Qualitative research is subjective, finding out what people think or feel where reality is socially constructed, the researcher is more of a detective looking for themes, data collected is mostly in the form of words (narratives), may generate theories from the data (inductive), small samples sizes and multiple perspectives are considered. Quantitative research is science based on objectivity, the belief in universal laws, the researcher is a scientist often testing theories and hypotheses (deductive), large sample sizes, data is collected as numbers and statistical tests are undertaken on the numerical data, researcher is interested in cause and effect, and relationships and results are generalised to the wider population.

5   Give an example of a qualitative research design and a quantitative research design. Qualitative research design could be focus groups – interviews or observations and a quantitative research design could be a randomised control trial (RCT) quasi-experiments or correlations.

6   Why is evidence-based practice important? It enables the use of research evidence to support decisions and professional practice.

7   What are the key aspects of informed consent to be considered when undertaking research? Participants who take part in any research study know what the study is about and what their participation in the research will involve. Informed consent involves voluntary participation, anonymity, confidentiality and the right to withdraw from the study.

FURTHER READING

Barker, J., Linsley, P. and Kane, R. (2016). *Evidence Based Practice for Nurses and Health Care Professionals* (3rd edn). London: SAGE.

Moule, P. (2018). *Making Sense of Research in Nursing, Health and Social Care.* London: SAGE.

Punch, K. (2013). *Introduction to Social Research: Quantitative and Qualitative Approaches* (3rd edn). London: SAGE.

Saks, M. and Allsop, J. (2014). *Researching Health: Qualitative, Quantitative and Mixed Methods* (2nd edn). London: SAGE.

REFERENCES

Babbie, E. R. (2013). *The Practice of Social Research* (13th edn). Belmont: Wadsworth Publishing Co. Ltd.

Braun, V. and Clarke, V. (2006). Using thematic analysis in psychology. *Qualitative Research in Psychology*, 3(2), 77–101.

Burke Johnson, R. and Onwuegbuzie, A. J. (2004). Mixed methods research: a research paradigm whose time has come. *Educational Researcher* 33(7), 14–26.

Crotty, M. (1998). The *Foundations of Social Research*. London: SAGE.

Department of Health (2005). *Research Governance Framework for Health and Social Care* (2nd edn). Available from: www.gov.uk/government/uploads/system/uploads/attachment_data/file/139565/dh_4122427.pdf.

Evans, D. (2003). Hierarchy of evidence: a framework for ranking evidence evaluating healthcare interventions. *Journal of Clinical Nursing* 12, 77–84.

Evans, J., Schneider, G. and Pinard, K. (2009). *The Internet – Illustrated* (6th edn). Boston: Course Technology Inc.

Gelling, L. (2015) Stages in the research process. *Nursing Standard*, 29(27), 44–49.

Gray, D, (2013). *Doing Research in the Real World* (3rd edn). London: SAGE.

Grix, J. (2001). *Demystifying Postgraduate Research from MA to PhD*. Birmingham: University of Birmingham.

Health Research Authority (2017). *UK Policy Framework for Health and Social Care Research*. Available at: www.hra.nhs.uk/planning-and-improving-research/policies-standards-legislation/uk-policy-framework-health-social-care-research/

Hek, G., Judd, M. and Moule, P. (2003). *Making Sense of Research: An Introduction for Health and Social Care Practitioners* (2nd edn). London: SAGE.

Ingham-Broomfield, R. (2016). A nurses' guide to the hierarchy of research designs and evidence. *Australian Journal of Advanced Nursing* 33(3), 33–43.

Kuhn, T. S. (1970). *The Structure of Scientific Revolutions* (2nd edn). Chicago: University of Chicago Press.

Kumar, K. (2011). *Research Methodology: A Step by Step Guide for Beginners*. London: SAGE.

Lacey, A. (2015). The research process. In D. Cormack, K. Gerrish and J. Lathlean (eds), *The Research Process in Nursing* (pp. 15–29). Chichester: John Wiley & Sons Ltd.

Lynch, S. M. (2013). *Using Statistics in Social Research: A Concise Approach*. New York: Springer.

Meadows, K. A. (2003). So you want to do research? 1: an overview of the research process. *British Journal of Community Nursing*, 8(8), 369–375.

Moule, P. (2018). *Making Sense of Research in Nursing, Health and Social Care*. London: SAGE.

Polgar, S. and Thomas, S. A. (2008). *Introduction to Research in the Health Sciences* (5th edn). Philadelphia: Elsevier Limited.

Polgar, S. and Thomas, S. A. (2013). *Introduction to Research in the Health Sciences* (6th edn). Philadelphia: Elsevier Limited.

Richards, K. (2003). *Qualitative Inquiry in TESOL*. Basingstoke: Palgrave Macmillan.

Ryan, G. (2018). Introduction to positivism, interpretivism and critical theory. Nurse *Researcher*, 25(4), 41–49.

Sackett, D. L., Rosenberg, W. M. C., Gray, J. A. M., Haynes, R. B. and Richardson, S. (1996). Evidence based medicine: what it is and what it isn't. It's about integrating individual clinical expertise and the best external evidence. *British Medical Journal* 312(7023), 71–72.

Steglitz, J., Warnick, J. L., Hoffman, S. A., Johnston, W. and Spring, B. (2015). Evidence-based practice. In *International Encyclopaedia of the Social & Behavioural Sciences* (2nd edn) (pp. 332–338). London: Oxford Elsevier.

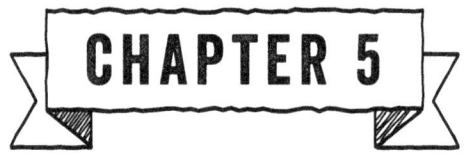

CHAPTER 5

THE LAW RELATING TO HEALTH AND SOCIAL CARE

INTRODUCTION TO KEY PRINCIPLES

Angela Smith and Julia Parkhouse

OVERVIEW

The initial part of this chapter will provide an introduction to some of the key legal principles underpinning the area of health and social care by critically examining how both criminal and civil law regulates the practice of those working within this field. For those working within the sector, the chapter will provide an overview of the rights and recourse patients and service users have by considering how the law operates in England and Wales. It will also consider other means by which health and social care professionals may be held accountable for their actions or omissions (inactions). More specifically, it will consider issues relevant to health and social care professionals who work on a daily basis with patients and service users. While this chapter primarily focuses on the law, many points of discussion are also relevant to ethical considerations. As such, students may wish to read this chapter alongside Chapter 17 which considers further legal and ethical considerations.

LEARNING OUTCOMES

By the end of this chapter you will be able to:

Discuss and evaluate the implications for a health and social care professional who may be held accountable for their actions or inactions

Identify and evaluate some of the key legal issues relating to caring for individuals within the health and social care sector

INTRODUCTION

Over the past century, the health and social care system in England and Wales has seen and benefited from medical advances. Additionally, patients and service users are now more informed in terms of their health and care needs, and are equally more aware of their rights than previously and willing to make their voices heard. Consequently, those working within the health and social care field need to be aware of how they may be held accountable for their actions, both personally and professionally. The fact is, there are a plethora of rules and regulations governing accountability and it is important that health and social care professionals are aware of these. This is because individuals may be held accountable for their actions (for what they do or fail to do) in a number of ways and not just held to account through the law and its systems. So, notwithstanding that the law does govern many activities (interactions and procedures), there are also other ways a health and social care professional may be held accountable. When considering the many ways in which a professional may be held accountable, in the area of health and social care law itself, there is a noticeable absence of legislation. This is irrespective of the judiciary (judges) calling for an informed parliamentary debate in many cases, and sometimes over a prolonged period of time (see, for example, the case of *Airedale NHS Trust v. Bland* [1993] AC 789, pp. 880B, 885E, 899F). Even where there is legislation, it still falls to an unelected judiciary to interpret and apply the detailed provisions of such legislation, and thus this chapter will predominantly focus on case law (where the judiciary have had no option but to decide cases, some of which are sensitive and raise ethical as well as legal concerns and where there may be a societal divide on the issue(s)).

Discussion within this chapter will refer to some of the key legal issues that professionals face every day when working within this field. However, while judicial decisions will be discussed throughout, learners should seek to take it upon themselves to further digest the full judgment from cases rather than rely on the section that we have chosen to discuss.

ACCOUNTABILITY

No health and social care professional is above the law, and we may all be held accountable for our actions. It is important that such professionals understand the importance of their actions (or omissions) and the consequences of falling below the set standards. There are numerous 'spheres of accountability' to ensure professionals discharge their professional duty. These spheres do not necessarily operate independently:

Legal accountability – civil and criminal law.

Professional accountability – health care professionals may be held accountable by their employer, by their regulatory body, by the Ombudsman.

Moral accountability – everybody has their own moral compass to which we adhere.

It is important that people working with patients and service users are answerable for their actions or omissions in order to provide such persons with a right of redress if something has gone wrong with their care.

LEGAL ACCOUNTABILITY

The legal system in England and Wales distinguishes between criminal and civil law. The consequences of being held accountable under the legal system varies depending on whether a person is being pursued for breaching civil or criminal law, although it is possible for an individual to be found liable under both limbs of the law. Encompassed within each of these aspects of the system is a variety of types of law, these being domestic legislation, European legislation and case law.

BOX 5.1   KEY POINTS ABOUT CRIMINAL LAW

- State intervenes in some matters – allegation investigated by police; prosecuted by Crown Prosecution Service
- Case heard in either the magistrates' court or the Crown Court depending on the seriousness of the offence, and either magistrates or a jury will hear the case and decide upon guilt
- Burden of proof is on the prosecution
- Standard of proof is guilty beyond 'reasonable doubt'
- If convicted, the criminal will be punished (by a fine, a community sentence or imprisonment)

BOX 5.2   KEY POINTS ABOUT CIVIL LAW

- Individual (the claimant) sues another (the defendant), usually for monetary compensation
- Case heard in either the County Court or the High Court, depending on the value and complexity of the case and a single judge will hear and decide the case
- Burden of proof is on the claimant
- Standard of proof based on 'balance of probability'
- If liable then there are options as to remedies (this could include monetary compensation, an injunction, specific performance of a contract)
- Aim of a civil remedy is not to punish but to put the claimant in the position they would have been in had the event not occurred

Within these categories of criminal and civil law, there is a variety of types of law that contribute as a whole to the English legal system, namely legislation, case law and European Union law.

BOX 5.3   LEGISLATION (ALSO KNOWN AS STATUTE AND ACTS OF PARLIAMENT)

- Law created by Parliament
- Rigorous review process in both Houses of Parliament (House of Commons and House of Lords) and then approved by the Crown.

- House of Commons is an elected body so enacted legislation is perceived to be the will of the people.
- Some relevant health and social care criminal law legislation includes: Mental Capacity Act 2005; Criminal Justice and Courts Act 2015 (relating to ill-treatment or wilful neglect of persons); Domestic Violence, Crime and Victims Act 2004 (relevant in the case of Baby P whereby it could not be established who had caused his death); Health and Safety at Work Act 1974 (relates to all aspects of patient and staff safety); Abortion Act 1967 (clarification of those allowed to conduct medical termination of pregnancy).
- Some relevant health and social care civil law legislation includes the Surrogacy Arrangements Act 1985 (provides clarity on the law on surrogacy arrangements within England and Wales); The Human Fertilisation and Embryology Act 1990 and 2008 (clarifies the law on assisted reproduction); The Care Act 2014 (England) and the Social Services and Well-being (Wales) Act 2014 (considers provision of care and support by Local Authorities to adults in need); Congenital Disability (Civil Liability) Act 1976 (allows a child to sue for injuries sustained prior to birth as a result of negligence).
- UK Parliament can also grant powers to other authorities to make law, known as secondary legislation. For example, Scotland, Wales and Northern Ireland have devolved governments who were granted their power through primary legislation enacted in London (The Scotland Act 1998, Northern Ireland Act 1998 and The Government of Wales Act 2006). Most forms of secondary legislation are through the format of Statutory Instruments (SI), also known as 'delegated' or 'subordinate legislation'. Generally, in any one year, there will be between 20–50 primary Acts of Parliament and between 1000–4000 SIs enacted.
- You can see how legislation is brought about by looking at www.parliament.uk/about/how/laws/acts/

However, in the field of medical law, there is limited legislation and even where legislation exists the judiciary need to interpret this to apply to individual cases. Consequently, the majority of law relevant to health and social care law is through case law.

BOX 5.4   CASE LAW (ALSO KNOWN AS JUDGE-MADE LAW AND COMMON LAW)

- Based on decisions previously made by judges.
- Based on established hierarchy within the court system of England and Wales whereby judges sitting in the higher courts have the greater power to overrule and reverse decisions of the lower courts.
- Decisions from the higher courts (Court of Appeal – civil division: Court of Appeal – criminal division; Supreme Court) bind lower courts through a system of precedent.

(Continued)

Once a decision has been made, then if the legal principle is similar, the lower courts should follow that earlier decision. If the facts of a later case differ then that court may distinguish the case on its facts and apply a different legal principle.

- Case law can be overridden by legislation as Parliament is the supreme law-making authority in the UK.
- Some relevant criminal law cases pertinent to health and social care include cases brought against 11 care workers at Winterbourne View for neglect or abuse of patients (BBC, 2012); R v. Cox [1992] 12 BMLR38 (convicted of attempted murder of his patient); R v. Brown [1994] 1 AC 212 (consent does not legitimise serious injury); R v. Catt [2013] EWCA Crim 1187 (convicted of administering poison with intent to procure a miscarriage).
- Some relevant civil law cases pertinent to health and social care include *Gillick v. West Norfolk and Wisbech Area Health Authority & Department of Health and Social Security Authority* [1985] 3 All ER 402 (discussed later in this chapter); *Bolam v. Friern Hospital Management Committee* [1957] 1WLR 582 (breach of a duty of care in respect of the tort of negligence); *Montgomery v. Lanarkshire Health Board* [2015] UKSC 11 (discussed later in this chapter).

BOX 5.5   EUROPEAN UNION (EU) LAW

UK joined the European Union in January 1973 (enacted through the European Communities Act 1972).

- Clarified in *R v. Secretary of State for transport ex parte Factortame Ltd (No. 2)* [1990] EUECJ Case C-213/89 that if a provision of domestic law conflicts with EU law then EU law will take priority and the domestic law has to be set aside.
- Majority of EU law relates to civil matters concerning trade and freedom of movement and so has limited applicability over matters concerning health and social care.
- When the UK eventually leaves the EU it will no longer have supremacy over UK law.

HUMAN RIGHTS ACT (HRA) 1998

While EU law takes supremacy over domestic law, it is not overly applicable in the health and social care field. However, one aspect of the English legal system that embraces all of the above discussions and is particularly relevant to the area of health and social care is that of the Human Rights Act (HRA) 1998. The European Convention on Human Rights (ECHR) was created in 1950 and came into effect in 1953. The UK was one of the founding signatories to the Convention (there are now 47 member states who have signed up to the Convention, compared to 28 member states of the EU). The UK has always agreed to be bound by the decisions of the European Court of Human Rights (ECtHR), although, given a Convention is not law, this was binding in honour only. The Convention rights were enshrined in UK domestic law in 2000 when the HRA 1998 came into effect. The rights contained within the Act mirror those within the Convention but as the Act is legally enforceable it gave UK citizens improved rights and remedies compared with those they had previously enjoyed under the Convention. Remedies include compensation for a breach of rights and can also result in a *declaration of incompatibility*. This is where the UK Parliament then has to enact domestic legislation in order to remedy the incompatibility; for example, in the case of Diane Blood and Joanne Tarbuck UK law was declared incompatible with Articles 8 and 14 leading to a change in the law so that deceased fathers may now be entered on their children's birth certificates (*Guardian*, 2003).

Some Articles particularly relevant in the health and social care arena include:

Article 2 – Right to life – see below.

Article 3 – Right not to be subjected to torture or to inhuman or degrading treatment or punishment. Please see the second part of Chapter 6 for a case example.

Article 5 – Right to liberty and security of person. Please see the second part of Chapter 6 for a case example.

Article 8 – Right to respect for his private and family life, his home and his correspondence. In *Evans v. Amicus Healthcare Ltd & Ors* [2004] EWCA Civ 727 (and subsequently referred to the ECtHR under *Evans v. UK* [2007] 6339/05 ECtHR 264) Natallie Evans argued that destruction of embryos breached Articles 2 and 8 and were incompatible with the Human Fertilisation and Embryology Act 1990. Her claim failed.

Please note that the Human Rights Articles can be accessed through the link www.legislation. gov.uk/ukpga/1998/42/contents and some defining cases can be found at https://rightsinfo.org/ infographics/fifty-human-rights-cases/.

ACTIVITY 5.1

Look at the case of Natallie Evans and consider why her claim failed before the courts. Consider the issues both legally and ethically and think about the situation from all three parties' point of view: the embryos that would be destroyed (right to life?); the mother; and the father.

Check the end of the chapter for an answer to this activity.

PROFESSIONAL ACCOUNTABILITY

Not all matters of dispute will be heard through the legal system. Allegations of misconduct/inappropriate behaviour/poor care, and so on can be heard through a variety of settings.

COMPLAINTS SYSTEM

Complainants can seek redress by complaining about the actions of an individual/body through the complaints system within the organisation itself (i.e. to the local NHS Health Board). Complaints are reviewed by the body that is being complained about and this may not be considered robust or satisfactory. It is necessary therefore to have a system whereby complainants may make their dissatisfaction with the service received known to an independent body, i.e. an ombudsman. Generally speaking, a complaint may only be heard by the ombudsman (Parliamentary and Health Service Ombudsman (England); Public Services Ombudsman for Wales; Scottish Public Services Ombudsman; Northern Ireland Public Services Ombudsman) once the complaints service of the provider has been exhausted. The role of the ombudsman is to independently investigate a complaint and to consider whether the complaint is upheld. If so, recommendations will be made to the offending body which may include: monetary payment to be made to the victim; an apology given; further training to be undertaken; a referral to be made to a professional body. Ombudsman reports are in the public domain, which in itself may be seen as an effective remedy in that it highlights an organisation's failures.

EMPLOYER

Staff are expected to work effectively and competently for their employer, who in return should provide a safe environment and relevant training. If an allegation is made against a member of staff, the employer has a duty to investigate the allegation. This may result in a disciplinary tribunal taking place, which ultimately may lead to sanctions against the employee, the most severe being dismissal.

PROFESSIONAL BODY

For those persons working in a professional capacity, registration has to be undertaken which is then renewed regularly with a professional body. For those working within health and social care, this may involve registration with the Nursing and Midwifery Council (nurses and midwives), the General Medical Council (doctors), Health and Care Professions Council (16 health and care professions including social workers, physiotherapist, paramedics). If an allegation is made against a registered professional, proceedings may be taken, which may, if founded, lead to sanctions. The most severe of those sanctions is removal from the relevant professional register so the professional will be unable to continue to practise.

MORAL ACCOUNTABILITY FOR ONE'S ACTIONS

Legal and ethical principles are often entwined. It is important to note that we all have our own moral compass to which we adhere. We are accountable to our own ethical code, and we have to be able to live with ourselves in the event of inappropriate or less than satisfactory behaviour towards another person, regardless of whether we are being held accountable in any of the more formal ways discussed above. Although this type of accountability is not measurable, it may still have a long-term detrimental effect on a person who has to live with the consequences of his/her actions for the remainder of their life.

CONSENT: ADULT AND CHILD

Consent is an integral aspect of the relationship between a health care professional and a patient. Without consent (permission) being given by a patient for treatment, any act of a professional may constitute both a crime of battery and a tort of assault. This section of the chapter will consider the underlying principles surrounding consent in respect of capable adults and children. The following section of the chapter will focus on adults who do not have decision-making capacity.

ADULT CONSENT

Aligning with the principle of autonomy, adults are entitled to make their own decisions as regards treatment and care, which also includes refusal to treatment. There are a variety of ways by which consent is given:

Implied – where the actions of a person implicitly gives permission (e.g. holding out one's arm to allow for blood pressure to be taken).

Express – this can be verbal or written (it should be noted that a signature does not necessarily constitute a valid consent).

Presumed – where a person has not opted out of a process e.g. relevant to Organ donation in England (Organ donation (Deemed Consent) Act 2019) and Wales (Human Transplantation (Wales) Act 2013).

However, certain provisos need to be considered when looking at consent.

An adult is a person over the age of 18 (see below for a discussion regarding those persons under 18).

The adult must be deemed to have mental capacity to give consent (further discussed below).

The consent should also be given without duress (undue influence/pressure) from another (*Re T* [1992] EWCA Civ 18).

Finally, consent should be informed. This issue has been the subject of much discussion over recent years. In *Montgomery v. Lanarkshire Health Board* [2015] UKSC 11 a pregnant woman was expecting a large baby. Despite her asking her doctor about the risks of giving birth vaginally, the doctor chose not to tell her the risks, on the basis that to do so would result in Mrs Montgomery requesting a Caesarean section, which her doctor considered not to be in the maternal interest. Unfortunately, the baby became stuck and as a result suffered severe harm. It was ultimately decided by the Supreme Court, and overruling the previous case of *Bolam v. Friern Hospital Management Committee* [1957] 1WLR 582, that 'material risks' need to be advised to patients when seeking consent.

CHILDREN AND CONSENT

As far as children are concerned, the law is confusing in respect of consent. As discussed in Chapter 17, children go through three stages of childhood in respect of the matter of consent, these being:

- Children of tender age – birth until they are deemed to be 'Gillick competent'.
- Gillick competent children.
- 16–17-year-olds.

Children of tender age are unable to give consent to treatment and therefore, generally, those persons with parental responsibility (PR) will give consent. In the majority of cases, the consent of one person with PR is sufficient, although there are some areas where consent of both parties will be required. These include sterilisation of a child, change of a child's surname, circumcision of a child and immunisation of a child. If a consensus cannot be reached between those with PR, or if the persons with PR disagree with the medical opinion, then the case could be decided by the court. In *Re B (a child) (immunisation* [2003] EWCA Civ 1148 (on appeal from *A & D v. B & E* [2003] EWHC 1376) the parents held different opinions in respect of immunisation. Accordingly, the court ordered immunisation, based upon the welfare of the child being the paramount consideration (s1 (1) Children Act 1989).

Gillick competent children: In *Gillick v. West Norfolk and Wisbeck Area Health Authority* [1985] 3 All ER 402 the House of Lords, through a split decision, set down guidance to establish relevant adolescent maturity which would allow a child under the age of 16 to give his/her own consent. The case itself asked for clarity when providing contraceptive advice to those minors below the age of 16 years. While sexual activity of children below the age of 16 is illegal, it was decided that provided a child has sufficient understanding and intelligence to enable him/her to understand fully what is proposed (Lord Scarman at p. 424) then that child can consent in their own right, irrespective of parental objection. It will be a matter of fact in each situation as to whether the child does have the understanding and intelligence, and this principle now applies in all areas of health and social care.

16–17-year-olds: Section 8(1) of the Family Law Reform Act 1969 provides that 16–17-year-olds are presumed to have capacity to make their own decisions in respect of health care. This presumption is, however, rebuttable (proved otherwise), although s8 (3) of the Act does not fully extinguish the rights of parents to consent on behalf of their child and equally maintains the ability of the court to intervene if necessary.

There will be occasions when children who are deemed 'Gillick competent' or are 16–17-year-olds will disagree with those holding PR and/or the medical profession. This is most likely to occur when such children refuse treatment. While the principles discussed above promote autonomy there is inconsistency when it comes to allowing children to refuse treatment. Whilst competent consent by minors cannot be overridden, the law provides for refusal to be overridden in two ways, by those with PR and by the court. In *Re L (a minor)* [1998] 2 FLR 810, a 14-year-old child refused blood products. The court considered that although she was intelligent, she was naïve as a result of her upbringing and as she grew in maturity would question her religion. She was not deemed to be Gillick competent, and treatment was ordered. Equally, even if she had been considered to be competent, her refusal could still have been overridden on the basis that 'no minor is a wholly autonomous individual' (Lord Balcombe in *Re W (A minor)(Medical treatment: Court jurisdiction* [1992] 3 LWR 758). In this case, the court vetoed the wishes of a 16-year-old girl (to not have treatment for her anorexia nervosa) and ordered transfer and treatment at a special unit.

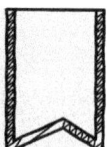

PAUSE FOR THOUGHT 5.1

Consider the various stages that a child goes through before they become an adult. Think of yourself and when you were allowed to start doing things/make decisions. Do some of these ages make sense? Why do they differ? When should a child be able to agree/refuse treatment? Should a 16-year-old child be allowed to refuse medical treatment even though they may die (compared to a 16-year-old entering the Army)?

Check the end of the chapter for an answer to this activity.

MENTAL CAPACITY ACT 2005 (MCA 2005)

If a person lacks capacity to make a decision about their care, the MCA 2005 and its Code of Practice show how they should be dealt with in a health and social care setting.

WHAT IS CAPACITY?

Mental capacity is the ability of a person to be able to make a decision for themselves. That person has to be able to understand the information, retain that information, use or weigh that information as part of the decision-making process and communicate their decision (whether by talking, using sign language or any other means) in respect of the relevant decision to be made (S3 (1) MCA 2005). An inability to be able to make a decision at the material time has to be due to an impairment of, or a disturbance in the functioning of the mind or brain (S2 (1) MCA 2005). Mental capacity is therefore patient, time and situation specific so whilst a person may be capable of making a decision in respect of medication they may be unable to make a decision regarding surgery (in the case of *Re Estate of Park* [1953] 2 All ER 1411 the Court of Appeal held that a person had capacity to make a decision to marry, but on the same day lacked capacity to make a will).

Mental incapacity may be permanent (e.g. severe brain injury, patients in a coma, patients with severe or advanced dementia) or temporary (e.g. persons who are intoxicated, under the influence of drugs, unconscious patients).

KEY PRINCIPLES OF THE MCA 2005

There are five key principles underpinning the Act that should be considered when dealing with any patient:

A person must be assumed to have capacity unless it is established that he lacks capacity (s1 (2) MCA 2005) – no assumptions should be made about a person's capacity based on age, appearance, behaviour, although this may trigger a concern, which should then be further investigated;

A person is not to be treated as unable to make a decision unless all practicable steps to help him to do so have been taken without success (s1 (3) MCA 2005) – assistance should be provided to ensure that language used is appropriate, that a person is given time to digest information, that pictures or sign language or an interpreter may be necessary in some situations;

A person is not to be treated as unable to make a decision merely because he makes an unwise decision (s1 (4) MCA 2005) – please see Activity 5.2 below for further discussion on this matter.

If it is decided, on the balance of probabilities, that the person lacks decision-making capacity at that time, for that specific decision, then the following principles come into effect:

An act done, or decision made, under this Act for or on behalf of a person who lacks capacity must be done, or made, in his best interests (s1 (5) MCA 2005). Discussed further below and in Chapter 17.

Before the act is done, or the decision is made, regard must be had to whether the purpose for which it is needed can be as effectively achieved in a way that is less restrictive of the person's rights and freedom of action (s1 (6) MCA 2005). This relates to the proportionality principle in that the law allows for interference in the life of another if it is for the best of reasons but only to the extent necessary. An example of this may be that if somebody has been injured in a car crash, is confused, bleeding profusely, in severe pain and with possible multiple fractures, the attending medical professional may deem them to lack capacity at that time to agree to any treatment.

Thus, it would be in that person's best interests to receive pain relief and for the bleeding to be stemmed. Once the pain has lessened and the patient regained capacity, then he can make a decision in respect of on-going treatment for his injuries.

WHO DECIDES?

Within the health and social care context, generally speaking, the health and social care professional providing care and treatment to the relevant person makes a determination of whether that person has or lacks capacity and, if so, determines and carries out what is in that person's 'best interests'. For simple matters, such as the provision of medication, it may be the administering nurse who makes the decision as to whether it will be in her patient's 'best interests' to receive the medication. For those patients with complex health and welfare needs a best interests meeting may be necessary to ensure that the patient's needs are fully considered. This may involve the medical team, social services, family members, carers and an Independent Mental Capacity Advocate depending on the circumstances.

In some instances, the decision will be made by a designated decision-maker. This could be a Lasting Power of Attorney with authority, or a Court appointed deputy with authority.

LASTING POWER OF ATTORNEY

There are two types of Power of Attorney – Health and Welfare; Property and Financial affairs.

- Power given by a person with capacity to enable another (or others) to make decisions on their behalf.
- Property and Financial affairs Power of Attorney can come into effect as soon as it is registered with the Office of the Public Guardian (i.e. the Attorney can make decisions on behalf of the donor whilst the donor still has capacity if this is what the donor wishes).
- Health and Welfare Power of Attorney only comes into effect when donor loses decision-making capacity.
- Attorneys obliged to act in the best interests of the donor. This power can be challenged and may result in Attorneys having their power revoked if they are not acting appropriately on behalf of the donor.

COURT-APPOINTED DEPUTY

Where the court believes that there is a need for ongoing decision-making powers for a person lacking capacity, it may under section s16 (2) MCA 2005 appoint a deputy to act for and make such decisions on behalf of the person.

ADVANCE DECISION TO REFUSE TREATMENT

In some instances the patient themselves may put their wishes in writing, to be carried out when they lose capacity. S24 (1) MCA 2005 allows for this in that it states that a person aged 18+ and with capacity to do so may make an Advance Decision to refuse treatment. Thus, at a later time when the person lacks decision-making capacity, professionals providing care and treatment to that person will know the specific treatments they do not want.

ACTIVITY 5.2

Consider the following scenario – based upon a real-life case – of *King's College Hospital NHS Foundation Trust v. C & V* [2015] EWCOP 80:

> C led a life that 'sparkled', characterised by impulsive and self-centred decision-making. She had four marriages, numerous affairs and spent money recklessly. Her life revolved around her looks, men and material possessions. Aged 49 she was diagnosed with breast cancer and underwent a lumpectomy and radiotherapy. She also suffered a relationship breakdown, leading to the loss of her business and home and resultant significant debt. C unsuccessfully attempted suicide (60 paracetamol tablets with champagne). She has been placed on dialysis, but maintains her desire to die. Those caring for her are cautiously optimistic of recovery. C, however, refuses further dialysis. The medical profession consider that C lacks capacity and wish to enforce treatment on her on the basis that it is in her 'best interests'. C wishes to be allowed to die.

Discuss.

Check the end of the chapter for an answer to this activity.

ACTIVITY 5.3   TEST YOURSELF

Having read this first part of the chapter please try to answer the following questions in order to test your knowledge:

1   Why are the legal and ethical principles discussed above considered to be so important within a health and social care setting?
2   Why do parents have the right (generally) to consent to treatment on their children?
3   Consider what should be taken into account when deciding whether or not to treat an adult who lacks capacity to agree to the treatment.

Check the end of the chapter for an answer to this activity.

CONCLUSION

This part of the chapter has considered and critically explored some of the key legal principles surrounding the area of health and social care. It is vital that those working within this area have such legal knowledge and understanding to inform and underpin their practice in the caring process that they are engaged within. Such knowledge and understanding will enable staff to practise effectively and within legal requirements. This part of the chapter has concluded with a discussion on mental capacity and is considered to be a natural break in the chapter so as not to confuse readers into assuming that a lack of mental capacity necessarily equates to a mental illness diagnosis or vice versa.

GO FURTHER ACTIVITY

For the future: In order to develop your knowledge of aspects of law and ethics we would direct the reader to undertake additional reading around these areas from specialist legal texts and the relevant research literature, as highlighted in the second part of this chapter.

ANSWERS TO CHAPTER 5 ACTIVITIES

——— Activity 5.1: Answer

Natallie Evans – Legally the case failed because the embryos had been created artificially through IVF. Both parties had contributed to their creation (eggs + sperm) and they had both signed a contract with the clinic whereby it was stated that continued consent to store the embryos would be required from both parties. They were therefore aware of this agreement. If Johnston refused consent to store the embryos then legally they would be destroyed.

From an ethical perspective it is perhaps not so simple:

Evans – this was her last chance to have her own biological child; she was not seeking assistance (financial or otherwise from Johnston);

Johnston – pressure to support child if brought into the world despite his wishes not to be involved; relationship had broken down, so if a child was brought into the world he would always be tied in some way to that unit;

Foetus – a foetus is not a human being and has no legal rights until it becomes a human being although some would say that life commences when a cell (let alone an embryo) is created.

——— Pause for Thought 5.1: Answer

Are the three phases of childhood that are applied to decision-making relevant in today's society? There are so many differing ages when children can do some things, e.g. join the army and get married (with permissions) at 16, learn to drive at 17, drink alcohol at 18 – what other anomalies can you think of? Should there be a distinction between agreeing/ refusing to allow treatment? Consider how a young person will suffer psychologically if they have been treated against their will when they feel able to make their own decision.

——— Activity 5.2: Answer

This answer is a summary of how the court reached its decision. The judge considered, based upon the evidence provided to the court, that C had the requisite capacity to make her own decision in respect of ongoing dialysis. Although he was aware of the implications of this decision (i.e. that C would die as a result) he made it clear that an individual with capacity is fully entitled to decide whether or not to accept treatment. This right extends to declining treatment even where, in the circumstances, that refusal will lead to death.

The judge acknowledged that the decision being made by C was an unwise decision – the fact that she considered growing old, the fear of living with fewer material possessions and the fear that her 'sparkle' would be lost outweighed the prospect of continuing life would alarm many people and would not be the view of many people in society. They may consider her decision to be unreasonable, illogical or even immoral. This in itself though does not evidence a lack of capacity. The court held that she was entitled to make her decision based on what was important to her, in keeping with her own set of values and personality and without conforming to society's expectations.

The court held that C had capacity and whilst the medical professionals should continue to persuade her of the benefits of receiving treatment, such treatment could not be given to C without her consent.

C continued to refuse treatment and died a few days after the judgment was given.

——— Activity 5.3: Test Yourself: Answer

1   Why are the legal and ethical principles discussed above considered to be so important within a health and social care setting?

Those staff working within any kind of health and social care setting will be working with and caring for some persons who may be considered to be vulnerable. The definition of 'vulnerable' was laid out in a consultation paper issued by the Lord Chancellor's office in 1997 and is a person who 'is or may be in need of community care services by reason of mental or other disability, age or illness; and who is or may be unable to take care of him or herself, or unable to protect him or herself against significant harm or exploitation' (Department of Health, n.d.). It is vital that those caring for them take this into consideration and treat them appropriately. Whilst all members of society may be held accountable for their actions in some ways it is vital that those working within the health and social care setting are trained and guided sufficiently well to the ethical and legal principles discussed in this chapter. By adhering to these principles this will ensure that

(Continued)

all service users, whether vulnerable or not, are provided with the care that they should receive. Equally, by adhering to these principles, all staff will be aware of and cognisant of their rights and duties in respect of the care that they provide.

2   Why do parents have the right (generally) to consent to treatment on their children?

The Children Act 1989 (CA 1989) gives detailed guidance as to how the law operates if there is dispute over how a child is brought up. Whenever a court is involved with such a question, then it is the court's responsibility to ensure that any decision made looks to the child's welfare as being of paramount consideration (s1(1)). However, usually the courts will not be a part of the process and it is necessary to consider who should make decisions on behalf of a child due to their lack of decision-making capacity. It has therefore been clarified in s2 CA 1989 as to who has decision-making authority. It is considered as a general principle that the parents of a child are the best people to make decisions on behalf of their children and this is reflected accordingly through the terminology 'parental responsibility'. Once a child is born, parental responsibility is automatically conferred upon the mother of the child and the father of the child if they were married at the time of the birth. If they are unmarried but subsequently marry then the father gains parental responsibility under the Family Law Reform Act 1987 although even if they remain unmarried but the natural father registers as the child's father on the birth certificate then he will automatically gain parental responsibility (since an amendment to the CA 1989 in 2003). It has to be acknowledged that parents will not always be in agreement as to the care and treatment of their child and thus it may be for the court to decide, again, taking the child's welfare as the paramount consideration. Similarly, whilst a child remains a minor until reaching the age of 18, the law acknowledges that the rights and duties of a parent should decrease as a child grows towards independence and thus should be given more decision-making authority if it is appropriate to do so. Please see Chapter 17 on the three stages of a child and how the rights and autonomy of a child to make their own decisions in respect of health increases as they progress towards full maturity.

3   Consider what should be taken into account when deciding whether or not to treat an adult who lacks capacity to agree to the treatment.

When an adult lacks decision-making capacity, it will generally be for the person who wishes to undertake treatment or care upon that person to decide whether or not that act would be in the person's best interests. For example, a nurse may make the decision as to whether it would be in that person's best interests to administer medication, compared to a consultation meeting (Best interests meeting) taking place in respect of whether to undertake heart surgery. Please refer to The Mental Capacity Act 2005 Code of Practice Chapter 5 (Office of the Public Guardian, 2007) for more detailed information.

When deciding whether an act should be done, the following provides a guide as to what should be considered but is not exhaustive:

The person for whom the decision is being made should be encouraged to take part, as far as is possible, in the decision-making process.

All of the circumstances that would be relevant to the person and their decision should be identified and considered.

The past and present wishes and feelings of the person for whom the decision is being made should be ascertained. These may have been expressed in a number of ways and to a variety of persons.

Any beliefs and values that the person had that may influence the decision.

Any other factors that the person would have been likely to consider if they had been in a position to decide for themselves.

Any kind of discrimination should be avoided when making a best interest decision.

Consider whether the decision needs to be made now or whether it can wait until (and if) the person regains capacity.

There should be no motivation to bring about a person's death and no assumptions should be made about quality of life.

If possible, consult with other persons for their views about what is in the person's best interests and to ascertain any information they have in respect of that person and how they may have arrived at a decision if they were in a position to do so. This could include anyone already named by the person to be consulted, carers, relatives or friends, any person appointed under a Lasting Power of Attorney and Court appointed Deputy, medical professionals, Independent Mental Capacity Advocates. Again this list is not exhaustive.

All of the above should be considered when weighing up whether or not the proposed treatment is in that person's best interests.

REFERENCES

Department of Health, n.d. No secrets: guidance on developing and implementing multi-agency policies and procedures to protect vulnerable adults from abuse. Accessed at: https://assets.publishing.service.gov.uk/government/uploads/system/uploads/attachment_data/file/194272/No_secrets__guidance_on_developing_and_implementing_multi-agency_policies_and_procedures_to_protect_vulnerable_adults_from_abuse.pdf

Office of the Public Guardian (2007). *Mental Capacity Act 2005 Code of Practice*. Accessed at https://assets.publishing.service.gov.uk/government/uploads/system/uploads/attachment_data/file/497253/Mental-capacity-act-code-of-practice.pdf

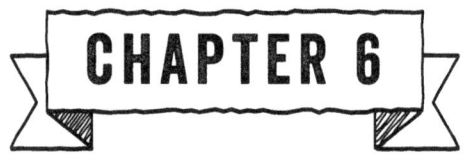

CHAPTER 6

THE LAW RELATING TO HEALTH AND SOCIAL CARE

FURTHER KEY PRINCIPLES

Angela Smith and Julia Parkhouse

OVERVIEW

Chapter 6 will consider further key legal principles underpinning the area of health and social care. It will provide an overview of the law related to mental health as well as confidentiality, both of which are relevant for those working within the health and social care setting in England and Wales.

LEARNING OUTCOMES

By the end of this chapter, you will be able to:

- Discuss and evaluate the law surrounding mental health issues and persons detained under mental health legislation.
- Identify and evaluate the key legal principles surrounding confidentiality for those working within the health and social care sector.

MENTAL HEALTH LAW

Before looking more closely at the law related to mental health, it is vital that those working within a health and social care setting are fully cognisant with the fact that just because a patient or service user may have a mental health illness it does not mean that person necessarily lacks mental capacity. Although there may be instances where this is so (e.g. severely unwell patients with a diagnosis of dementia at an advanced stage of their illness or other severely unwell mental health patients), in some instances a mental health diagnosis still means that mental capacity should be assumed. Thus, a patient with dementia may be perfectly able to make a decision (although this may fluctuate and will be time and decision specific); similarly, a person with a diagnosis of a psychotic illness may have the mental capacity to make decisions. On the other side, a person with no formal mental health diagnosis may well lack capacity, again being time and decision specific. For example, an unconscious patient would lack capacity while unconscious, or a person under the influence of drugs (whether legal or illegal) may lack capacity to make a decision while under the influence. Nonetheless, in both previous examples, in order to determine if the patient lacks the requisite capacity to make a decision, they would still need to satisfy the criteria under the Mental Capacity Act 2005. This means they would need to have an impairment of the mind or brain or a disturbance affecting their own mind or brain (temporary or permanent), and the impairment or disturbance impact upon their ability to make a decision, and this would be limited by any Advance Decision refusing medical treatment or Lasting Power of Attorney (MCA 2005, MCA CoP 2007).

The remaining discussion will therefore focus on mental health as opposed to mental capacity.

There are numerous Acts relating to mental health as it is pertinent to many other areas of activity within society. Some of the relevant Acts include:

- Mental Health Act 1983 (MHA 1983)
- Mental Health Act 2007
- Mental Health (Wales) Measure 2010 (supported by a Code of Practice) – note in England the Care Programme Approach is non-statutory guidance
- Mental Health (Assessment of Former Users of Secondary Mental Health Services) (Wales) Regulations 2011
- Mental Health (Care Co-ordination and Care and Treatment Planning) (Wales) Regulations 2011
- Police and Crime Act 2017 (extensions to s135/136 of MHA 1983)

The MHA 1983 remains the main piece of legislation and it focuses on entry into, care in and discharge from institutions, and is supported by the Mental Health Code of Practice (separate Code for England and for Wales). It is a significant piece of legislation made up of a number of Parts and Schedules including the following:

- Part I: the Application of the Act
- Part II: Compulsory Admission to Hospital and Guardianship
- Part III: Patients Concerned in Criminal Proceedings or under Sentence
- Part IV: Consent to Treatment
- Part IVA: Treatment of Community Patients Not Recalled to Hospital
- Part V: Mental Health Review Tribunals

In addition to the provisions of the above referenced legislation, those suffering from mental illness may commit crimes and be subject to criminal proceedings. So, in addition to the MHA 1983 which makes provision under Part III, the legislation listed below therefore relates to procedures in the sphere of criminal activity:

- Criminal Procedure (Insanity) Act 1964 (as amended)
- Police and Criminal Evidence Act 1984
- Criminal Procedure (Insanity & Unfitness to plead) Act 1991
- Powers of Criminal Courts (Sentencing) Act 2000
- Coroners and Justice Act 2009

It is also of note that the key common-law case of *R v. M'Naghten* (1843) 10 CL & Fin 200, HL still provides the legal definition of insanity. Based upon this definition it would mean that a person who may be suffering from the symptoms of epilepsy, diabetes or sleepwalking may be classified as insane if they commit a crime at that time. In the case of *R v. Sullivan [1983] 2 All ER 673* the defendant suffered from epilepsy. While having a seizure he kicked a friend and caused him significant injury. Although charged with grievous bodily harm, it was judged that the correct defence to put forward was that of insanity as the epilepsy had impaired his reason, memory and understanding. Further, in the case of *R v. Burgess [1991] 2 All ER 769* the defendant, while sleepwalking, again caused injury to a friend. When charged with actual bodily harm, the Court of Appeal held that the correct defence was that of insanity as the sleepwalking was a result of an abnormality of brain function, and thus a disease of the mind within the context of the *McNaghten* rules.

ACTIVITY 6.1

Peter, aged 24, but with a mental age of 10, has been arrested for the murder of a child in the area. He is detained by the police, not allowed a solicitor, not allowed to see his mother and held for three days. After intense questioning, Peter confesses, although later retracts this as he claims he only confessed so that he could see his mother.

Consider whether Peter's rights have been violated and whether his mental disability should be taken into account at the trial. You may wish to look at the Police and Criminal Evidence Act 1984 and also refer to the case of Stefan Kiszko.

Check the end of the chapter for an answer to this activity.

THE HUMAN RIGHTS ACT 1998

The Human Rights Act 1998 is also relevant to mental health. Some relevant examples include:

Article 5: In accordance with Article 5(1), no one should be dispossessed/deprived of their liberty/freedom unless it is in accordance with the law. In some cases, the MHA 1983 provides the lawful basis to detain patients as it may be necessary to restrict or remove a person's liberty if they pose a danger to themselves or others. This is because the person is suffering from a mental disorder to such an extent the criteria for detention is satisfied. However, please note before an application for admission under the MHA 1983 is made the least restrictive options and alternatives should be considered and explored so detention under the Act is essentially a last resort because of the interference with the rights and freedom of individuals. One landmark decision that was handed down in respect of this Article is in the case of R v. Bournewood Community Mental Health NHS Trust ex parte L [1998] UKHL 24 3 All ER 289 (and subsequently referred to the ECtHR under HL v. UK [2004] 45508/99 ECHR 471). In this case, L, who had a severe mental health disability, was informally admitted to a mental health hospital (Bournewood) as a result of his disruptive behaviour at the day centre he was attending. Although his carers applied for his discharge this was refused and the House of Lords agreed that his detention was lawful based on the common-law principle of necessity. However, the decision was successfully challenged in the ECtHR and it was held that the informal detention of a person lacking mental capacity in a psychiatric hospital did not contain proper safeguards and therefore breached this Article. As a result of this case UK domestic law was changed and the Deprivation of Liberty Safeguards implemented. The Mental Health Act 2007 was the vehicle that was used to amend the Mental Capacity Act 2005 bringing about the introduction of these Safeguards.

The Deprivation of Liberty Safeguards are a significant part of the MCA 2005 and ensure that persons in hospitals or care homes and who lack mental capacity to make decisions in relation to their care and treatment are not unlawfully or inappropriately deprived of their freedom. Through the Safeguards legal process, hospitals and care homes seek authorisation to deprive a patient of their liberty. However, these Safeguards are considered complex and controversial and without going into the detail legislation in the form of the Mental Capacity (Amendment) Act 2019 received Royal Assent in May 2019 introducing a new system to replace the existing Deprivation of Liberty Safeguards (DoLS). It is expected the new system will be implemented in October 2020 and although not directly referred to in the new legislation, the new system is referred to as the Liberty Protection Safeguards (LPS) and will be accompanied by its own Code of Practice which is presently being drafted and it is anticipated this Code will bring clarification on issues related to the new scheme. The LPS also provides a process for authorising a deprivation of liberty where a person lacks the mental capacity to consent to care and treatment arrangements that amount to a deprivation under Article 5(1) of the ECHR. Presently, DoLS only applies to patients aged 18 or over in hospitals and care homes and an order of the Court is required to authorise a 16- or 17-year-old be deprived of their liberty. The new LPS will apply to those aged 16 and over (mirroring other provisions under the MCA) and they will apply in other settings such as supported living and private settings and may be used to authorise transportation provisions and attendance at a day centre. There are other changes being introduced to simplify the legal framework under the assurance of improved outcomes for those persons who will be subject to the new provisions.

Article 3 provides protection from mental and physical torture or inhuman or degrading treatment or punishment. In the case of R (on the application of Wilkinson) v. Broadmoor Hospital, Responsible Medical Officer & Ors [2001] EWCA Civ 1545 a mental health patient was held in Broadmoor, a secure mental health institution. The patient refused to consent to an injection of anti-psychotic drugs and had to be forcibly restrained to administer them. Although he made a claim under Article 3, it was held that this Article would not be breached if treatment for the mental health condition was given against the patient's will provided that it was a medical necessity.

Article 8 provides protection of a person's private and family life, his home and his correspondence. In the case of Re AB (Termination of pregnancy) [2019] EWCA Civ 1215 it was stated that termination of pregnancy 'absent a woman's consent is a profound invasion of her Article 8 rights' (King, LJ at para. 24). In this instance the Court of Appeal reversed the decision made by the Court of Protection which had sanctioned a termination of pregnancy on a 24-year-old woman with learning difficulties who lacked capacity to make a decision. The court held that any such interference with these rights was only acceptable if the procedure would be in that person's best interests and it was not satisfied that in this instance a very late and intrusive termination would be in the woman's best interests.

THE MENTAL CAPACITY ACT 2005

The Mental Capacity Act 2005 is also relevant to mental health. For some persons with a mental health illness there may be a concern in relation to their capacity to make a decision about their care and treatment or where they are going to live. It should not, however, be assumed that because somebody is diagnosed with a mental health condition that they do not have capacity to make decisions.

MENTAL HEALTH ACT 1983

As indicated above, the law relating to mental health is substantial and cannot be covered in any depth in this commentary, thus the focus is on some of the issues related to compulsory admission into a mental hospital under sections 2 and 3 of the Act. Further reading is recommended for wider understanding of this area of mental health law.

ADMISSION FOR ASSESSMENT; ADMISSION FOR TREATMENT

These are two key features of the MHA 1983 in that they may result in a person's liberty being restricted in light of their mental state. Looking at these Sections of the Act:

S2 MHA 1983 relates to admission for assessment. Under this section of the Act, a person may be compulsorily admitted to a mental hospital for assessment. This is provided the person concerned meets the grounds (criteria) set out in the Act, namely, that he or she is suffering from a *mental disorder* of a *nature or degree* which warrants the detention of that person for at least a limited period, and that he or she needs to be detained in the interests of his own health or safety or with a view to the protection of other persons. This period cannot exceed 28 days under this section of the Act. The patient has a right of appeal against his/her detention to the Mental Health Review Tribunal within 14 days and can also request the Hospital Managers for their discharge from detention under the Act. Please note in this instance, hospital managers are not those who manage the hospital on a day-to-day basis, but a specially appointed panel independent of the hospital. Additionally, the patient's *nearest relative* may also order the discharge of a patient detained under this section (see s 26 of the MHA 1983 for the definition of and functions of the nearest relative as this is a legal term under the MHA and not the same as next of kin who has no rights under the Act). The *nearest relative* needs to give the hospital managers 72 hours' notice of their intention to discharge and throughout this period the patient's Responsible Clinician can issue a 'barring notice' preventing the nearest relative from exercising this power for six months if they consider the patient would be likely to act in a manner dangerous to others or themselves. Please note acting in a manner dangerous to others or themselves is considered to be greater than those factors required to be detained under the Act in the first instance (dangerous is not defined in the Act and it is given its every day meaning and the word danger is not set out in the criteria for admission).

S3 MHA 1983 relates to admission for treatment. A person may be compulsorily admitted to a mental hospital for treatment, provided that he is suffering from a *mental disorder* of a *nature or degree* which makes it appropriate for him to receive medical treatment in a hospital, that it cannot be provided unless he is detained under this Section and appropriate medical treatment is available for him. A person can initially be detained for up to six months (s20) although this can be extended. The same rights of appeal apply as per Section 2 for the patient save for the 14-day limit and the patient can apply to the Tribunal anytime within the six-month period. The *nearest relative* may also order the discharge of the patient under this section as per Section 2 discussed above.

Looking at some of the above points:

No individual may be detained unless he/she is suffering from a 'mental disorder'. According to the Act (as amended by MHA 2007), this is defined as *any disorder or disability of the mind* (s1 (2)). This definition is wide and provides experts with a wide discretion to identify conditions within its scope. A person with a learning disability will only be included within this definition if their disability is associated with abnormally aggressive or seriously irresponsible conduct on his part (s1(2A)). Similarly, dependence on alcohol or drugs is excluded from the definition; it is not considered to be a disorder or disability of the mind (s1 (3)) for the purpose of detention; however, a person with such a dependence may come within the Act if also suffering from another mental disorder which necessitates action under the Act including any such disorder arising out of their dependence. Notably, having a diagnosis of a mental disorder does not in itself amount to sufficient grounds for detention under the Act.

Nature or degree? In the case of *R v. Mental Health Review Tribunal for South Thames Region Ex p. Smith* [1998] EWHC 832 the court refused to discharge the patient and said that the words 'nature or degree' within the Act may be looked at separately and distinctly. This means that the chronic nature of illness is also relevant to the decision whether to discharge the patient even though the degree of the illness (by being currently static) was not relevant. The key word is therefore 'or'.

Medical treatment. Treatment in this context relates to treatment for the mental health condition as opposed to any physical condition. For example, in the case of *Re C (Adult: Refusal of treatment) [1994] 1 WLR 290* it was held that despite the fact that a patient was being detained in a secure mental hospital in respect of his condition of paranoid schizophrenia he had sufficient capacity and was entitled to make his own decision as to whether to agree or refuse amputation of his gangrenous foot. Whilst therefore the law is clear that an adult with decision-making capacity is entitled to refuse treatment for a physical condition on the basis of patient autonomy, this does not apply if the patient is compulsorily detained under the MHA 1983 and receiving treatment for their mental disorder (subject to some exceptions – see sections 57, 58 or 58A). Under s63 the consent of a patient is not required for any medical treatment given to him for the mental disorder from which he is suffering if the treatment is given by or under the direction of the approved clinician in charge of the treatment. There may be interrelated conditions whereby it will be necessary to consider whether the condition is a consequence of the mental illness (which, if not, cannot be treated under this Section without patient consent) or a symptom or manifestation of the mental illness (which can be treated under this Section without patient consent). For example, it has been decided that refusal to eat by those patients with a diagnosis of anorexia nervosa is a symptom/manifestation of their mental health illness and they could therefore be treated (force fed) against their will as it is considered to be the mental health condition that is being treated (*A NHS Foundation v. Ms X [2014] EWCOP 35, MHLO 96*).

CONFIDENTIALITY

Confidentiality and data protection are vital within a health and social care setting. From a practical perspective, maintaining confidentiality means that health and social care professionals do not disclose information to others; they do not gossip about patients and information is kept secure. It is important that individuals entering a health and social care setting feel secure in the knowledge that their personal and sensitive information will not generally be disclosed to others. This helps to build and develop trust within the relationship, resulting in a full picture of the patient and their lives, enabling effective care and treatment to be provided.

Those working within the health and social care setting have a three-fold duty of confidence to their patients: a duty under their contract of employment; a duty under their professional code of conduct; and a duty under the law. As far as the duties under the contract of employment and code of conduct are concerned, please revisit the beginning of this chapter and consider how health and social care professionals may be held accountable for their actions and, more specifically here, what could happen if they breach the duty of confidentiality.

DUTY OF CONFIDENTIALITY IMPOSED BY LAW

The legal system imposes a duty of confidentiality upon professionals under the General Data Protection Regulation 2016 and Data Protection Act 2018, the Human Rights Act 1998 and the common law (as discussed earlier, where the judiciary decide cases). However, no law imposes an absolute right of confidentiality. While it is important to maintain confidentiality, there will be some instances where disclosure of information has to be made (i.e. there is a duty to disclose), whereas in other instances disclosure may be made, provided it can be justified (i.e. a power to disclose).

Not all information provided to others imposes a duty of confidentiality on the practitioner. A breach of confidentiality only arises if three components are present:

1   The information given is of a personal and intimate nature (this will be present in a health and social care aspect where people are divulging private information in respect of their health and personal circumstances).
2   The information was given in circumstances imparting an obligation of confidence (this applies in the patient/health professional context in that people expect the information they divulge to be used for specific purposes as opposed to gossiping).
3   There is a possibility that the person giving the information will suffer as a result from the breach of confidentiality. This was relevant in the case of *Venables & Anor v. News Group Newspapers & Ors* [2001] EWHC QB 32 whereupon injunctions were granted to ensure that no information in respect of the convicted killers of James Bulger was released by the media upon their release from detention. In this instance it was apparent that Thompson and Venables may have suffered harm from those seeking revenge for the murder although even if no specific detriment it would still be in the public interest to support the enforcement of confidentiality.

(AG v. Guardian Newspapers Ltd (No 2) [1988] UKHL 6)

EXCEPTIONS TO MAINTAINING CONFIDENTIALITY

There are certain situations when confidentiality breaches are viewed as acceptable but do not fall within one of the Duty or Power categories. These include:

It is accepted that confidentiality needs to be breached in order to provide ongoing care, although patients should be made aware, and information only shared between those directly caring for that patient. If a patient refuses this sharing of information then their wish should be respected and they should be made aware of the limits this may put on their care and treatment. This means that staff should not disclose confidential patient information through inappropriate means such as gossiping, and should only access information for the patients in their care. For example, a nurse was struck off by the Nursing and Midwifery Council for revealing to an ex-patient (with whom she was having an affair) that his partner had undergone an abortion 19 years earlier (TeessideLive, 2006). In another case, a paramedic was dismissed from his job and received a caution from the Health and Care Professions Council for posting a picture on Facebook of a patient's skull with three nails embedded in it (due to the unusual circumstances of this case it meant that the patient may be identifiable) (TeessideLive, 2009). Similarly, when advice is sought about a patient's care and treatment with a colleague it should be done in private so that confidentiality is not inadvertently breached. All patient information and records need to be private and physically secure.

If permission is given from the patient to disclose information to others then this is acceptable, although consent should be in writing. This may be required if a patient is pursuing legal action against someone and medical records are required to evidence the claim. Only information that is strictly necessary to the claim should be released.

The Department of Health advises that there are a number of exceptions allowing disclosure to appropriate sources without patient consent, including:

- Where the patient is incapable or unwilling to know details; in these circumstances disclosure to a relative or carer may be deemed appropriate.
- Under the provisions of the Mental Capacity Act 2005 disclosure may need to be made to others when determining a best interest decision; to an independent Mental Capacity Advocate; to an Attorney under a Lasting Power of Attorney; to a Court appointed deputy.
- Where there is suspected abuse of dependent elderly and children under Local Authority protection procedures.
- To parents in respect of young persons (but note the principles of Gillick competence and the right of the child to make their own competent decisions without parental interference).

EXCEPTIONS REQUIRED BY LAW (I.E. A DUTY TO DISCLOSE)

There are certain Acts whereby disclosure of information has to be made. These include (but note this list is not exhaustive):

- Public Health (Control of Disease) Act 1984; Public Health Protection (Notification) Regulations 2010; Health Protection (Notification)(Wales) Regulations 2010 (requirement to notify relevant Local Authority of Notifiable Diseases or Infections or Contamination which presents, or could present significant harm to human health).
- Abortion Act 1967 and Abortion Regulations 1991 (information to be provided to the Chief Medical Office for statistical purposes).
- Aids (Control) Act 1987 (statistical purposes).
- Births and Deaths Registration Act 1953 – requires births and deaths to be registered.
- A doctor, optometrist or other health care professional should notify the DVLA of concerns if an individual cannot or will not advise the DVLA in respect of their fitness to drive. Patients should be advised that the DVLA will be advised. The GMC and DVLA offer guidelines on this matter.
- Terrorism Act 2000 (information in respect of suspected acts of terrorism must be reported to the police).
- Disclosure to a court. There is a distinction between legal privilege (whereby all communications between a client and his/her lawyer are protected and cannot be disclosed without permission of the client) and that of the doctrine of confidentiality. This means that all other disclosures (for example disclosures to the clergy, and to health care professionals) can be ordered to be disclosed by a court if it is considered necessary in the interests of justice. Thus, in the case of *Attorney General v. Mulholland* [1963] 1 All ER 767, a journalist was ordered to reveal his sources of information. The courts do, however, take the principle of confidentiality very seriously and will only order disclosure of information as is necessary for the purposes of deciding the case at hand.

POLICE

There is no general duty to report alleged crime to the police but there are exceptions to this principle (e.g. there is a duty to report suspected terrorist activity). There is also a duty to provide access to medical records as specified in a warrant issued under the Police and Criminal Evidence Act 1984. Similarly, under s172 Road Traffic Act 1988 (as amended by s21 Road Traffic Act 1991) a person is obliged to provide information that would lead to identification of a driver in respect of a road traffic offence, to the police, if required to do so. In the case of *Hunter v. Mann* [1974] 1QB 767 a doctor was successfully prosecuted for failing to disclose information to the police. His defence that to do so would breach the patient's right to confidentiality was not accepted. Although there is no general duty to report alleged crime to the police (although see discussion below in respect of public interest), a person cannot require their confidential disclosure to be maintained if they have admitted wrongdoing. In the case of *R v. Wilson* [1996] Crim LR 573 the defendant branded his initials upon his wife's buttocks. She developed an infection and the doctor reported the incident to the police on the basis that this was potentially a crime (actual bodily harm under s47 Offences Against the Person Act 1861). Whilst the case focused on the issue of her consent (which was found to have been valid as the branding was considered to be akin to tattooing and cosmetic enhancement) it is of interest that the breach of confidentiality by the doctor was acceptable in this situation.

EXCEPTIONS NOT REQUIRED BY LAW BUT WHERE DISCLOSURE MAY BE MADE IF IT IS JUSTIFIED

There will be instances where it is felt that disclosure should be made, but where this needs to be justified. These exceptions are contained within the Human Rights Act 1998, the General Data Protection Regulation 2016 and Data Protection Act 2018 and within the common law case of *W v. Egdell* [1990] 1 All ER 835:

In this case, W was detained in a secure hospital as a consequence of being convicted of manslaughter. He applied for conditional discharge from his detention and was granted authorisation to obtain an independent psychiatric report in respect of his mental health, which he hoped would support his application. Dr Egdell was instructed to provide this report. The report did not support W's case for either discharge or for a transfer to a regional secure unit, and ultimately W withdrew his application. However, despite W not giving consent, Dr Egdell then sent a copy of the report to the hospital where W was being detained, and then pressed the hospital to forward a copy to the Home Office (stating that if they did not do so then he would). The hospital complied with this request.

W sued Dr Egdell for breach of confidentiality. The Court of Appeal held that although the law recognises an important public interest in maintaining professional duties of confidence, it has to treat such duties 'not as absolute but as liable to be overridden where there is held to be a stronger public interest in disclosure' (Bingham LJ). Accordingly, W's claim was unsuccessful.

Thus, this case confirmed that confidentiality may be breached on the basis that there is a public interest defence and therefore the breach is justified. Examples of when it may be in the public interest to disclose information would include: disclosure for the public good; disclosure in the interests of justice; disclosure to prevent a civil wrong; disclosure to protect a third party; disclosure to prevent or detect a serious crime. It will be a matter for the individual to consider and to think of the consequences of making such a disclosure.

However, it should be noted that while disclosure may be justified, it was made clear in the case of *X v. Y* [1988] 2 All ER 648 as to the criteria that need to be satisfied in order to justify disclosure. In this case, general practice doctors were believed to be practising despite the fact that they had contracted AIDS. Although the argument for disclosure by the newspaper was based on informing a debate on this matter, the injunction was granted, thereby ensuring that the doctors' identities remained confidential. The court considered that there has to be a balancing act between the public interest in maintaining confidentiality against a countervailing public interest which favours disclosure. Each case will differ depending on the facts. As far as guidance is concerned when this balance is being weighed, the following needs to be shown in order to favour disclosure:

- The risk (i.e. resulting from non-disclosure) is real, immediate and serious.
- That risk will be substantially reduced by disclosure.
- That disclosure is no greater than is reasonably necessary to minimise the risk.
- That the consequent damage to the public interest protected by the duty of confidentiality is outweighed by the public interest in minimising the risk (Mr Justice Rose).

ACTIVITY 6.2

Consider the following scenario:

Judy has come to your surgery and, after she leaves, you discover her handbag which contains a large quantity of ecstasy.

What will you do with this information? Are you obliged to inform the police? Are you empowered to inform the police? Consider also if the drug was instead a small quantity of cannabis.

Check the end of the chapter for an answer to this activity.

ACTIVITY 6.3   TEST YOURSELF

Having read this chapter please try to answer the following questions in order to test your knowledge:

1   Why might the concepts of mental health and mental capacity be considered to be both separate yet linked to one another?
2   Why is it necessary to have specific legislation in respect of those persons suffering from mental illness?
3   Consider and discuss some of the issues surrounding the legal position on when confidentiality may be waived if in the public interest.

Check the end of the chapter for an answer to this activity.

CONCLUSION

This chapter has considered some of the key legal principles surrounding the area of health and social care. The key implications of not complying with the topics discussed within this chapter should now be evident to the reader. It is of major importance that anybody entering the sphere of health and social care avails and updates themselves on a regular basis with the requirements for practising within the confines of the law. By doing so this will mean that patients and service users are cared for effectively but equally means that staff recognise the duty of care that they owe to all those under their care, and comply accordingly.

ANSWERS TO CHAPTER 6 ACTIVITIES

——— Activity 6.1: Answer

As a result of several miscarriages of justice, including the case of Stefan Klitzo, it was acknowledged that the police were not treating those people under suspicion of committing offences fairly. Accordingly, in 1984 the Police and Criminal Evidence Act 1984 and its accompanying Codes of Practice gave detailed advice in respect of the treatment of those persons arrested, questioned and detained for alleged crimes. This now means that young persons (those under 17) and those persons considered to be vulnerable (such as Peter in the example) should not be interviewed unless in the presence of an 'appropriate adult'. This is in addition to their right to a solicitor. Further, any confession obtained through oppression (and again, one may consider that the behaviour of the police in this scenario towards Peter is oppressive) then this may be considered to be inadmissible in court.

——— Activity 6.2: Answer

In respect of both drugs – The police have no general right of access to health records. This is not a suspected act of terrorism, is not a road traffic accident, and the police do not have a warrant. There is therefore no obligation to disclose this information to the police, and in the absence of patient consent, is there a robust argument for informing the police? Is it in the public interest to disclose?

Ecstasy – There would be a public interest in preventing or detecting a serious crime here. Supplying a Class A drug is a serious offence and thus disclosure is justified. However, although disclosure is justified, it should be limited to the minimum necessary to meet the relevant purpose and the patient should be informed of the disclosure (unless informing the patient would defeat the purpose of the investigation, allow a potential criminal to escape or put staff at risk).

Cannabis – This is less clear. Although cannabis is a Class B drug (with a maximum sentence of 5 years for possession and 14 years for supply), the patient only has a small supply in her handbag, and may be using it for recreational/pain relief purposes as opposed to supplying it to others. Consideration has to be taken of the impact such disclosure would have on the patient and the wider community, and also the element of trust between patient/health care professional that will be lost if disclosure is made. It would be for the health care professional to decide whether disclosure is in the public interest and further, whether it can be justified.

——— Activity 6.3: Test Yourself: Answer

Mental Health and Mental Capacity concepts are considered to be separate yet they are linked to one another with both having a protective element. With regards to Mental Health, the compulsory powers that exist under the Act provide a legal framework within which persons with enduring and serious mental health conditions who are considered a risk to themselves or others, can be dispossessed of their liberty and assessed and treated (if necessary) in the absence of their consent. Under the Mental Capacity Act the main issue is that the person lacks decision-making capacity. The broad framework provided by this Act ensures health and social care providers do all they can to enable the patient to make a decision in the first instance but if unable to do so, thereafter make a decision on that person's behalf. This Act is concerned with the protection of the patient and not others.

It is necessary to have specific legislation because of the vulnerability of those persons suffering from mental illness. Mental Health legislation is protective and is required in certain circumstances so those persons who are suffering with serious mental health issues receive the necessary care and treatment possibly without their consent in order to prevent them from potentially causing harm to themselves or others. Equally, the introduction of the Deprivation of Liberty Safeguards into the Mental Capacity Act 2005 via the 2007 Mental Health Act protects those individuals aged 18 or over, who lack the capacity to make decisions for themselves in relation to their care and treatment, who are or may become deprived of their liberty in a hospital or care home setting.

Importantly, trust is an essential element of the relationship between a health and social care professional and the patient and embedded in this, is the duty of confidentiality. However, in certain circumstances this duty is not absolute and disclosure in the public interest is one of these circumstances. Disclosure in the Public Interest is to be considered when the welfare and rights of the public may be at risk and need to be protected and enhanced. While a decision to disclose in the public interest is considered on a case by case basis but may be made where it is considered necessary to prevent a serious and imminent threat to national security, public health, to protect the life of an individual or a third party or to prevent or detect a serious crime. It will be a matter for the individual to consider and to think of the consequences of making such a disclosure.

FURTHER READING

In order to develop your knowledge around aspects of law and ethics we would recommend you to undertake additional reading around these areas from specialist legal texts and the relevant research literature, as listed below:

Brazier, M. and Cave, E. (2016). *Medicine, Patients and the Law*. Manchester: Manchester University Press. An overall view of legal issues relating to healthcare matters.

British and Irish Legal Information Institute. Available at www.bailii.org. Allows access to British and Irish case law and legislation, EU case law, Law Commission reports and other law-related British and Irish material.

Jones, M. (2015) *Mental Health Act Manual.* London: Sweet & Maxwell. A comprehensive text on all mental health issues.

Judicial Office International Team. The Judicial System of England and Wales: A visitor's guide. Available at www.judiciary.uk/wp-content/uploads/2016/05/international-visitors-guide-10a.pdf. Gives a comprehensive account of how the English legal system works in practice.

The Stationery Office (2007) Mental Capacity Act Code of Practice. Available at https://assets.publishing. service.gov.uk/government/uploads/system/uploads/attachment_data/file/497253/Mental-capacity-act-code-of-practice.pdf. This provides clear guidance as to how the MCA should be interpreted and gives scenarios that students can work through.

REFERENCES

TeessideLive (31 January 2006). Struck off. Available at: www.gazettelive.co.uk/news/local-news/struck-off-3783556 (accessed 20 June 2019)

TeessideLive (11 July 2009). Paramedic disciplined after X-ray picture posted on web. Available at: www.gazettelive.co.uk/news/local-news/paramedic-disciplined-after-x-ray-picture-3716790 (accessed 20 June 2019)

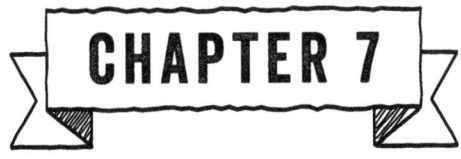

REFLECTIVE PRACTICE AND CRITICAL THINKING

Sally Riggall

OVERVIEW

This chapter will explore some of the core attributes which are necessary to a health and social care professional on their journey in becoming a skilled, intuitive, reflective practitioner. None of these attributes are innate, which is good news, because this means we can develop the necessary qualities and hone them to enhance our practice. Core attributes will be explored, including resilience (i.e. how tough we are and whether we can bounce back from adversity with a positive attitude); self-knowledge (i.e. how well we understand how our upbringing, background and unconscious processes have shaped our views, methods of communication and ways of managing ourselves); and how far we might become perceptive, critical practitioners. A skilled practitioner recognises that developing all of these areas is a life's work. If we ever reach the point where we think we understand everything there is to know about ourselves and about others, then we would have to ask ourselves what we are missing, what is just out of reach? What have I missed? How can I improve next time? This chapter will invite you to develop your knowledge and understanding of yourself in ways which will help you to become a more self-aware and consequently resilient practitioner. The final section of the chapter will explore critical thinking and will introduce you to two different methods of developing good, critical, reflective practice. The topics discussed in the chapter may not appear to be immediately evident in practice. However, effective, engaged, self-aware practitioners are almost certain to be using aspects of all of the areas explored here.

LEARNING OUTCOMES

By the end of this chapter you will be able to:

- Explain the role of self-knowledge in being a reflective and critical practitioner
- Define what makes a resilient practitioner and understand the role resilience plays in being a reflective practitioner
- Describe some of the unconscious processes which affect our professional behaviour and assess ways of bringing these into conscious awareness

(Continued)

- Explain how different models of critical reflection can be used to help us to develop into reflective practitioners
- Evaluate our own journey in becoming reflective practitioners

INTRODUCTION

Health and social care work in the current climate operates under a highly pressured environment with heavy caseloads and where time is limited. Consequently, the main emphasis is often on completing tasks with service users in the shortest possible time. However, critical commentators have argued that the most effective practitioners are those who are self-aware and reflective and who devote time to developing themselves as well as focusing on tasks. Munro (2011, p. 86) argues that the current managerialist approach consists of collecting information and making plans at the expense of creating and sustaining effective relationships with service-users where individuals are engaged with and listened to by practitioners who have the capacity to reflect on their own practice, to learn from it and to manage their own emotions. Munro highlights the necessity of practitioners being in touch with their inner thoughts and feelings and their unconscious processes which can be made conscious via self-reflection and supervision. Such critical practice analyses this intuitive way of working and can translate into a deeper understanding of what might be really happening in service users' lives. Gaining such insight assists health and social care practitioners in working collaboratively with service users and it is also crucial in the development of practitioner resilience.

Reflective and critical practice begins during our training and continues throughout our careers, whichever aspect of health and social care we choose to specialise in. Indeed, reflective practice is located clearly within continuing professional development (CPD) which is specified as being essential in the Code of Conduct for Healthcare Support Workers and Adult Social Care Workers in England (Skills for Care, 2013). The recommendation here is that all practitioners participate in CPD to strive to improve the quality of health care, care and support and to achieve the competence required for their roles.

A good way of developing reflective writing skills is to keep a reflective journal. Bassot (2016) suggests that whilst reflective practice helps us to explore our experiences, critically reflective practice involves us engaging with deeper elements which are just below the surface, such as our emotional responses to events and interactions and challenging some of the assumptions we make about ourselves and those we engage with. She argues that a reflective journal is a tool that enables us to record such events and explore ways of working by applying reflective models. Also, because writing creates a permanent record, we can return to our learning in the future. A learning journal also helps us to identify patterns in our thinking, feelings and behaviour and to document our developing skills.

WHY DEVELOPING RESILIENCE THROUGH REFLECTIVE PRACTICE IS AN IMPORTANT QUALITY

Developing resilience has become important on the agenda in health and social care training in recent years; for example, Grant (2012) found that 20 per cent of social workers leave the profession every year while Revalier (2017) found that over 50 per cent of social workers are planning to leave their job. The figure is equally disturbing for nursing: from October 2016 to September 2017, 35,363 nurses and midwives left the profession (NMC, 2017) and there were 40,000 vacancies (Royal College of Nursing, cited in House of Commons Health Committee Report, (2017). Current vacancies for all health workers across the entire NHS is now 100 500, or 9.1 per cent of the workforce (NHS Improvement, 2018).

Many health and social care workers planning to leave their profession cite stress as a critical factor. Considine et al. (2015, p. 216) define resilience as 'the personal capacity to adapt to change and manage internal and external stressors'. Being able to do this in the face of the considerable pressures practitioners face on a day-to-day basis is a real challenge. Munro (2011) comments on the need for practitioners to develop resilience and states there are support mechanisms that can really help. She argues that good management and supervision are critical factors in enhancing resilience and reducing burn-out in staff and good reflective practice is an essential vehicle in this process. We will explore how to develop resilience later in the chapter.

First, it will be useful to try and define what a resilient practitioner might look like. Grant and Kinman (2014) in their research have identified a number of characteristics that resilient people possess including the following:

- A high level of self-awareness, self-efficacy and self-esteem
- Emotional literacy – recognising and attending to own and others' feelings and moods
- Social confidence
- Flexibility and the ability to be adaptable to change
- Optimism, enthusiasm and a positive outlook on life, work and the future
- A high level of interpersonal skills including empathy
- A willingness to be open and to learn from new experiences
- Good, critical, reflective skills
- Hardiness, persistence and the ability to recover quickly when circumstances are difficult
- Knowledge of and ability to access internal and external resources

Many of these characteristics are similar to Maslow's definition of self-actualisation which were interpreted by Hough (1994, p. 45):

- The ability to tolerate uncertainty and resist pressure
- Autonomy and self-reliance
- The ability to be objective and perceive clearly what is really happening
- Being open in expression and to new thoughts and approaches
- Acceptance of self and others including strengths and weaknesses
- The ability to look outside of self to problems in the wider world
- Being spontaneous in thought and action and maintaining a sense of humour
- Having the ability to establish and maintain deep interpersonal relationships
- Being aware of and interested in social and community issues
- A willingness to experiment with new ideas and ways of working
- Having an appreciation of nature and everyday events

All of the above are areas we can personally reflect on and engaging with our motivations in such a deep manner helps us to really develop our practice.

ACTIVITY 7.1

Read the lists above and rate yourself on a scale of 1–4 for each of the characteristics of resilience listed. 1 should relate to you possessing little of this characteristic, whilst 4 relates to you being strongly developed in this characteristic. How much resilience do you think you already possess? You are unlikely to feel confident in all areas, so what do you need to work on? How might this self-knowledge aid you in being reflective within your practice?

Check the end of the chapter for an answer to this activity.

FACTORS OF RESILIENCE

The list above focuses on a number of elements: aspects of our personalities, our attitude to the world and to others, and also how we see and respond to outside influences. Developing resilience requires a focus on two areas, both of which may overlap with each other. The first factor we need to understand is to identify the different facets of our personality, our interpersonal style, our history, our ways of seeing the world and our values and understand how all of these areas can impact on ourselves and others. Howe (2008, p. 11) names this as emotional intelligence and defines it as 'the ability to understand both our selves and other people as emotional beings'. Howe then sees two aspects to this concept: our *interpersonal* intelligence (i.e. how well we can tune in to and understand other people's emotions and motivations); and our *intrapersonal* intelligence (i.e. how knowledgeable we are of ourselves, and how we can use this knowledge to enhance our relationships with others). Reflective practice helps us to develop both of these equally important elements.

INTRAPERSONAL INTELLIGENCE AND ITS EFFECT ON RESILIENCE

UNCONSCIOUS PROCESSES AND TRANSFERENCE

How well do we really know and understand ourselves? How do others really experience us and how do we learn about the effect we might be having on them? The more we know about those areas which are neither visible nor known to us, the more resilient we will become. Until we become aware of how we function and act with others, these unconscious processes can detrimentally affect our relationships with service users and other professionals.

There is much to learn from psychodynamic theory here. Freud (1916) was one of the originators of this approach and he states the unconscious is that which is concealed and not accessible to us. He states that it consists of feelings we found uncomfortable from early childhood events which we go on to repeat throughout our lives in our relationships with others. In other words, we transfer these feelings onto those we work with without being aware that we are doing so. Transference, then, is the process by which we are unconsciously influenced by our past experiences in the shaping of our thoughts, feelings and behaviours in current situations. A service user may remind me of a significant person from my childhood and then I react to them in a similar way; for example, they may remind me of my mother when they look at me disapprovingly and I respond by feeling anxious and wanting to please them. Murdin (2010) argues that the past always leaves traces and these traces affect what is happening in the present. She says 'the transference trace will appear like a muddy footprint on a white carpet' (Murdin, 2010, p. 8). In other words, our unconscious processes, located from the past and extended into the present, can stain our relationships and cause conflict and stress.

Transference also occurs in service users and they may react to their practitioner in a similar way. Jacobs (2010) argues that we often remain unconscious to these processes until someone brings it to our attention. This is why being willing to engage in reflective practice during supervision can really help us to explore these deeper aspects of ourselves. Supervision offers us the opportunity to receive feedback on our interactions with others, reflect on our engagement skills and improve our practice in the future. However, it is worth noting that supervision is often time-limited and may focus more on decision-making rather than on practitioners' emotions. In these instances you may need to find another supportive worker who you trust to engage with for this level of self-exploration.

CASE STUDY 7.1

Anna (40) is a practitioner in an Adult Services team. She grew up in a small, tightly knit family. Her mother was a single parent and Anna never knew her father. When she was 20, her mother became ill with cancer and died a year later. She was also close to her grandmother who was 75 when Anna's mother died and who lived for another 15 years after her daughter's death. Anna was her sole carer. Anna's grandmother also had a son (James) who left the area when he was 18 to live 200 miles away in Cardiff. Anna remembers her Uncle James (who she experienced as opinionated and uncaring) visiting her and her mother a few times when she was a child and once after her mother died but he kept his distance and refused to have any contact with Anna's grandmother, although he did attend her funeral (which Anna organised).

This week Anna meets for the first time Owen, the 45-year-old son of Kenneth, who Anna has had referred to her. Kenneth is finding it difficult to cope on his own at home after the death of his wife. Owen is not local and has made a long round trip to visit. As soon as Owen starts to talk, Anna folds her arms, removes eye contact and is aware she is struggling to listen to him. She feels intense dislike towards him and also feels he is not going to offer any support at all for his father and she has to catch her breath with the ferocity of emotions which overwhelm her. In the meantime, Owen stops talking to Anna, feeling she is not hearing what he has to say and that his meeting with her has been a waste of time.

Afterwards, in supervision with Aylin, Anna explores what happened and how uncomfortable she felt. With Aylin's help and support, Anna realises that it was the point she first heard Owen speak that triggered her strong feelings. Owen has a similar accent to her Uncle (Owen has lived for decades in the same area). She has transferred her feelings of rejection, of being unsupported and let down by her Uncle James onto Owen, believing he will act in the same manner with his own father. As soon as she realises this transference has occurred, she is able to see that Owen is a different person and her difficult emotions are lifted. She also realises that she has never fully acknowledged how hurt and alone she felt all the years she cared for her grandmother without her uncle's help and support.

It can be seen from the case study that transference can evoke strong and immediate feelings which can overwhelm the person experiencing them. From Owen's point of view, his first meeting with his father's support worker consists of engaging with someone who will not give him eye contact and who seems sullen and uninterested. It is not a good start. Both parties are likely to experience a raised pulse and other symptoms of stress and both are likely to dwell on the experience afterwards when they get home. With Anna learning more about her transference response from her discussions with and feedback from her supervisor, her resilience will have become more solid and she will be able to meet again with Owen and move their relationship onto a better footing. Self-knowledge and being willing to reflect are key factors here, and if a similar situation arises again, Anna will be better prepared, having reflected on and worked through this aspect of her past.

COUNTER-TRANSFERENCE

When a transference takes place, the response of the other person is said to be counter-transference (Murdin, 2010). Transference is where the feeling and behaviour is initiated and counter-transference is the response to it. In the above example, Owen's response to Anna's transference is to shut down. He views her as uninterested in him and possibly in his father too. Anna's manner with him may remind Owen of other figures of authority who have acted in a similar way and he may react in an old, familiar way.

Reflection on counter-transference responses to a service user's words and/or behaviour can really help the practitioner develop their engagement and thus improve their resilience. In the next example, counter-transference is explored:

- Amy is a health practitioner leading a group of people who meet once a month and who care for partners or family with Parkinson's disease. After the session, Frank asks to talk to Amy on her own. Frank insists on standing up during their meeting and he interrupts Amy whenever she speaks. Frank then tells her his wife has said she wants to leave him and that 'I can't talk sense into her – I have no idea why she wants to go'. She can see Frank's foot tapping and that his hands are clenched and again as she tries to speak, Frank says, 'I look after her and provide her with everything she needs and look how she treats me'. Amy's response is now to remain quiet, even though she has things she wants to say and she feels defeated, unheard and quite disempowered. Amy is able to recognise this as her own counter-transference response to Frank and wonders if Frank's wife may be feeling the same in response to his manner and she stores this thought, wondering if there might be the right moment to gently challenge Frank to help him gain some insight into why his wife might be wanting to leave.

The above example demonstrates that if Amy can identify and engage with her own feelings and thoughts that ensue from her interactions and thus bring them into conscious awareness, she can utilise these to develop her responses. Also, by being able to use her 'self' in this manner, she is not going to leave the session with the feelings that arose for her in the middle of the interaction (defeated, unheard and dejected) because she is able to place them where they belong: as a counter-transference response. Without this insight, she would be likely to carry on feeling these negative emotions for the remainder of the day and beyond. Understanding the transference and her own counter-transference response, then, develops the practitioner's resilience and maintains her well-being.

Another technique which can be very helpful during sessions is to think: 'If my supervisor was to ask me at this moment what is really going on for the service-user and for me, what would I say to her?' Casement (1985) named this process 'the internal supervisor' and it is a useful way of identifying transferences and counter-transferences that might be occurring during the session. In Amy's case above, she could have asked herself this question and this would have helped her to identify her own responses to Frank's demeanour.

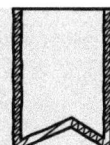

PAUSE FOR THOUGHT 7.1

Think of a recent interaction which was difficult for you. What unconscious processes were going on for you? Who might you really have been relating to (underneath)? What transferences and counter-transferences did you recognise?

Check the end of the chapter for an answer to this activity.

METHODS OF UNCOVERING OUR UNCONSCIOUS PROCESSES

It is all well and good learning that we have unconscious processes which can impact on our communication and resilience. However, if we have to wait until we are confronted with them during service-user meetings in order to learn from them then our self-knowledge is going to arise via a series of short, sharp shocks. Luckily, there are models, theories and exercises from which we can draw which can help us to pre-empt the process. One such model is the Johari Window which will be explored next.

JOHARI'S WINDOW

In 1961 Joseph Luft and Harry Ingham (Luft, 1961) developed the Johari Window (an amalgamation of their first names) as a forum for examining our own behaviour in relation to others. The Johari Window enables us to bring into conscious awareness those aspects of ourselves which are just out of reach for us, and by so doing we can improve the quality of engagement with others and increase our resilience. It is a good aid to reflecting on ourselves and our practice at a deep level. Johari's Window comprises four segments (see Figure 7.1).

	Known to Self	Not Known to Self
Known to Others	**Open Area** **Area of Free Activity** I know these things about me and I know that you know them too.	**Blind Area** You know these things about me but I am, as yet, unaware of them. They include positive and negative aspects.
Not Known to Others	**Avoided or Hidden Area** I know these things about me but do not wish you to know them	**Area of Unknown Activity/Mystery** This area represents the potential within me, which no one, including myself, is as yet aware of. It includes my untapped skills and talents and hidden resources and dreams.

Figure 7.1 Johari's window

Examples of aspects of ourselves that might appear in each segment might be as follows and we can place ideas in the Blind Area in order to check them out with others. Imagine this is the Johari Window of Ben (Figure 7.2), a ward supervisor at a city hospital.

OPEN AREA	BLIND AREA
• I am 180 centimetres tall • I like to keep active and play a number of sports regularly • I believe that a physically healthy body also leads to good mental health • I like reading books which make me think about the human condition • I hate injustice • I hate animal cruelty and am a vegetarian • I become emotional when others are upset, especially children • I have a phobia about spiders • My political views are left wing, I believe strongly in the NHS and would not want to work in private health care • I like to think that I am broad-minded and that nothing shocks me • I get irritated when other people are late • I panic when I think I am going to be late • I like to be in control	• I am not sure whether I stand up straight • Do I come across as obsessive? • Do others experience me as judgemental when they do not have the same attitude to fitness and health? • Do I see people who do not read books as inferior to me? • What are my prejudices and how do they manifest in my verbal and non-verbal behaviour? • Do I recognise when patients are scared and upset about their illness and treatment? • How accommodating am I of others' failures, especially the staff on my ward? • How judgemental am I of others' political views? • Am I jaded? Is it all becoming routine? • Do I become inappropriately irritated and jeopardise working relationships? • What negative consequences are there to my obsessive behaviour? • How effective am I in placing other people in control and at the centre of decision-making – especially patients?
AVOIDED OR HIDDEN AREA	AREA OF UNKNOWN ACTIVITY/MYSTERY
• This is my very private area. When engaging with patients it includes not sharing the following: • Details of my relationships with my partner and family • Aspects of my past and upbringing which brought me difficulties and pain • Various events which have happened to me throughout my life • My sexuality • The assumptions I make which I do not like to admit to with regard to gender, culture, disability, sexuality, age and class.	• People tell me I have good management skills and that my ward is one of the best run in the hospital. Perhaps I could explore this as a career option. • I have recently begun a part-time class in photography and received some fabulous feedback from the tutor and classmates, and wonder whether I might be successful in photography competitions.

Figure 7.2   Johari window of Ben

Each pane of the Window will change shape as we develop more understanding of ourselves, with the Open Window increasing in size as we gain greater conscious knowledge of ourselves (see Figure 7.3).

Luft (1961) states that when we ask others for feedback we decrease our Blind Area and increase our Open Area, and in so doing we develop more truth about ourselves and are able

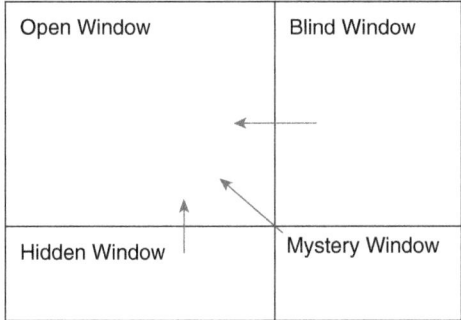

Figure 7.3   Developing the open area

to reach out more deeply to others. When exploring our Blind Area with another person, we find out how our behaviour, thinking and emotions impact on others. Once this becomes part of our conscious awareness, this learning can be brought into our Open Area: 'I know this about me and I know that you know this about me too.' In Ben's case, he could ask for feedback from his colleagues about how they experience him as a ward supervisor: do they find him irritable or particularly obsessive and if so could they give him examples to illustrate? If his colleagues confirm they experience Ben in this way, these aspects of his personality are then brought into his Open Area: Ben knows this about himself and knows others know it too. The more willing Ben is to explore and reflect on aspects of his Blind Area, the more self-aware he will become, and consequently be a better practitioner. The more we know about ourselves, our strengths, areas for development, how our non-verbal communication and verbal responses affect others; how our values and attitudes impact on each service user we engage with then the closer we edge to becoming a skilled practitioner.

Analysing these four aspects of ourselves in this way is a very good way of reflecting on ourselves and our practice. Supervision is a fine place to explore all aspects of our Johari Window and so develop an increased level of understanding about how our intrapersonal processes impact on our interpersonal communication.

ACTIVITY 7.2

Draw your own blank Johari's Window and then write statements in each area. You may just wish to remain aware of your Hidden Area without writing anything down here. Try and make the statements as specific as you can and do not be afraid to write down traits about yourself in your Blind Area about which you wish to receive feedback. Your Open Area is likely to be quite small to start with, but the aim is to increase your own self-knowledge and thus the size of this area. Choose someone you trust and who will be honest with you to help you explore your Blind and Mystery Areas. Conveying honest feedback is a skill in itself and you may have to be able to 'read between the lines' of the comments you receive. Finally, armed with your new self-knowledge, re-visit and expand your Open Area.

Check the end of the chapter for an answer to this activity.

BRINGING IT ALL TOGETHER: CRITICAL REFLECTION

It can be seen from the examples in this chapter so far that the more we understand ourselves, our conscious and unconscious processes then the greater our ability will be to form and maintain good-quality relationships with service users and to communicate and engage effectively. Developing this understanding and maintaining the curiosity to do so are some of the building blocks of critical reflection: the more I am in touch with what I am thinking and feeling and how I am behaving then the more likely I am to be able to choose ways of working which are professional and accountable. Rutter and Brown (2015) argue that critical reflection is the process of focusing on and evaluating our experiences in such a way that we can develop new understandings of our thinking and ways of working. Developing and utilising our self-awareness is integral to this process. Feltham (2010) suggests that the highest level of critical thinking and reflection involves approaching everything practitioners are involved in analytically and with some scepticism in order to investigate possible alternatives. This way of critical reflection can be applied to our practice: the way we utilise theory, how our values affect our practice, the way we use our professional powers and how we manage risk; how wider influences affect what is happening to ourselves and our service users such as inequalities and poverty and their direct effect on our service users or organisational policy which impacts on workers' caseloads.

Understanding our strengths as well as areas for development is also important. Critical reflection means being able to analyse what was good about our practice too. When an action has gone well, we need to recognise what we did and how we did it just as clearly as when something goes awry. When reflecting on good practice, we need to understand how we engaged: what did we say and do which was good? Developing insight into our strengths helps us to draw from these skills and to build on good ways of working in future interactions. It also enables us to share best practice with colleagues.

A common difficulty for health and social care students when first writing about their practice is to write descriptively rather than critically. Learning how to become critically reflective as opposed to being purely descriptive is a challenge, but these skills can be easily developed by utilising one of several models which are available to aid critical reflection. Here, two will be described and applied.

MODEL 1

John Hilsdon's (2012) 'Model to Generate Critical Thinking' is the first model to be explored as a method of moving from description to critical reflection. This model takes a step-by-step process:

1   First be descriptive
2   Next be analytical
3   Finally be evaluative

Hilsdon suggests the following approach:

- Who was there? (Descriptive)
- What did s/he say? (Descriptive)
- What did I say? (Descriptive)
- Why did I respond in that way? (Analytical/reflective)
- How did each of us feel as a result? (Analytical/reflective)

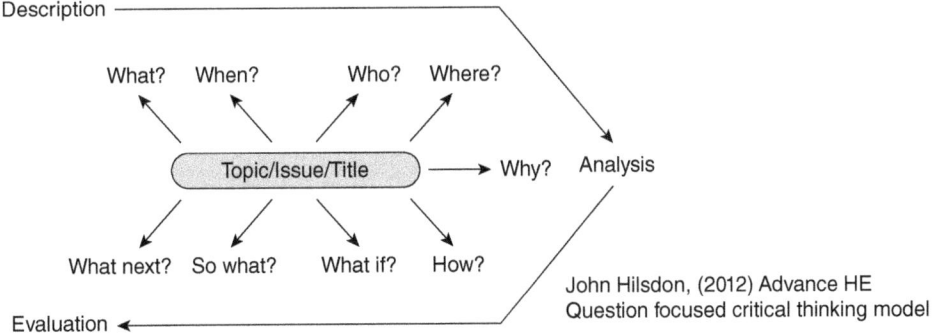

Figure 7.4 Hilsdon's model to generate critical thinking

Source: Hilsdon (2012). Reproduced with kind permission from John Hilsdon.

- What if I had chosen my words more carefully? (Analytical/reflective)
- So what? Would that have made a difference to the outcome? (Reflective/evaluative)
- Where can I go from here in my interactions with this person? (Reflective/evaluative)

EXAMPLE

In this example, Paul, a student nurse on placement on a gerontology ward, has been asked to write about an interaction he had with Mr and Mrs H, who are both in their eighties. Mr H has severe arthritis and is in hospital at the moment receiving a new drug therapy. His wife looks after him at home but is finding it increasingly difficult to cope.

Paul: During the course of the conversation, I thought about my own grandfather, who also had arthritis and how he eventually went into a home. It was the best thing for him and for everyone. I asked them both if they had considered Mr H going into residential care and at this point everything seemed to go wrong. Mrs H said this was absolutely not going to happen and how could I have suggested it. She said they had been married for nearly 60 years and they were not going to be parted now. She asked if there was another nurse on duty who could look after Mr H. I knew I had made a big mistake but did not really know how to get back on track and when I left them, Mrs H was still distressed.

Applying Hilsdon's model, Paul is better able to reflect on how he could have handled the interaction differently (see Table 7.1).

Table 7.1 Applying Hilsdon's model to Paul

Who was there?	Mr and Mrs H were both present along with myself as the nurse in training.
What did she say?	Mrs H said she was finding it increasingly difficult to cope.
What did I say?	I asked if they had considered residential care for her husband.
What did she say?	Mrs H said: 'This is absolutely not going to happen and how could you even suggest it? We have been together for nearly 60 years and we are not going to be parted now.'

(Continued)

Table 7.1   (Continued)

Why did I respond in that way?	Mr H reminded me of my own grandfather, who also had arthritis and who finally entered residential care when my grandmother could no longer cope. I made an error in thinking that what was right for my family would be right for Mr and Mrs H.
How did each of us feel as a result?	Mrs H felt distressed at the thought she could ever be parted from her husband and she was indignant that I had thought this might be a solution. She was angry with me for not recognising her love and commitment to her husband and I also think she felt who was I to sit at the bedside and make such a distasteful suggestion without getting to know them both first.
	I felt despair for saying something which was so unthinking and remorseful for the impact my statement had on Mrs H. Although I had not meant it as a suggestion, I could see that it had been taken as such and I was sorry about this. I also felt completely inadequate and afraid of the response of my supervisor when I told her.
What if I had chosen my words more carefully?	I should not have allowed my own experiences with my grandfather to influence my communication. I have learned in class that I am not here to make suggestions, but rather to find out from service-users what they think, feel and need. I forgot my theory base as soon as I started the conversation. If I had thought more carefully about models of communication, I would have taken more time to build a relationship with both Mr and Mrs H and to really listen to them – and demonstrate I was listening. Doing this would have helped me to enter their world and it would have been apparent that they did not want to be parted. I should have asked them what would help them the most to manage Mr H's condition.
So what? Would that have made a difference to the outcome?	I feel this would have made a real difference to the outcome. By remembering I am there to help patients remain at the centre of decision making wherever possible, and to find out their needs (Egan, 2018), I would have strengthened our relationship and worked alongside them rather than being seen as someone to tell them what to do.
Where can I go from here in my interactions with this person?	I need to go back and try to repair the relationship with Mr and Mrs H. I need to be congruent and empathic and say to them both that I am sad that I was unable to begin our relationship on a better footing and that I can see that although Mrs H is feeling exhausted, she wants to find a way of supporting her husband in their own home and that I can put them in touch with the hospital social worker to plan this. I hope that by being honest about my feelings about the first conversation and by demonstrating a greater level of empathy then we can begin again.

Hilsdon's model assists in breaking down what happened during an interaction into smaller parts which can be analysed with increasing depth. It enables the practitioner to consider how the actual words used in communication can impact on the other person and it invites a critically reflective response.

PAUSE FOR THOUGHT 7.2

Think of 'a time I learned something vital about my practice'.

Follow Hilsdon's model and increase the level of analysis and evaluation as you progress through the different questions. How has this model increased your awareness of yourself and your skills? How successful is it in assisting you to think of ways in which you could have changed your practice?

Check the end of the chapter for an answer to this activity.

MODEL 2

The second model which can assist the practitioner to be critically reflective is Summerscales' Cycle of Reflective Practice (2006, unpublished). Summerscales has built on some of the concepts from Kolb's Experiential Learning Cycle (1978, cited in Kolb, 2015) in developing the following model for reflective practice in social work and health and social care (Figure 7.5).

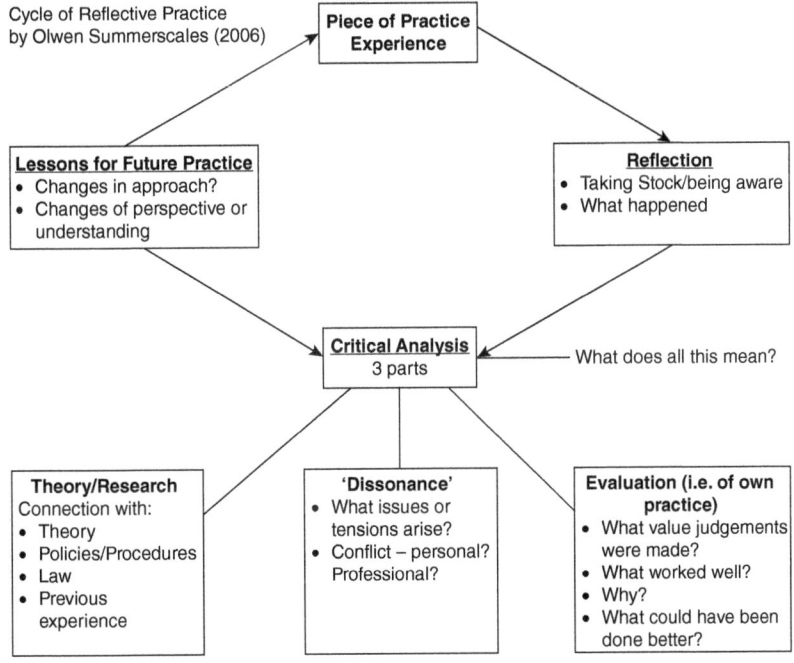

Figure 7.5   Summerscales' model for critical thinking

Source: Summerscales (2006). Reproduced with kind permission from Summerscales.

Summerscales' model, like Hilsdon's, can assist the practitioner to reflect in detail on the quality of their engagement with others. This model focuses on different elements and encourages theory, statute and policy to be incorporated into reflections too.

In the following example, Meena, a social worker in training, was set a task to visit a single mother in her house to discuss a referral made by a local school concerning her daughter's recent change in behaviour. She writes the piece of practice experience which suffices for the uppermost square of the model:

> I made sure I had my identification to hand when I knocked on the door at 1pm. A woman answered and I introduced myself and asked if I could come in. Once I was inside it became clear that the person who answered the door was not the person I had come to see – she was seated in the living room. The house was cold and X was sitting on the sofa in her pyjamas. She looked unkempt and sad. I then introduced myself to X and asked her if it was ok to talk to her in front of the other person. She said yes so I told her why I was visiting. X said there were no problems with her daughter and she didn't see why a visit from Children's Services was necessary. I replied that we had to act on the referral from the school. At this point X sat back in her chair and folded her arms and repeated that everything was fine and that she did not want any interference from social workers. I asked her some questions about her daughter but she gave me one-word answers and it was clear we were not getting anywhere. At one point, the other person (X's sister, who was visiting) urged X to 'tell her what your daughter thinks about your new boyfriend'; however, X remained silent.

This first part of the model is written in a purely descriptive manner. Reflection takes place in the next stage. If the student was to continue using Summerscales' model, her reflective piece may look like Table 7.2.

Summerscales' model enables us to first describe our practice and then to analyse and reflect on it. The second box of reflection, where we take stock, moves us on from being purely descriptive to starting to think about what went well and what did not go so well. The third box enables us to critically analyse these reflections and to really learn from them. By systematically bringing in the three elements of critical thinking here – evaluation, dissonance and theory – and breaking these down further into their specific sections (values, conflicts, theory and policy, etc.), the practitioner is invited to develop real insight into the strengths and areas for development in their practice. Statements in the final box, exploring lessons for future practice, then become precise and specific: the practitioner is clear about what they need to do differently (or the same) next time and, more importantly, this way of working helps them to focus on how they will do this.

One of the issues with using models to reflect on practice is that they can become prescriptive: 'do this first, then ask yourself this question, then that question … and then finish by …' A frequent problem with this approach is that the stated order might not necessarily fit the occasion being analysed. As with all models which are designed to help us to develop and strengthen our skills, we draw from them in ways which make sense and which enable us to learn about ourselves, the way we work now and the way we could work more effectively in the future.

PAUSE FOR THOUGHT 7.3

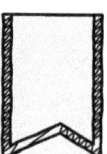

Think of an interaction you have had with another person (or people) recently which left you feeling that you could have used your skills in a different or more productive way. Follow Summerscales' model, teasing out more exactly what it was that went well and not so well. Explore each element of each box and finish with some specific goals and actions to work on next time.

Check the end of the chapter for an answer to this activity.

Table 7.2 Applying Summerscales' model

Reflection

Taking stock • **What happened?**	I organised myself beforehand and thought about how I would introduce myself at the door and thought about how I would introduce myself at the door quietly so that neighbours would not be aware of my presence. However, I failed to establish the identity of the person who answered the door and this could have led to a breach in confidentiality. I felt the visit did not go well and I did not establish a good working relationship with X. She seemed upset that the visit was taking place and I found it hard to engage her in any conversation about her daughter. I thought it unusual that she was still in her pyjamas at 1 p.m. Her sister gave me a cue but I was too focused on my questions to the mother to recognise this until after I had left.

What does all this mean?

Critical analysis:

• **Evaluation of own practice** • **Inclusion of theory/research/ policy/law/previous experience** Dissonance: * **What issues and tensions arise?** * **Conflict – personal/ professional**	I was not really aware at the time that I was making value judgements, but looking back, I was thinking, 'Why hasn't she got dressed today and why isn't the house any warmer – especially as she has a visitor?' I now wonder if it was a struggle for her to get herself out of bed and ready and this is making me wonder why she is feeling so down. What worked well was the way I lowered my voice at the door and managed to negotiate my way in. I was able to work with Children's Services' Policy and Procedures and show my identification badge discreetly and my confident and polite tone helped me to be invited in. There were many things I could have improved. First of all I should have checked the identity of the person who answered the door. Then, I forgot the principles of relationship building we have learnt about in class. Ruch et al. (2010) emphasise that a good professional relationship is central to good practice but I launched straight into the referral from the school without any attempt at building a relationship with X first. I could have recognised that she was reluctant to see me and tried to convey an understanding of what that might be about (Egan, 2018) by saying that I could see it was difficult for her to receive a visit from me and that it could feel an intrusion. This would have helped to develop the relationship. I could also have used empathic responding more (Rogers, 1961) by paraphrasing what X said rather than asking her question after question. I think that my constant questions closed her down (Egan, 2018) and she sat there, eyes downcast, just waiting for the next one. By focusing on the questions I wanted to ask, I missed the comment from X's sister. Had I been more engaged in what both of them were saying and demonstrated this by using some reflective responses (Howe, 2013) then I feel they would have felt more comfortable in talking to me and I would have been better able to tune in to their verbal and non-verbal disclosures. This would have helped me to develop a more detailed picture of what might be happening with X's daughter. My professional skills were in question in that I failed to check the identity of the person who answered the door. I noticed that X was still wearing her pyjamas, looked unkempt and that the house was cold but I failed to recognise any meaning behind these pointers. I could have checked out whether or not she was alright and this would have given her an opportunity to say if she was not. I was also aware that X, by giving one-word answers to my questions, was signalling that she was not willing to engage at all and I failed to recognise that asking more questions compounded the problem.

(Continued)

Table 7.2 (Continued)

	The less she said, the more I became directive by questioning, and as Egan (2018) suggests, responses such as these ignore the service user's key messages and feelings that have been expressed. This flawed interaction left both of us feeling more and more tense and resulted in me feeling inadequate with my skills and perhaps X feeling distrustful of me and my motives. It was not a good start and I wished I could have rewound the session and started again.
Lessons for future practice:	
• Changes in approach? • Changes of perspective/ understanding?	I need to learn from my mistakes and to build on the good practice I did use. I will make another appointment with X and listen more. Egan (2018, p. 102) offers a saying: 'The person who says too much says nothing.' I dominated the first conversation with my questions so it is important next time to put into my own words what X and her sister said. I could begin with a summary of the previous session. Egan (2018) states that by beginning with a summary, it puts the ball back in the service-user's court and invites more clarity. I could include in my summary awareness of my own thoughts and feelings when we met; for example, *'When I visited I felt worried about you: I noticed you weren't dressed, and you looked sad, almost defeated, as if everything required so much more energy than you had.'* I would wait and see what X's response was to this, allowing any silences to continue, knowing this would be enabling to X in her thinking (Hough, 1994). However X responds I would try and reflect back the meaning of her response to her to help her feel heard. I also need to choose the right moment to summarise and probe on what X's sister said, and Egan (2018) states this would need to be delivered in a non-judgemental manner and with empathy if it has a chance of being engaged with. For example, I could say: 'What has been going around in my head since we met is what your sister said about your daughter's response to your new boyfriend.' This statement might be enough for X to make a response, but if she doesn't, I will add a probing statement: '... and I am wondering what she might have meant when she said this.'

CONCLUSION

This chapter has explored some of the core attributes that health and social care workers need to develop in becoming engaged, skilful, resilient and reflective practitioners. First, we need to begin the journey of understanding who we are and how the traits which make up our unique personalities influence our thinking, feelings and behaviour. Being armed with this greater level of insight into ourselves helps us to reflect on how we might be perceived by service users, colleagues, managers and other professionals and to consequently develop more effective ways of engaging and working with others at a deeper level. The more skilled we become in each of these areas, the greater the chances we have of developing higher levels of resilience, which is an essential attribute in the pressurised atmosphere of health and social care that exists today. Some of the themes introduced in this chapter, such as using supervision, empathy, self-awareness, communication and engagement skills, resilience and critical practice, will be explored further in later chapters. At this stage in the book, however, it is important to recognise that everything discussed so far can be looked upon as work-in-progress on the road to becoming a skilled practitioner.

GO FURTHER ACTIVITY

'Learning by doing' is highly applicable to developing skills in reflective practice. In order to continue on your journey, the following activities are suggested:

- Keep a reflective journal where you document key interactions and note what you have learned about your use of theory, your skills and yourself.
- Practise using one or more of the models discussed in this chapter for your reflections.
- Find someone you trust who will help you to reflect on your learning and provide you with feedback and encouragement.
- Engage in some further reading as detailed below.

ANSWERS TO CHAPTER 7 ACTIVITIES

——— Activity 7.1: Suggested Answer

After rating yourself, you are likely to have different scores for each of the different elements and your ratings are there to help you to think about where you might possess most and least resilience. Let us imagine you have given a score of 2 to the characteristic of

(Continued)

'social confidence'. You might well feel shy when you are meeting people for the first time but if you engage well with people you already know, then you will have some resilience already with this characteristic. To develop your resilience further (especially in new situations), it would be useful to devise an action plan to assist you. Your action plan will be individual to you, however an example might be:

1   On my next bus journey, I will smile at the bus driver and the person sitting next to me (and note their engagement with me afterwards).
2   I will make myself have a conversation with someone who I wouldn't usually engage with, such as a supermarket checkout operator by asking them how they are doing, and then paraphrase back to them so they know I am really listening.
3   I will reflect on the effect of my interactions by observing the other person's verbal and non-verbal responses. I will also note how I feel when my interactions have prompted a good response from others (to deepen my social confidence).

———— Pause for Thought 7.1: Suggested Answers

The worked example within the chapter should help you to begin to analyse your own unconscious processes. Be aware that these can take many forms and will be individual to each of us. Anything from the five senses (sight, sound, smell, taste and touch) can trigger a transference. For example, if a service user uses the same perfume as my favourite, aged and quite frail aunt, the perfume might unconsciously remind me of her. I might automatically then become protective towards, and do things for the service user in the same way as I do for my aunt (transference). If I am then doing things for the service user that he or she is capable of doing for themselves, then their counter-transference response (to my transference) might be to become dependent on me.

Another example is where the service user might have a similar physical characteristic to someone who is important in your own life, such as height, a certain mannerism such as the raising of one eyebrow, a way of talking, a particular accent, or a particular look. The list is endless and if you find you are feeling uncomfortable in an interaction, it is worthwhile to ask yourself: who does this person remind me of and why am I reacting to them in this way? Supervision is an excellent forum for exploring these issues.

———— Activity 7.2: Suggested Answer

Your Window will be unique to you. Try and be as specific as you can with your statements, especially those in your Blind Area that you want to find out more about. For example, you might write initially that you want to know how you are experienced by others. A more specific statement would be to wish to know what your facial expressions are like when someone tells you something you do not agree with; or what mannerisms you use with your hands and arms when you are talking. Really think about what you would like to check out with others: the better you know yourself, the deeper will be your engagement skills with others. Once you have a better understanding from discussing your Blind Area, you can bring your reflections into your Open Area. For example, in your Open Area now might be the statement 'I know that if someone says something to me that I do not agree with, I tend to fold my arms and remove eye contact and this is something I need to work on.'

—— Pause for Thought 7.2: Suggested Answer

The worked example within the chapter should give you some ideas for how you can use the model to reflect on your own skills. First, describe an incident or particular interaction which had an impact on you. Then start to look at your role in the interaction. What did you say and what impact did this have on the other person? What made you interact in this way? Perhaps there was some transference going on here and you could reflect on this. Or maybe, you were thinking about something else and missed something crucial that the service use told you. There are many factors which would have affected your response and the more accurate you can be in your reflection here, the better practitioner you will be next time. How did this leave you both feeling and what was the impact of this on both of you? When focusing on your own emotions, can you accurately name them? For example, if you realised the service user was angry about something you said, did you feel embarrassed/de-skilled/scared/dejected/unaffected or something else?

The analytical aspect here is to really think about what you could have done differently. For example, if you realised the service user was angry with you, what steps could you have taken here? Reflection could include 'I could have apologised for being insensitive and acknowledged that my words were inappropriate (using congruence). I could then have tried to paraphrase the message they were trying to convey and which I had missed: 'I can see the last thing you want is to be parted and we need to find a way of supporting you in your own home.' This would have acknowledged I was in the wrong and conveyed that I wanted to put this right.'

Asking yourself how the model has helped you to increase awareness of yourself and your skills is a good way of adding contents to the Open Area of your Johari's Window. Again, the more you know your strengths and weaknesses and the way you move forward when you have made mistakes all develop your resilience and assist you in becoming a better practitioner in the future.

—— Pause for Thought 7.3: Suggested Answer

Again, the worked example within the chapter should help you to formulate your own reflections using the model. For your critical analysis, answer each of the questions from the three boxes (evaluation of your own practice; theory/research which underpinned your interaction; and dissonance: the conflicts, issues and tensions for you. Finally, write a specific action plan for your future practice.

Think of an interaction you have had with another person recently which left you feeling that you could have used your skills in a different or more productive way. Follow Summerscales' model, teasing out more exactly what it was that went well and not so well. Explore each element of each box and finish with some specific goals and actions

(Continued)

to work on next time. For example, you might want to develop your listening skills. You could make this much more specific by thinking exactly what it is you want to work on and develop a goal such as the following. 'I wish to be able to read between the lines: to identify what the service user is implying but not necessarily saying directly and to say this back to the service user in a reflective statement. I will ask a friend if I can practise this with them first and I intend to incorporate it into my professional practice within one month.' Writing a goal in this specific way means you will be more likely to achieve it because you will know exactly what you need to do and will recognise when you have achieved it.

FURTHER READING

Bolton, G. (2018). *Reflective Practice: Writing and Professional Development* (5th edn). London: Sage.

Howatson-Jones, L. (2016). *Reflective Practice in Nursing* (3rd edn). London: Sage.

Howe, D. (2008). *The Emotionally Intelligent Social Worker*. Basingstoke: Palgrave Macmillan.

Luft, J. (1961). The Johari Window: a graphic model of awareness in interpersonal relations. *Human Relations Training News* 5(1), 6–7.

Rutter, L. and Brown, K. (2015). *Critical Thinking and Professional Judgement for Social Work* (4th edn). London: Sage.

REFERENCES

Bassot, B. (2016). *The Reflective Journal* (2nd edn). Basingstoke: Palgrave.

Casement, P. (1985). *On Learning from the Patient*. London: Routledge.

Considine, T., Hollingdale, P. and Neville, R. (2015) Social work, pastoral care and resilience. *Pastoral Care in Education* 33(4), 214–219.

Egan, G. (2018). *The Skilled Helper, a Client Centred Approach* (2nd edn). Andover: Cengage Learning EMEA.

Feltham, C. (2010). *Critical Thinking in Counselling and Psychotherapy*. London: Sage.

Freud, S. (1916) Lecture 7: the manifest content of dreams and the latent dream-thoughts. In J. Strachey and A. Richards (eds) (1962), *Freud: 1. Introductory Lectures on Psychoanalysis*. Reading: Pelican.

Grant, L. (2012). Enhancing wellbeing in social work students: building resilience in the next generation. *Social Work Education* 31, 605–621.

Grant, L. and Kinman, G. (2014). *Developing Resilience for Social Work Practice*. London: Palgrave.

Hilsdon, J. (2012). *Critical Thinking: What is the Question?* Advance HE Knowledge Hub Online. Available at: www.heacademy.ac.uk/knowledge-hub/critical-thinking-what-question (accessed 7 January 2019)

Hough, M. (1994). *A Practical Approach to Counselling*. London: Pitman.

House of Commons Health Committee (2017) *The Nursing Workforce: Second Report of Session 2017–19*. House of Commons. Available at: https://publications.parliament.uk/pa/cm201719/cmselect/cmhealth/353/353.pdf (accessed 19 November 2018)

Howe, D. (2013). *Empathy: What It Is and Why It Matters*. Basingstoke: Palgrave Macmillan.

Howe, D. (2008). *The Emotionally Intelligent Social Worker*. Basingstoke: Palgrave Macmillan.

Jacobs, M. (2010) *Psychodynamic Counselling in Action* (4th edn). London: Sage.

Kolb, D. A. (2015). *Experiential Learning: Experience as the Source of Learning and Development* (2nd edn). Upper Saddle River, NJ: Pearson Education.

Luft, J. (1961). The Johari Window: a graphic model of awareness in interpersonal relations. *Human Relations Training News* 5(1), 6–7.

Munro, E. (2011). *The Munro Review of Child Protection: Final Report: A Child-Centred System*. London: The Stationery Office. Available at: https://assets.publishing.service.gov.uk/government/uploads/system/uploads/attachment_data/file/175391/Munro-Review.pdf (accessed 7 November 2018)

Murdin, L. (2010). *Understanding Transference*. Basingstoke: Palgrave Macmillan.

NHS Improvement (2018). *Performance of the NHS Provider Sector for the Quarter Ended 31 December 2018*. London: NHS. Available at: https://improvement.nhs.uk/documents/4942/Performance_of_the_NHS_provider_sector_for_the_quarter_ended_31_Dec_2018.pdf (accessed 16 July 2019)

Nursing and Midwifery Council (2017). Increasing number of nurses and midwives leaving profession 'highlights major challenges faced by health and care sectors'. News and updates. www.nmc.org.uk/news/news-and-updates/increasing-number-nurses-midwives-leaving-profession-major-challenges (accessed 19 November 2018)

Revalier, J. M. (2017). *UK Social Workers: Working Conditions and Wellbeing*. Independent publication of Bath Spa University. Available at: www.basw.co.uk/system/files/resources/basw_42443-3_1.pdf (accessed 19 November 2018)

Rogers, C. (1961). *On Becoming a Person: A Therapist's View of Psychotherapy*. London: Constable.

Ruch, G., Turney, D. and Ward, A. (2010). *Relationship-based Social Work*. London: Jessica Kingsley.

Rutter, L. and Brown, K. (2015). *Critical Thinking and Professional Judgement for Social Work* (4th edn). London: Sage.

Skills for Care (2013). *Code of Conduct for Healthcare Support Workers and Adult Social Care Workers in England*. Leeds and Bristol: Skills for Care and Skills for Health. Available at: www.skillsforhealth.org.uk/images/services/code-of-conduct/Code%20of%20Conduct%20Healthcare%20Support.pdf (accessed 31 May 2019)

Summerscales, O. (2006). *Reflective Writing as a Tool for Professional Development*. MA thesis, University of Birmingham.

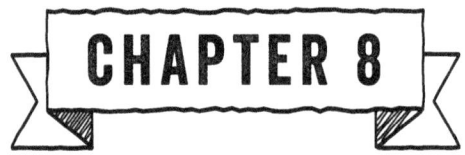

CHAPTER 8

PHYSIOLOGICAL EFFECTS OF AGEING IN THE OLDER ADULT

John Knight

OVERVIEW

This chapter will explore the current knowledge of how ageing affects the anatomy and physiology of the human body and examine how ageing can predispose older people to a variety of age-related diseases. Wherever possible scientific and medical terminology will be kept to a minimum and the implications of ageing to health and social care will be explored.

LEARNING OUTCOMES

By the end of this chapter you will be able to:

- Explain how an ageing population is likely to place increasing demands on health and social care resources
- Describe how ageing is associated with anatomical and physiological changes that can negatively impact on health
- Explain how ageing is associated with a variety of common age-related diseases
- Describe how lifestyle can influence ageing and how leading a healthy lifestyle can reduce many of the physical and psychological problems associated with ageing

INTRODUCTION

Throughout the chapter, a variety of short, multiple-choice questions will allow the reader to assess their knowledge of the subject material.

The United Nations estimates that between now and 2050 the population of older people (classified as 60 or older) throughout the world will more than double to around 2.1 billion individuals (United Nations, 2015). Since ageing is associated with reduced mobility and an increased risk of a wide variety of diseases this will place a massive financial and logistical strain on global health and social care services necessitating much forward planning of resources. Better nutrition and advances in health care have significantly increased lifespan in the UK with many individuals enjoying healthy active lifestyles into their eighties and beyond. The ageing process is multifaceted and influenced by a wide variety of genetic and environmental factors; for this reason two people of the same age may differ significantly in both their outward appearance and physical health status. Multiple genes have been demonstrated to influence the rate of ageing and susceptibility to a variety of age-related diseases, with new genes linked to ageing being continually discovered. Humans currently have no control over the genes they inherit from their parents although with rapid advances in genetics this may soon change. Ageing is also influenced by exposure to environmental factors including food and airborne pollutants/toxins, bacteria and viruses. Exposure to some environmental factors that are known to accelerate ageing can be avoided such as choosing not to smoke tobacco products and avoiding or limiting the exposure to direct ultraviolet radiation (sunlight). Differences in hormones and internal physiology typically results in gender differences and in many developed countries women typically outlive men on average by around seven to ten years. Adopting a healthy lifestyle with regular aerobic exercise and a healthy diet appears to reduce the physical effects of ageing with some studies showing that regular physical activity and a nutrient dense diet may actually slow the ageing process itself. Despite a progressively ageing world population our current understanding of the ageing process remains incomplete and limited.

AGEING OF THE CARDIOVASCULAR AND RESPIRATORY SYSTEMS

The cardiovascular system consists of the heart (cardio) and blood vessels (vascular) and is responsible for circulating around 4.5 litres (8 pints) of blood around the average body. It is often referred to as the major transport system since blood facilitates the movement of oxygen and nutrients (e.g. glucose and amino acids) to all regions of the body whilst simultaneously carrying metabolic waste products such as carbon dioxide to the lungs and urea and uric acid to the kidneys for elimination. Blood also acts as the medium for circulating hormones such as insulin around the body; these chemical signals play a crucial role in homeostasis which is defined as the ability to maintain a stable internal environment. Since blood is a warm fluid, as it circulates it distributes and helps to dissipate heat thereby ensuring that our core body temperature is maintained at around 37 degrees Centigrade (Martini et al., 2018).

Unfortunately, with increasing age the cardiovascular system becomes less effective and circulation of blood less efficient. Since all parts of the human body have a requirement for oxygen and nutrients the ageing of the cardiovascular system has a negative impact on virtually all major organs and tissues contributing to ageing throughout the body.

BLOOD VESSEL CHANGES

There are three major types of blood vessel:

- *Arteries*: These are thick-walled muscular blood vessels with most carrying oxygen rich blood under high pressure away from the heart.
- *Capillaries*: These are the smallest blood vessels which permeate most regions of the body and act to distribute oxygenated blood from the arteries to the organs and tissues.
- *Veins*: These are thin-walled blood vessels which carry deoxygenated blood under low pressure from the tissues towards the heart.

All blood vessels show age-associated changes but these variations are particularly apparent in the arteries. Humans are born with arteries that are flexible and elastic with clean interiors free from deposits. Young arteries are compliant and when blood is ejected from the heart their elastic walls stretch allowing a smooth efficient flow of blood. With advancing age, the arteries begin to stiffen as a result of *collagen* fibres being progressively deposited in their walls (Harvey et al., 2016) and many older people will also show deposition of fatty deposits which can reduce the diameter of the blood vessel. This process of arterial stiffening is frequently referred to as 'hardening of the arteries' and is a common feature of old age. Note the reduced internal diameter (lumen) of the blood vessel in Figure 8.1.

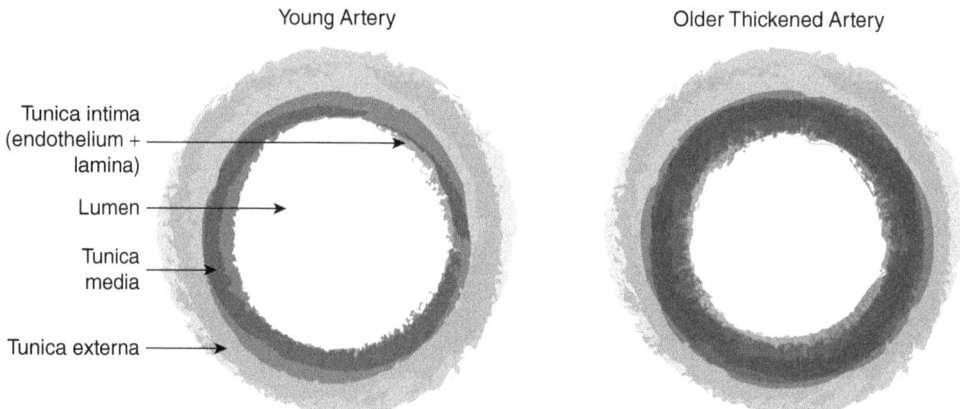

Young Artery   Older Thickened Artery

Tunica intima
(endothelium +
lamina)

Lumen

Tunica
media

Tunica externa

Figure 8.1   Arterial thickening

ACTIVITY 8.1   THE NATURE OF COLLAGEN

We have just examined how increases in collagen deposition contribute to stiffening of blood vessels in advancing age. Changes in collagen composition throughout the body are a key feature of the ageing process and the exercise below is designed to familiarise you further with this major structural component of the body.
Using online resources or textbooks answer the following questions:

1   What type of material is collagen?
2   In what form is collagen produced?
3   Which cells produce collagen?
4   Where is collagen found and what is its purpose?

Check the end of the chapter for an answer to this activity.

FATTY DEPOSITS (ATHEROSCLEROSIS)

The build-up of fatty deposits (fatty plaque) inside of arteries is termed atherosclerosis and is the most common form of blood vessel disease worldwide. Older people with a history of smoking, hypertension or diabetes are particularly likely to suffer atherosclerotic occlusion since the toxins found in tobacco smoke, high blood pressure and high levels of sugar in the blood are all known to damage the delicate lining of blood vessels. This trauma triggers a build-up of fat and reduces the internal diameter (lumen) of the vessel. Atherosclerotic occlusion of the coronary arteries which supply blood to the heart muscle (myocardium) is termed coronary artery disease (CAD) and this often causes worrying central chest pain (angina). Unfortunately, these fatty deposits increase the risk of blood clots which can completely block a coronary artery resulting in a heart attack (myocardial infarction). During a heart attack the blockage caused by a clot results in portions of the muscular wall of the heart dying. Unsurprisingly, heart attacks are a major cause of mortality and become more common with increasing age.

AGEING OF THE HEART

Since ageing is associated with a stiffening of the arteries the heart has to work harder and pump with greater force to push blood through hardened and potentially narrowed blood vessels. The heart is a muscle and like any other muscle in the body if it has to work harder it grows bigger (think of weightlifters). The ventricles of the heart typically increase in thickness by around 30 per cent between the ages of 20 and 80 with thickening associated with enlargement and redistribution of muscle fibres which changes the shape and physical appearance of the heart (Knight and Nigam, 2017a).

PALPITATIONS AND HEART ARRHYTHMIAS

The heart has an in-built natural pacemaker termed the sinoatrial node (SAN) which sets the basic beat rhythm of the heart. With age the pacemaker cells that make up the SAN begin to die and the SAN becomes fibrosed by the deposition of collagen fibres; these changes increase the risk of palpitations and other rhythm disturbances (Csepe et al., 2015). Palpitations are often perceived as a 'skipped beat' or irregular/racing heart rate and whilst most are harmless they can cause immense anxiety, particularly when experienced for the first time or for prolonged periods. Sometimes more serious arrhythmias may be triggered in older people, the most common of which is termed atrial fibrillation (AF). AF occurs when the upper chambers of the heart contract very rapidly and in an unco-ordinated manner which can lead to dizziness, breathlessness and more seriously can trigger blood clots (thrombi) which may travel upwards from the heart to the brain causing a cerebrovacular accident (stroke). For this reason patients with persistent AF are normally prescribed anticoagulation therapies, such as warfarin, to reduce the chances of clots forming.

AGEING AND BLOOD PRESSURE

As a result of the structural changes to the heart and the stiffening of the blood vessels, ageing is usually associated with an increase in blood pressure. Blood pressure is recorded using a cuff which is usually placed on the upper arm before being inflated. Blood pressure is measured in mm of mercury (mmHg) with a typical healthy reading being around 120/80 mmHg. The upper reading is referred to as the systolic reading and the lower figure the diastolic reading;

- *Systolic blood pressure*: This corresponds to contraction of the heart (systole) and records the blood pressure when blood is being ejected from the heart into the arteries.
- *Diastolic blood pressure*: This corresponds to relaxation of the heart (diastole) and records the blood pressure when no blood is being ejected.

In most individuals their systolic blood pressure usually increases with age. In men an average systolic reading of 126mmHg is typical at age 25 years but this often rises to around 140mmHg at age 60. Today cheap automatic digital blood pressure recorders are available to allow patients to monitor their blood pressure at home and more expensive, calibrated versions of these have gradually replaced the potentially dangerous mercury-containing devices used in hospitals and GP surgeries. Consistently raised blood pressure can impose increased wear and tear to the internal structure of the heart potentially damaging the heart valves; the thin flaps of tissue that ensure that blood flows in the correct direction. It is also associated with damage to the eyes which may result in blindness, progressive kidney damage and increased risk of brain haemorrhages (strokes with bleeding). Many older patients are on long-term medications to help control their blood pressure and bring it within normal limits.

POSTURAL HYPOTENSION

Although blood pressure generally rises with age, older people are also at increased risk of their blood pressure suddenly dropping when they stand up which can result in fainting, falls and injury. This phenomenon is termed postural hypotension and is reported to affect around 30 per cent of people over 65 years of age (Low, 2008).

In healthy young people the drop in blood pressure that occurs when standing is detected by blood pressure sensors (baroreceptors) in the walls of the arteries and the body responds by increasing the heart rate and constricting the blood vessels (Martini et al., 2018). This helps maintain the blood pressure ensuring adequate blood flow upwards to the brain. Age-associated hardening of arteries may interfere with the ability of baroreceptors to record a drop in blood pressure on standing increasing the risk of postural hypotension. It is always good advice to remind older people to rise to a standing position from their beds and chairs slowly to allow the body to adapt to gravity-induced fluid shifts and reduce the chances of postural hypotension and fainting.

AGEING OF THE RESPIRATORY SYSTEM

The ability of the cardiovascular system to deliver oxygen to the tissues is further compromised by age-related changes that occur to the respiratory system. In youth, the ribcage is relatively supple and elastic since the front portion (costal region) is composed largely of flexible cartilage. With age there is a gradual increase in calcification of these cartilaginous regions which over many years gradually turn to bone resulting in a progressive increase in the rigidity of the chest wall (Forman and Kent, 2014). Older people may also show a gradual narrowing of the cartilaginous disks between the vertebrae of the spine, which is one of the reasons people appear to shrink and lose height as they age. These changes to the thoracic spine may also result in an abnormal spinal curvature, termed kyphosis, which is very common in old age and reduces the volume of the thorax (Roghani et al., 2017). The major breathing muscles are the diaphragm and intercostals (muscles between the ribs) and these gradually lose strength with age and this, together with the stiffening of the chest wall and the reduced volume of the thorax, can make breathing progressively difficult.

AIRWAY CHANGES AND INCREASED RISK OF RESPIRATORY TRACT INFECTION

With every breath inhaled dust, pollutants and infectious agents, such as bacteria and viruses, are introduced into the respiratory tract. Elaborate mechanisms are present which help clear foreign particulate material. The upper respiratory tract is lined by cells with tiny, fragile mobile hair-like structures termed cilia. When air is inhaled particles stick to mucus which is then lifted upwards towards the back of the throat and swallowed before being sterilised in the hydrochloric acid of the stomach. Since this mechanism can be visualised as being similar to a mechanical staircase it is referred to as the 'mucociliary escalator'. Unfortunately, with age this mechanism slows and becomes less effective potentially increasing the risk of inhalation of particles and lead to infection (Bailey et al., 2014). Smoking progressively damages the mucociliary escalator, paralysing and destroying the delicate cilia thereby compounding the effects of ageing. However, it is known that once a person (of any age) gives up smoking some ciliary function is gradually restored and the mucociliary escalator can again begin to clear particulates from the airway (American Cancer Society, 2018). It is always advisable for health care workers to encourage people of all ages to quit their cigarette habit to improve their respiratory health.

ACTIVITY 8.2

1   Smoking is not only damaging to lung tissue but is known to accelerate the ageing
     process in different regions of the body. Using online resources research the effects of
     smoking on the cardiovascular system and the skin.
2   Recently the introduction of e-cigarettes has led to an explosion in 'vaping'. Again
     using online resources research the perceived benefits of vaping over traditional
     cigarette smoking. Are there any documented health issues associated with vaping?

Check the end of the chapter for an answer to this activity.

REDUCED COUGHING REFLEX

Inhaled particulate debris usually triggers an explosive coughing reflex to dislodge and expel any irritants. In older people the sensory receptors that monitor the airways tend to become less sensitive and so a coughing reflex may not be initiated. Even when coughing is triggered reduced respiratory muscle strength and increased rigidity of the chest wall can reduce the clearance of inhaled pathogens and particulate materials. Reduced coughing reflexes increase the chances of pathogens and irritants reaching the deep lung tissues raising the risk of respiratory tract infections which are unfortunately the most common cause of death from infection in older patients (WHO, 2016).

EMPHYSEMA AND COPD

Poor clearance of particulate material in older people can lead to irritants and mucus collecting in the delicate alveoli (air sacs) of the lung which may begin to collapse and break down resulting in emphysema. This is particularly common in older people that have been long-term smokers; here the irritation associated with inhaling the toxins and particulates in cigarette smoke results in chronic inflammation within the airway and large-scale alveolar damage and collapse. These effects are collectively referred to as chronic obstructive pulmonary disease (COPD) which is one of the most common respiratory diseases in the older population. Since the alveoli of the lungs are where gas exchange takes place COPD is associated with low oxygen levels and difficulty in breathing. In the UK around 1.2 million people are thought to suffer COPD (NHS, 2018) and in its later stages patients often become dependent on oxygen cylinders which can limit their mobility and social interactions.

Ageing of cardiovascular and respiratory systems reduces the ability to undertake exercise. In standard walk tests (which measure the distance that can be walked in six minutes) individuals aged 80 typically walk around 200 metres less than individuals aged 40 (Janssens, 2005).

ACTIVITY 8.3   MULTIPLE CHOICE QUESTIONS

1   Which of the following is true about ageing of the heart:

   a   The heart normally beats slower with age.
   b   The heart normally decreases in size with age.
   c   Palpitations become more common with age.
   d   Heart problems become less common with age.

2   A build-up of fatty deposits in the internal lining of a blood vessel is referred to as:

   a   Multiple sclerosis
   b   Atherosclerosis
   c   Exocytosis
   d   Myelinisation

3   Feeling faint when standing up quickly occurs usually as a result of:

   a   Postural hypotension
   b   Postural hypertension
   c   Hypertension
   d   Tachycardia

4   What usually happens to the chest wall during normal ageing?

   a   It gradually stiffens and becomes less flexible as cartilage is replaced with bone.
   b   It gradually becomes more flexible as bone dissolves away.
   c   Nothing, the chest wall is one of the few areas of the body unaffected by ageing.
   d   There is a reduction in the total number of ribs as ribs gradually fuse together in old age.

5   The mucociliary escalator:

    a   Is composed of cartilage.
    b   Has cells with mobile hair-like projections termed cilia.
    c   Is found lining the heart.
    d   Is found lining blood vessels such as arteries.

Check the end of the chapter for the answers to this activity.

AGEING OF THE MUSCULOSKELETAL SYSTEM

Ageing is associated with a loss of muscle and bone mass and strength that significantly increases frailty and contributes to reduced mobility in older people. Both loss of muscle mass and bone mass will be explored further.

LOSS OF MUSCLE MASS

Loss of lean muscle mass is common in old age and is clinically referred to as sarcopaenia. Peak muscle size and power is reached in young adults in their twenties and thirties before gradually declining. From the mid-forties onwards skeletal muscles that allow conscious physical movement atrophy (shrink) and lose strength (Larsson et al., 2019). Reduced muscle mass contributes to frailty with associated weakness, fatigue and an increased susceptibility to adverse events such as falls (Fragala et al., 2015). Age-related sarcopaenia can also impact on everyday living in older people with reduced strength making routine tasks such as preparing meals or keeping the home clean more difficult and exhausting. The movable joints of the body are supported and reinforced by the surrounding muscles, hence muscle wastage can contribute to the changes in posture that are characteristic of old age and increase the risk of age-related joint diseases such as osteoarthritis. Loss of muscle mass is caused by a variety of factors including reduced levels of anabolic (muscle-building) hormones such as growth hormone and testosterone-like hormones which decrease in middle and old age. Typically, a loss of 3–8 per cent of lean muscle mass is seen per decade after the age of 30 and, since muscle burns many calories, unless diet is adjusted excess calories may be stored as fat (Knight and Nigam, 2017b).

LOSS OF BONE MASS AND OSTEOPOROSIS

Into middle age, bone density decreases in both men and women with losses accelerating into old age. Typically, a person aged 80 will have around 50 per cent less bone mass compared to their peak in young adulthood (Colón et al., 2018; Lau and Adachi, 2011). Bone is a dynamic tissue and is continuously being built and broken down. The bone-forming cells of the skeleton are termed osteoblasts and these cells are increasingly active when the skeleton is stressed by the weight of the upright active body. Older frailer individuals tend to spend less time engaged in physical activity and as a result their skeleton is placed under less stress reducing osteoblast activity and decreasing bone density (Nigam et al., 2009).

Loss of bone mass primarily reflects a loss of the mineral calcium phosphate from bones which display a porous and spongy appearance that is classically indicative of osteoporosis. Two forms of osteoporosis are recognised. Type 1 is seen in menopausal and postmenopausal women, and occurs as a result of a decline in the levels of female sex hormones. Oestrogen in particular plays a key role in maintaining bone density in females by stimulating calcium deposition, some postmenopausal women that suffer osteoporosis are prescribed hormone replacement therapy (HRT) to supplement the depleted oestrogen and improve bone health. However, many forms of HRT are known to increase the risk of certain malignancies including breast and uterine cancer, and so HRT may not be suitable for individuals with a family history or other risk factors for these forms of cancer. Type 2 osteoporosis is usually referred to as senile osteoporosis and affects both men and women. This form of the disease appears to be caused by reductions in the number and activity of the bone-forming cells (osteoblasts) although the exact causes of type 2 osteoporosis is currently poorly understood. The vertebrae of the spine are particularly vulnerable to osteoporosis and may develop tiny fractures which weaken the individual bones. Over many years these weakened vertebrae can begin to collapse under the weight of the body. This together with the compression of the soft cartilaginous interverte-bral discs (described above) frequently result in spinal deformities in old age such as kyphosis (Roghani et al., 2017). Osteoporosis also increases the risk of fracture of bones throughout the body with studies of older populations in Europe, USA, Japan and Australia in 2010 revealing that around 6.7 per cent of older adults could expect a fracture related to osteoporosis in any given year (Wade et al., 2012).

JOINT CHANGES

Osteoarthritis is recognised as both an age-related and 'wear and tear' disorder and is the most common joint pathology (arthropathy) in the world. In older people the cartilages in weight-bearing joints such as the knees, hips and lower spine can gradually deteriorate over the years resulting in painful bone-to-bone contact. In the UK it is estimated that osteoarthritis is responsible for joint pain in around 8.5 million people (NICE, 2015). With increasing age the composition of the ligaments that surround and support the joints can also change and lose elasticity leading to increased joint stiffness. Stiffness and pain in the joints can impact on the quality of life of older people and may be particularly apparent on waking in the morning or following long periods of resting (Richardson et al., 2014). Joint stiffness is often regarded as a normal consequence of ageing with many older people complaining of how 'it takes me a while to get moving in the mornings'.

AGEING OF THE SKIN

Since the skin covers the outside of body the effects of ageing are most visually noticeable here. It is common knowledge that the skin loses elasticity, develops wrinkles and becomes thinner with age. The skin is actually the largest organ in the human body covering around 1.6 square metres and weighing around 4–5 kilograms (Marieb and Hoehn, 2015). This organ has multiple functions including acting as a physical barrier to infection, regulating body temperature and preventing water loss.

There are two major layers to the skin:

- *Epidermis*: This is the outer layer consisting of cells rich in the tough protein keratin. Keratin is such a dense protein that once produced, cells become progressively impermeable to oxygen and gradually die off. This means that the outer layer of the skin is composed entirely of dead tissue with the cells at the surface continually flaking off taking with them any surface pathogens such as bacteria. The epidermis forms the major mechanical barrier to infection in humans.
- Dermis: This is the lower and thicker layer of skin that contains many of the structural components of the skin such as blood vessels, hair follicles, sweat glands and sensory receptors for touch temperature and pain. The dermis also contains sebaceous glands which produce an oily secretion (sebum) that softens hair and skin and has antibacterial properties.

The ageing of both the cardiovascular and respiratory systems (described earlier) results in less oxygenated blood arriving at the skin. It has been estimated that blood flow to the skin decreases by around 40 per cent between the ages of 20 and 70 and contributing to skin ageing and reduced tissue healing (Bentov and Reed, 2015). Fibroblasts are one of the most active cell types within the dermal layer of the skin. These cells get their name because they produce a variety of different fibres including collagen and elastin which provide a supporting framework to the lower skin layer. With reductions in oxygen supply, fibroblasts become less active and production of collagen progressively declines. With less supporting collagen the skin becomes looser and gradually the fine wrinkles that are indicative of old age begin to appear (Cipriani et al., 2016).

Multiple environmental factors are known to cause extrinsic ageing of the skin including environmental pollutants, poor diet, smoking, skin trauma and extended exposure to the ultraviolet (UV) light of the sun (photo-ageing). These factors are known to directly damage the DNA in skin cells increasing the risk of skin cancers and triggering the production of damaging free radical molecules which promote skin ageing. It is generally accepted that fairer skin ages faster than darker skin types and it has been estimated that over 80 per cent of ageing of the facial skin is due to the cumulative effects of UV exposure (Flament et al., 2013). Unlike the fine wrinkles that occur through normal ageing, extrinsic damage is characterised by much deeper wrinkling, the appearance of spider veins and a rougher skin texture with an irregular pigmentation which often results in a mottled appearance.

Thinning of the skin becomes very noticeable in older people with the skin often taking on a translucent appearance reminiscent of tracing paper with underlying veins appearing, larger darker and more prominent. It is estimated that the dermal layer of the skin decreases in thickness by around 20 per cent in old age (Nigam and Knight, 2017).

Gradual thinning of the skin increases the risk of mechanical damage with older people more susceptible to cuts, grazes and skin abrasions. Frailty and reduced mobility in old age is frequently associated with increased time spent sitting down and lying in bed; this increased immobility in conjunction with a thinner skin significantly increases the risk of pressure ulcers in older people (Jaul et al., 2018). Loss of skin integrity often necessitates regular visits from nurses and health care support workers to apply and reapply dressings to open wounds. Since the immune system is less effective in older people and wound healing is slower any open skin wounds are more likely to become infected and it is not uncommon for infected skin lesions to quickly progress into life-threatening sepsis. For these reasons fastidious skin care is essential in later years and patients with mobility problems may also benefit greatly from specialised air mattresses which can help prevent and treat pressure ulcers.

Under the dermal layer of the skin is a layer of fatty tissue termed the hypodermis. This subcutaneous layer plays an important role in insulating the body to prevent heat loss and also acts as a cushion helping to protect the skin and underlying structures from mechanical damage following trauma. Unfortunately, with age the thickness of the hypodermis decreases and as a result older people are more at risk of heat loss and hypothermia. For this reason it is essential to ensure that the accommodation in which older people reside is adequately heated throughout the year.

Growth of finger and toenails slows with age and since nails remain on the nail bed for longer they often become much thicker and may begin to curl (Tobin, 2016). Ram's horn nails occur when the toenails begin to grow around the toe; unfortunately these have the potential to begin to cut into the skin and flesh beneath. Many older people find thickened nails, particularly toenails, impossible to cut and so regular visits to/from a chiropodist may be necessary to prevent overgrowth and reduce the risk of infection from ram's horn or other forms of in-growing toenails.

AGEING OF THE NERVOUS AND SENSORY SYSTEMS

In most areas of the body, ageing cells and tissues are replaced as a result of continual cell division. However most of the neurons (nerve cells) that make up the nervous system lack the capacity to divide and once lost cannot be replaced. Brain tissue atrophies (shrinks) as we age (Figure 8.2) with around 0.5 per cent brain volume lost every year of life (Fotenos et al., 2005). In an average 90-year-old the mass of the brain will have typically declined by around 11 per cent compared with early adulthood (Wyss-Coray, 2016). With increasing age, neural tissue typically accumulates a variety of toxic materials including the metals aluminium and iron, and may gradually change to a darker colour due to the accumulation of pigments which stain the brain tissue (Youssef et al., 2016).

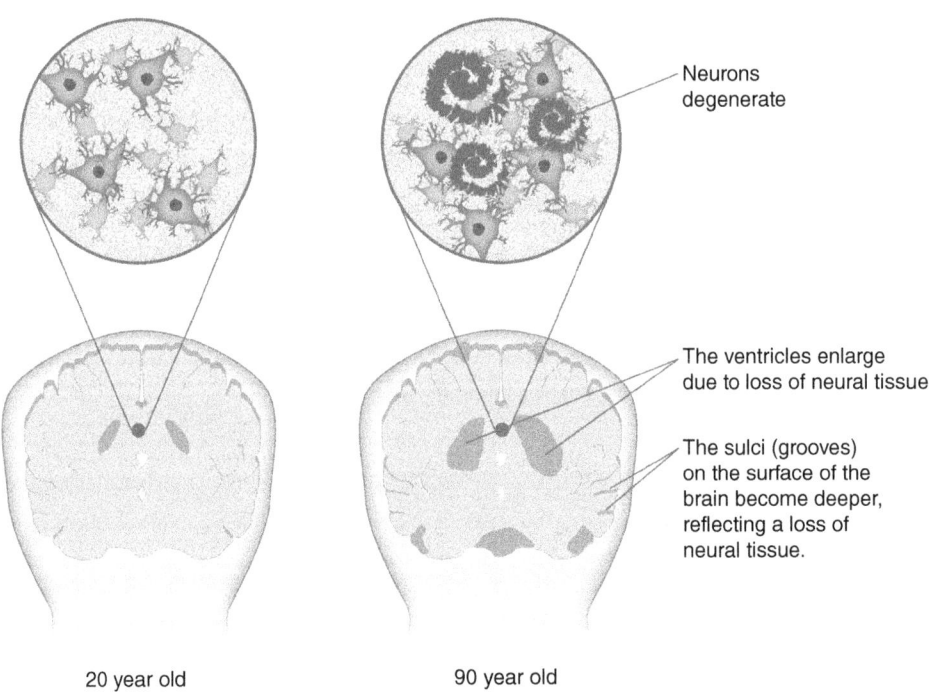

Neurons degenerate

The ventricles enlarge due to loss of neural tissue

The sulci (grooves) on the surface of the brain become deeper, reflecting a loss of neural tissue.

20 year old   90 year old

Figure 8.2   Age-related changes to the brain

The cardiovascular and respiratory changes described earlier in this chapter decrease the flow of oxygenated blood to the brain. A gradual reduction in cerebral blood flow is observed throughout life (Tarumi and Zhang, 2018) which equates to around a 27 per cent decline over 70 years of life (Chen et al., 2011).

Reductions in blood flow, loss of neural tissue and associated brain shrinkage have a cumulative impact on cognition in older people.

COGNITIVE CHANGES COMMONLY EXPERIENCED IN OLD AGE

- *Decreased verbal acuity*: It is very common for individuals aged 70 plus to notice a decrease in their verbal communication skills. This is often initially experienced in trivial ways such as finding it difficult to choose appropriate words to finish a sentence. There is evidence that many older people find this very frustrating and sometimes embarrassing and this can reduce social interactions. The hippocampus is a key area of the brain linked to learning of new skills and this undergoes dramatic shrinkage with age (Adler et al., 2018). As a result, many older people report learning of new languages becomes increasingly difficult.
- *Loss of short-term memory*: This is probably the most famous of the cognitive changes associated with old age. Most older (and even middle-aged) people experience the minor inconveniences of misplacing a set of car keys or forgetting to buy a key item at a supermarket. Unlike dementia normal age-related memory lapses tend to not affect life skills, such as the ability to cook food, get dressed in the morning or look after a home. However, since dementia is so common in the population, many older people find minor memory lapses very worrying and so reassurance is very important since worry and stress are both known to be associated with poorer recall. Although long-term memory is generally more stable and in the absence of disease much better maintained throughout life, remembering the exact sequence of a series of events and their timings (episodic memory) often declines with age (Nyberg, 2017).
- *Age-related depression*: Many of the brain chemicals (neurotransmitters) associated with feelings of well-being and happiness such as serotonin are thought to decrease with age (Ogle, et al., 2013). This may contribute to an increase in depression in older people. Recent figures for England indicate symptoms of depression are experienced by around 22 per cent of men and 28 per cent of women over the age of 65 with up to 40 per cent of residents in residential care affected (Age UK, 2017). The physical changes that occur to the ageing body that have been described in this chapter may themselves contribute to both anxiety and depression. Increased frailty in old age as a result of circulatory, musculoskeletal decline and common joint diseases such as osteoarthritis can limit mobility. Since exercise itself is associated with an increase in feel-good chemicals such as serotonin and endorphins, housebound or bedridden older people are more likely to experience a low mood. Depression can also reduce social interactions and can increase feelings of isolation.
- *Reduced reaction times*: Age-associated changes within the brain and spinal cord can reduce reaction times increasing the risk of injury. For example, the ability to quickly hold onto a handrail when beginning to slip on a staircase. Such reactions may be further diminished by the loss of muscle and stiffening of joints associated with old age. These changes undoubtedly contribute to the increased rate of injury from falls and other accidents in the older population.

BRAIN RESERVE

The average human brain contains over 100 billion interconnected neurons and this huge number of cells ensures that the brain has a built-in redundancy (the brain reserve) which even in the face of normal age-related neural losses and brain shrinkage allows cognitive function to be maintained throughout life. Research indicates that older people should be encouraged to increase their mental activity, for example by reading more and actively participating in games and when possible sports. Such activities, particularly those which promote greater social interactions, are thought to help reduce the decline in cognitive performance associated with ageing (Lee and Kim, 2016).

VISUAL CHANGES

The eyes are supported by a layer of retro-orbital fat which gradually shrinks with age and as a result the eyes visibly sink deeper into the eye sockets of the skull. This can cause the eyelids to be pulled away from the front of the eyeball creating an airspace resulting in poor wetting and lubrication of the eyeball. The rate of tear production also decreases with age and so older people can be prone to 'dry eye syndrome' which affects up to 14 per cent of the over 65s (Wigham et al., 2017).

PRESBYOPIA

Presbyopia is the term applied to the gradual age-related decrease in the ability to focus on objects up close. It is most obviously manifest in problems with reading, particularly the fine print in books and newspapers. Presbyopia occurs due to the lens of the eye gradually becoming thicker with age and losing its flexibility so that it is no longer able to focus light effectively. This phenomenon usually begins to be problematic in the fourth decade of life and becomes noticeable when a reader has to hold the text further and further away from the eyes to bring it into focus, so eventually reading glasses will be required. In some older people the progressive thickening of the lens will result in it becoming cloudy and opaque indicating the formation of a cataract which will usually require surgical removal to restore clear vision (Sreelakshmi and Abraham, 2016). Although ageing is the major risk factor for the formation of cataracts there are multiple other risk factors including smoking, high blood pressure, diabetes, excessive alcohol consumption and use of certain medications such as corticosteroids (Raju et al., 2017).

AGE-RELATED MACULAR DEGENERATION (ARMD)

Some older people suffer permanent visual changes including complete blindness as a result of ARMD. This condition occurs as a result of death of the cells (called cones) that are responsible for high-quality colour vision. Two major types of ARMD are recognised. Dry ARMD is the most common form accounting for round 90 per cent of cases and is characterised by a slow loss of vision in both eyes. The remaining 10 per cent of cases are referred to as wet ARMD and this is characterised by a leakage of a watery fluid into the photosensitive part of the eye (the retina) and the progressive growth of abnormal blood vessels. This wet form is far more aggressive and usually results in more severe and rapid loss of vision. Unfortunately, there are few treatment options available for both forms of ARMD which currently accounts for half of all visual impairments in people over the age of 75 (AMD.org, 2017).

HEARING CHANGES

The outer fleshy part of the ear termed the pinna or auricle gradually enlarges with age and often displays increased external hair growth, with these changes particularly noticeable in men. The ear canal becomes increasingly dry as the glands that produce ear wax (ceruminous glands) become less active. This drier environment encourages hardening of earwax in the outer ear canal which can interfere with hearing and often necessitates regular syringing of the ear.

PRESBYCUSIS (AGE-RELATED HEARING LOSS) AND TINNITUS

Sense of hearing is at its peak acuity at around ten years of age before progressively declining with age. Presbycusis is the term applied to age-related hearing loss and is usually associated with a gradual degeneration of the sensory cells and neurons within the inner ear. The cumulative effects of exposure to loud noises throughout life is thought to contribute to age-related hearing loss although poor blood flow, exposure to environmental toxins and inheritance of faulty genes that predispose to deafness all influence the rate at which it develops (Wigham et al., 2017). Hearing loss at frequencies associated with speech is particularly problematic in older people and can restrict verbal interactions (Parham et al., 2011). Age-related hearing loss is also associated with tinnitus where a variety of intrusive phantom sounds such as buzzing, humming, ringing or whooshing noises are perceived (British Tinnitus Association, 2017). Tinnitus can cause much distress and is also associated with disturbed sleep patterns and depression.

CHANGES TO SENSE OF BALANCE

The inner ear has an elaborate system of fluid-filled channels (the vestibule and semi-circular canals) in which are located the sensory organs associated with balance. Progression into old age is associated with a loss of up to 40 per cent of the sensory cells within the semi-circular canals (Allen et al., 2016). These losses are not only associated with poor balance but may result in dizziness and falls. Problems with balance are exacerbated in older people by reduced reaction times and losses in skeletal muscle mass and strength (see above).

CHANGES TO SENSE OF SMELL AND TASTE

Sense of taste is intimately associated with sense of smell (olfaction). With age there is a progressive decline in the olfactory sensors within the nose with many older people having a significantly reduced sense of smell (Attems et al., 2015). Not only does this reduce and impair the sense of taste, but loss of olfaction can also reduce the ability of older people to recognise dangerous odours such as smoke from a house fire or fumes from a petrol spillage. Fortunately, commercially available detectors are cheap and can be installed in the homes of older people to alert them to dangers such as smoke or gas leaks. Reductions in sense of smell and taste can reduce the enjoyment of food leading to reduced food intake and increasing the risk of weight loss. Unfortunately, to enhance flavour in their food many older people may resort to adding increasing amounts of salt which, although it may make food more palatable, can raise blood pressure and increase the risk of cardiovascular disease.

ACTIVITY 8.4   MULTIPLE CHOICE QUESTIONS

1   Loss of lean muscle mass that is commonly seen in older people is referred to as:

    a   Anaemia
    b   Polycythaemia
    c   Sarcopaenia
    d   Thrombocytopaenia

2   Ageing is commonly associated with:

    a   An increase in muscle mass
    b   A decrease in bone mass
    c   An increase in bone mass
    d   An increase in muscle strength

3   Which of the following is true of the skin when it ages?

    a   It becomes thinner
    b   It has less underlying fat
    c   It has reduced blood flow
    d   All of the above are true

4   Which of the following is true of the ageing brain?

    a   It gradually shrinks with age
    b   The number of neurons (nerve cells) increases with age
    c   Ageing of the brain eventually will always result in dementia
    d   All of the above are true

5   Ageing of the eye is commonly associated with:

    a   Decreased pressure within the eyeball
    b   Overproduction of tears
    c   Problems reading text up close
    d   A thinning and increase in the flexibility of the lens

Check the end of the chapter for the answers to this activity.

CONCLUSION

Although the ageing process is inevitable there are many things that people can do through-out their life to reduce the physical and psychological issues associated with growing older. It is clear that the ageing of the cardiovascular and respiratory systems has a major knock on effect in promoting the ageing of other body systems. Fortunately, many of the factors and lifestyle choices required to maintain a healthy and optimally functioning cardiovascular and respiratory system are well understood. The heart, blood vessels and lungs all benefit from regular aerobic exercise. This does not have to mean running a marathon or cycling in a 50-kilometre road race. Research indicates that 20–30 minutes of regular aerobic exercise which can raise the heart rate and breathing rate can provide significant health benefits such as maintaining cardiac muscle mass, lowering blood pressure and improving respiratory function as well as increasing muscle mass and bone density and lifting mood (Abou Elmagd, 2016).

Lifestyle choices also play a key role with a nutrient-dense balanced diet that is low in sodium (salt), refined sugars and sticky saturated fats widely promoted as being beneficial to health. Smoking is clearly extremely damaging to the lungs and promotes fat deposition in the arteries raising the risk of coronary artery disease and heart attacks. Unfortunately, many older people today were born at a time when the dangers of smoking were poorly understood and tobacco products were actively promoted which helps explain the huge numbers of older people currently suffering from smoking-related diseases such as heart disease, lung cancer and COPD.

Ensuring a healthy cardiovascular and respiratory system throughout life can help reduce the effects of ageing on other areas such as the skin and nervous system. As the only major organ continually exposed to the environment the skin is extremely vulnerable to pollutants and in particular the photo-ageing effects of ultraviolet light. The use of sun-block applied to the skin is proven to not only reduce the ageing of the skin but also reduce the risk of skin cancer. In terms of quality of life, a major issue is the increase in frailty that is associated with ageing. With increasing age bones become less dense and the risk of osteoporosis, spinal deformity and bone fracture increases. Loss of muscle in older people is associated with weakness and a tendency to remain immobile in bed or seated in chairs for longer periods of time. This can result in a vicious circle of increasing frailty since immobility itself is associated with reductions in both muscle and bone mass. As with the cardiovascular and respiratory systems light aerobic exercises such as walking a dog at a brisk pace for 20–30 minutes are shown to increase muscle mass and strength and also increase bone density reducing the risk of fracture and osteoporosis.

Ageing of the nervous system and changes in cognition are less well understood. Ageing is certainly associated with shrinkage of the brain size and reductions in the number of nerve cells. However, in the absence of dementia there are so many neurons (the brain reserve) that most cognitive skills are generally well maintained throughout life. Ageing itself is recognised as a natural part of the human life cycle. As we have seen throughout this article, cumulatively, the current evidence suggests that eating a balanced diet and taking regular exercise can reduce many of the negative physical and psychological effects associated with the ageing process thereby enhancing the quality of life throughout the entirety of the human lifespan.

GO FURTHER ACTIVITY

This chapter has examined some of the complex changes that occur within the human body as it ages. To help consolidate the information you have just learnt you are encouraged to:

1   Reflect on which of these changes are inevitable
2   Reflect on which of these changes can be modified or slowed down by lifestyle changes
3   Using online resources explore how diet and dietary modification may affect the ageing process
4   Research the effects of sun exposure on the ageing of skin and eyes – are there any perceived benefits for extended sun exposure?

Check the end of the chapter for the answers to this activity.

ANSWERS TO CHAPTER 8 ACTIVITIES

———— Activity 8.1: Answers

1   Collagen is a protein, indeed it is the most common protein in the human body.
2   The amino acids (building blocks of proteins) that form collagen are usually found linked together and wound into a triple helix (triple spiral) to form fibres.
3   The major cell type that produces collagen is the fibroblast, these cells are found throughout the body. The term fibroblast was coined because these cells produce structural fibres in the body including collagen fibres and elastic fibres.
4   Collagen is found throughout the body as a general purpose structural protein than 'knits' organs and tissues together providing strength and reinforcement. Collagen is particularly common in connective tissues such as cartilage and bone. It also forms the major component of tendons and is found at high concentrations in the skin. When the human body is injured collagen fibres are used to repair and close wound sites and for this reason scar tissue is also very rich in collagen.

———— Activity 8.2: Answers

1   Smoking damages the lining of arteries provoking atherosclerosis (fatty deposits) which reduces blood flow and increases blood vessel hardening and blood pressure, Regular smokers also have blood that clots more readily increasing the risk of stroke and heart attacks.

Smoking is known to cause premature ageing of the skin by a variety of mechanisms, including reducing collagen levels leading to increased sagging and wrinkling (smoker's wrinkles). Since smoking increases the risk of fatty deposition in blood vessels (atherosclerosis) blood flow to the skin is reduced and the skin can begin to look sallow with many smokers having a yellowish grey complexion. Smoking also reduces wound healing meaning that cuts and grazes to the skin take longer to resolve. For additional information visit: www.nhs.uk/smokefree/why-quit/smoking-health-problems

2   Vaping is thought to be an effective method of weaning off traditional combustible tobacco products such as cigarettes, cigars and pipes. Vaping through the use of e-cigarettes is thought to carry a fraction of the risk of traditional tobacco products since the nicotine is inhaled in the form of a vapour which is free of the combustible particulate materials and tars that are known to play the dominant role in damaging lung tissue. Using e-cigarettes many people have been able to quit cigarette smoking and improve their respiratory health. However, the long term effects of vaping are yet to be clearly established and some of the solvents used in creating the vapour that is inhaled are thought to be potentially damaging in the long term. See the following link for further information on the use of e-cigarettes to stop smoking. www.nhs.uk/live-well/quit-smoking/using-e-cigarettes-to-stop-smoking/

———— Activity 8.3: Multiple Choice Questions: Answers

1   Which of the following is true about ageing of the heart

c   Palpitations become more common with age

2   A build up of fatty deposits in the internal lining of a blood vessel is referred to as:

b   Atherosclerosis

3   Feeling faint when standing up quickly occurs usually as a result of:

a   Postural hypotension

4   What usually happens to the chest wall during normal ageing

a   It gradually stiffens and becomes less flexible as cartilage is replaced with bone

5   The mucociliary escalator

b   Has cells with mobile hair-like projections termed cilia

———— Activity 8.4: Multiple Choice Questions: Answers

1   Loss of lean muscle mass that is commonly seen in older people is referred to as:

c   Sarcopaenia

2   Ageing is commonly associated with

b   A decrease in bone mass

3   Which of the following is true of the skin when it ages

d   All of the above are true

4   Which of the following is true of the ageing brain

a   It gradually shrinks with age

5   Ageing of the eye is commonly associated with

c   Problems reading text up close

———— Go Further Activity: Guided Answers

1   Many of the age-associated changes to the human body are inevitable and little can be done to avoid these. For example, age-related changes to hearing and eyesight happen to everybody and no life-style changes can prevent loss of auditory acuity or the gradual hardening of the lens of the eye that will necessitate the use of reading glasses.

(Continued)

2   Many of the changes that we have explored can certainly be slowed by simple changes to lifestyle. For example, reducing salt (sodium) and saturated fat consumption, can improve blood vessel health and help reduce blood pressure. Abstaining from smoking will reduce the risk of blood vessel hardening due to fatty deposits (atherosclerosis) increasing blood flow to all major organs and tissues. Abstaining from smoking will also prevent the toxins from combustible tobacco products accelerating ageing of lung tissue and the skin.

3   There is much information on how calorific restriction may be beneficial in slowing the process of ageing. However most of the evidence for this comes from animal studies where animals with significantly reduced calorific intakes appear to have longer life spans. The current evidence in humans is limited but calorific restriction does tend to be associated with significant reductions in cardiovascular disease and diabetes, see the following link for further details: www.nia.nih.gov/health/calorie-restriction-and-fasting-diets-what-do-we-know Eating a balanced diet that is rich in vitamins and minerals is associated with better health parameters in older people and avoiding junk food particularly fried foods and excessive use of alcohol is associated with a reduction in damaging molecules termed free radicals which are known to accelerate ageing, see the following link for further details: www.medicalnewstoday.com/articles/318652.php

4   Since the skin is continually exposed to the external environment it is particularly vulnerable to extrinsic damage. Sunlight is particularly damaging to human skin, it is the ultraviolet component of sunlight that is associated with 'photoageing' since prolonged exposure can damage the cells of the skin and result in reduced collagen fibres. Since collagen is the major structural protein of the dermis loss can reduce dermal support leading to sagging and wrinkling. UV light can also cause significant damage to the DNA of our skin potentially leading to mutations and skin cancer. See the following link for further details: www.skincancer.org/healthy-lifestyle/anti-aging/what-is-photoaging. Since the damaging effects of UV light are today well known many people avoid excessive sun exposure although this approach is sensible in terms of skin health it has led many people to become deficient in vitamin D. Vitamin D is commonly known as the 'sunshine vitamin' since the skin can begin to manufacture this vitamin when exposed to direct sunlight. Vitamin D is essential to bone health since it is needed to absorb both calcium and phosphate which form the mineral component of bones. Vitamin D also plays a key role in normal muscle and immune function. Unfortunately it is the same ultraviolet light that is known to damage human skin that is essential to the biosynthesis of vitamin D. However, recent research indicates that the use of sun-blocks that are applied to protect the skin are not associated with vitamin D deficiency. Vitamin D can also be acquired through the diet and as a fat-soluble vitamin, dairy products, fatty cuts of meat and oily fish are particularly good sources, vegetable sources include spinach, kale and okra. See the following link for further details: www.skincancer.org/healthy-lifestyle/vitamin-d/damage

FURTHER READING

Farley, A., McLafferty, E. and Hendry, C. (2011). The *Physiological Effects of Ageing: Implications for Nursing Practice*. Wiley-Blackwell: Oxford.

Knight, J. and Nigam, Y. (2017). Anatomy and physiology of ageing 1: the cardiovascular system. *Nursing Times* 113(2), 22–24.

Knight, J. and Nigam, Y. (2017). Anatomy and physiology of ageing 2: the respiratory system. *Nursing Times* 113(3), 53–55.

Knight, J. and Nigam, Y. (2017). Anatomy and physiology of ageing 5: the nervous system. *Nursing Times* 113(6), 55–58.

Knight, J. and Nigam, Y. (2017). Anatomy and physiology of ageing 11: skin. *Nursing Times* 113(12), 51–55.

Knight, J., Hore., N and Nigam, Y. (2017). Anatomy and physiology of ageing 10: muscles and bone. *Nursing Times* 113(11), 60–63.

Knight, J., Wigham, C. and Nigam, Y. (2017). Anatomy and physiology of ageing 6: the eyes and ears. *Nursing Times* 113(7), 39–42.

REFERENCES

Abou Elmagd, M. (2016). Benefits, need and importance of daily exercise. *International Journal of Physical Education, Sports and Health* 22, 22–27.

Adler, D. H. et al. (2018). Characterizing the human hippocampus in aging and Alzheimer's disease using a computational atlas derived from ex vivo MRI and histology. *Proceedings of the National Academy of Sciences of the United States of America* 115(16), 4252–4257.

Age UK (January 2017). Later life in the United Kingdom. Factsheet. www.ageuk.org.uk/health-well-being

Allen, D. et al .(2016). Age-related vestibular loss: current understanding and future research directions. *Frontiers in Neurology* 7, 231.

AMD.Org (2017). Dry AMD The Macular Degeneration Partnership. Available at: www.amd.org/what-is-macular-degeneration/dry-amd/

American Cancer Society (2018). Benefits of quitting smoking over time. www.cancer.org/healthy/stay-away-from-tobacco/benefits-of-quitting-smoking-over-time.html

Attems, J. et al. (2015). Olfaction and aging: a mini-review. *Gerontology* 61, 485–490.

Bailey, K. L. et al. (2014). Aging causes a slowing in ciliary beat frequency, mediated by PKCε. *American Journal of Physiology-Lung Cellular and Molecular Physiology* 306(6), 584–589.

Bentov, I. and Reed, M. J. (2015). The effect of aging on the cutaneous microvasculature. *Microvascular Research* 100, 25–31.

British Tinnitus Association (2017). What is tinnitus? www.tinnitus.org.uk/what-is-tinnitus

Chen, J. J. et al. (2011). Age-associated reductions in cerebral blood flow are independent from regional atrophy. *NeuroImage* 55(2), 468–478.

Cipriani, E. et al. (2016). Wrinkles: origins and treatments. *Advances in Cosmetics and Dermatology* 2(1), 1–7.

Colón, C. J. P. et al. (2018) Muscle and bone mass loss in the elderly population: advances in diagnosis and treatment. *Journal of Biomedicine* 3, 40–49.

Csepe, T. A. et al. (2015). Fibrosis: a structural modulator of sinoatrial node physiology and dysfunction. *Frontiers in Physiology* 6, 37.

Flament, F. et al. (2013) Effect of the sun on visible clinical signs of aging in Caucasian skin. *Clinical, Cosmetic and Investigational Dermatology* 6, 221–232.

Forman, J. K. and Kent, R. W. (2014). The effect of calcification on the structural mechanics of the costal cartilage. *Computer Methods in Biomechanics and Biomedical Engineering* 17(2), 94–107.

Fotenos, A. F. et al. (2005). Normative estimates of cross-sectional and longitudinal brain volume decline in aging and AD. *Neurology* 64, 1032–1039.

Fragala, M. S., Kenny A. M. and Kuchel, G. A. (2015). Muscle quality in aging: a multi-dimensional approach to muscle functioning with applications for treatment. *Sports Medicine*, 45(5), 641–658.

Harvey, A. et al. (2016). Vascular fibrosis in aging and hypertension: molecular mechanisms and clinical implications. *Canadian Journal of Cardiology* 32(5), 659–668.

Janssens, J. P. (2005). Aging of the respiratory system: impact on pulmonary function tests and adaptation to exertion. *Clinics in Chest Medicine* 26, 469–484.

Jaul, E. et al. (2018). An overview of co-morbidities and the development of pressure ulcers among older adults. *BMC Geriatrics* 18, 305.

Knight, J. and Nigam, Y. (2017a). Anatomy and physiology of ageing 1: the cardiovascular system. *Nursing Times* 113(2), 22–24.

Knight, J. and Nigam, Y. (2017b). Anatomy and physiology of ageing 10: muscles and bone. *Nursing Times* 113(11), 60–63.

Larsson, L et al. (2019). Sarcopenia: aging-related loss of muscle mass and function. *Physiological Reviews* 99(1), 427–511.

Lau, A. N. and Adachi, J. D. (2011). Bone aging. Chapter 2 in Y. Nakasato and R. L. Yung (eds), *Geriatric Rheumatology: A Comprehensive Approach*. Springer Science+Business Media: New York.

Lee, S. H. and Kim, Y. B. (2016). Which type of social activities may reduce cognitive decline in the elderly? A longitudinal population-based study. *BMC Geriatrics* 16(1), 165.

Low, P. A. (2008). Prevalence of orthostatic hypotension. *Clinical Autonomic Research* 1, 8–13.

Marieb, E. N. and Hoehn, K. N. (2015). *Human Anatomy and Physiology*. Upper Saddle River, NJ: Pearson.

Martini, F. H. et al. (2018) *Fundamentals of Anatomy & Physiology* (11th edn). NJ: Pearson.

NHS (2018). Improving outcomes in chronic obstructive pulmonary disease (COPD). www.england.nhs.uk/rightcare/2018/01/08/improving-outcomes-in-chronic-obstructive-pulmonary-disease-copd/

NICE (2015). Osteoarthritis – summary. https://cks.nice.org.uk/osteoarthritis #!topicsummary

Nigam, Y. et al. (2009). Effects of bedrest 3: musculoskeletal and immune systems, and skin. *Nursing Times* 105, 23.

Nigam, Y. and Knight, J. (2017). Anatomy and physiology of ageing 11: the skin. *Nursing Times* 113(12), 51–55.

Nyberg, L. (2017). Functional brain imaging of episodic memory decline in ageing. *JIM* 281(1), 65–74.

Ogle, W. O. et al. (2013). Potential of treating age related depression and cognitive decline with nutraceutical approaches: a mini-review. *Gerontology* 59, 23–31.

Parham, K. et al. (2011). Challenges and opportunities in presbycusis. *Otolaryngology – Head and Neck Surgery* 144(4), 491–495.

Raju, M. et al. (2017) Investigating risk factors for cataract using the Cerner Health Facts database. *Journal of Eye & Cataract Surgery* 3(19). doi: 10.21767/2471-8300.100019

Richardson, J. C. et al. (2014). 'Keeping going': chronic joint pain in older people who describe their health as good. *Ageing & Society* 34(8), 1380–1396.

Roghani, T. et al. (2017). Age-related hyperkyphosis: update of its potential causes and clinical impacts-narrative review. *Aging Clinical and Experimental Research* 29(4), 567–577.

Sreelakshmi, V. and Abraham, A. (2016). Age related or senile cataract: pathology, mechanism and management. *Austin Journal of Clinical Ophthalmology* 3(2), 1067.

Tarumi, T. and Zhang, R. (2018). Cerebral blood flow in normal aging adults: cardiovascular determinants, clinical implications, and aerobic fitness. *Journal of Neurochemistry* 144(5), 595–608.

Tobin, D. J. (2016). Introduction to skin aging. *Journal of Tissue Viability* 26(1), 37–46.

United Nations Department of Economic and Social Affairs, Population Division. World Population Ageing (2015). Report ST/ESA/SER.A/390. www.un.org/en/development/desa/population/publications/pdf/ageing/WPA2015_Report

Wade, S. W. et al. (2012). Sex- and age-specific incidence of non-traumatic fractures in selected industrialized countries. *Archives of Osteoporosis* 7, 219–227.

WHO (2016). The top 10 causes of death. www.who.int/news-room/fact-sheets/detail/the-top-10-causes-of-death

Wigham, C. et al. (2017). Anatomy and physiology of ageing 6: the eyes and ears. *Nursing Times* 113(7), 39–42.

Wyss-Coray, T. (2016). Ageing, neurodegeneration and brain rejuvenation. *Nature* 539, 180–186.

Youssef, S. A. et al. (2016). Pathology of the aging brain in domestic and laboratory animals, and animal models of human neurodegenerative diseases. *Veterinary Pathology* 53(2), 327–348.

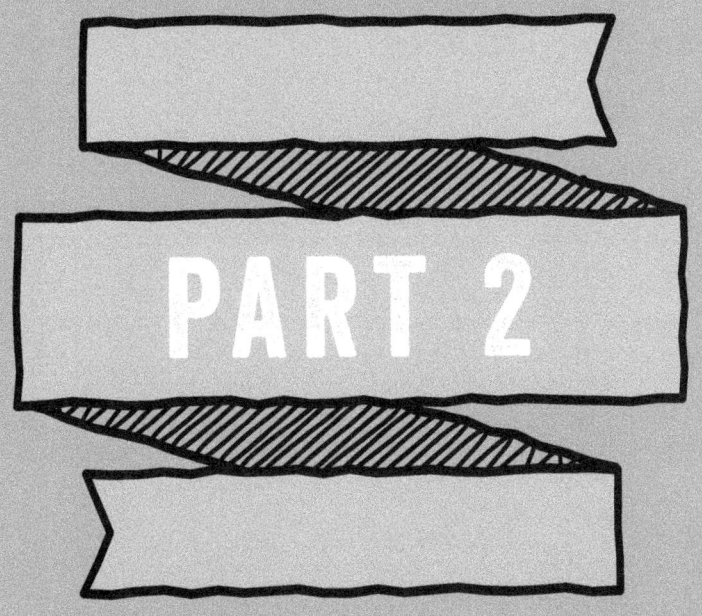

PART 2

HEALTH AND SOCIAL CARE IN ACTION

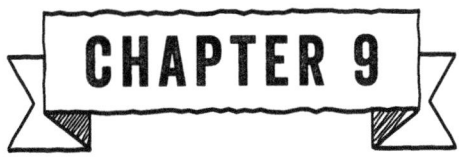

CHAPTER 9

SAFEGUARDING CHILDREN AND ADULTS

Charlotte Chisnell and Caroline Kelly

OVERVIEW

This chapter aims to provide students of health and social care and related studies with a foundational knowledge of safeguarding children and adults in the United Kingdom. While safeguarding is commonly stated to be everyone's business, health and social care services have key roles and responsibilities in this area of practice. In the UK, there is now a widespread consensus that the state should intervene when abuse or neglect occurs. However, safeguarding can be complex and challenging for the services involved.

LEARNING OUTCOMES

By the end of this chapter you will be able to:

- Describe key aspects of safeguarding children and adults in the UK
- Understand legal frameworks for safeguarding adults and children
- Explain the significance of inquiries that have influenced practice
- Describe theories and approaches relevant to safeguarding children and adults

INTRODUCTION

The chapter will set the context for safeguarding, consider how this has evolved and discuss the key terminology used. It will also outline the current legislative and policy frameworks in the UK and some of the inquiries and reviews that have influenced their development. A comparative overview of safeguarding policies across the devolved nations will also be included. Themes related to inter-professional and inter-agency working and listening to the voice of the child or adult who is at risk will be considered. There will also be a discussion of structural factors associated with safeguarding such as inequality and discrimination and the impact of issues such as substance misuse, domestic abuse and mental health. Exercises focusing on the recognition of safeguarding concerns, the identification of risks of abuse and ways to respond within the remit of health and social care roles are included to raise awareness of priorities. The chapter also aims to develop knowledge and understanding of theories and approaches relevant to safeguarding children and adults.

Developments in child and adult safeguarding have occurred within different contexts and timescales. Despite these differences safeguarding aims to protect children and adults with additional needs from harm, to ensure that care is consistent and achieve best possible outcomes. This chapter will consider key developments and current frameworks for children's safeguarding before discussing the way in which responses to safeguarding adults have emerged and key priorities for practice in this area. While there are notable differences in legal and policy frameworks, there are also a variety of themes that are relevant to safeguarding across the lifespan. These themes will be explored further in concluding the chapter.

SAFEGUARDING CHILDREN

THE HISTORICAL CONTEXT OF SAFEGUARDING CHILDREN

Developments in safeguarding policy and reforms to social work practice have been influenced by high-profile cases, which have invariably highlighted deficiencies in protecting children and adults at risk of abuse. We will begin by looking at the historical construction of protection and how responses to abuse and neglect have led to the current system for safeguarding.

THE HISTORICAL CONTEXT OF CHILD PROTECTION

One key debate that has dominated child-protection practice is being able to determine the balance between a child's absolute right to be safe, parental rights and the state's responsibility to protect a child's best interests. The awareness of the need to protect vulnerable children slowly grew during the twentieth century with the introduction of a more collective responsibility for the provision of services. This era of social democracy saw a shift in political ideology and led to the creation of the welfare state. There was a growing political awareness that children could be vulnerable. During the 1970s and 1980s (Corby et al., 2012), the recognition of abuse as a social issue led to the development of child-protection policy and procedures including the at-risk register (Parton and Williams, 2017). In 1998, working in partnership with families became a key policy driver during New Labour's government and initiated the transition from an emphasis on protection to the current safeguarding agenda, which aims to protect a child's health and well-being, and promote their right to be free from abuse and neglect (Corby et al., 2012).

INQUIRIES

The relationship between social work and child protection also began to change following increased public awareness of the concept of child abuse and the view that professionals had failed to protect children. Sidebotham (2012) identified failure to interpret, record and share information as key themes that have consistently appeared in serious case reviews, and such themes have been a consistent feature in child deaths during the past 70 years. During the 1970s and 1980s there was an intense public and media interest in the perceived failings of social work agencies in several child deaths. In 1973 Maria Colwell was murdered by her stepfather, despite the fact that there had been 50 visits made to the family by social services. An inquiry into her death concluded that there were a number of failures including a lack of communication and poor liaison between the agencies involved.

In 1984 Jasmine Beckford was killed by her stepfather although she had been in the care of Brent social services for two and a half years before she died. By 1985 a further 29 inquiries had been held into child deaths that had resulted from abuse (Chisnell and Kelly, 2019).

As a consequence of these cases and the subsequent public inquiries resources began to be diverted to the investigation of abuse as opposed to a focus on prevention. The other key development at this time was the enactment of the Children Act 1989 which continues to be the main piece of legislation to support families and protect children.

VICTORIA CLIMBIÉ

On 25 February 2000 Victoria Climbié died after being systematically tortured by her great-aunt and her great-aunt's partner; she had 128 injuries but died from hypothermia. At the time of Victoria's death, she was known at two social services departments, paediatricians, police officers, the church and other organisations. A public inquiry headed by Lord Laming identified comprehensive failings of the protection system, including widespread organisational ineffectiveness (Laming, 2003). As a direct response to the death of Victoria Climbié the safeguarding agenda moved to placing the responsibility on social workers to work in partnership with other professionals to prevent abuse and to promote the welfare of children.

BABY PETER

Baby Peter died in 2007; he was murdered by his mother's boyfriend. He suffered broken ribs, removed fingernails, bruising to his head and face, a broken spinal cord, injuries to his chest, bruises, wounds, bite marks and a missing tooth. Before his death, a number of social workers and health professionals knew him. Despite the inquiry into Peter's death, which highlighted professional faults and recommended reforms to the safeguarding system, there continues to be criticism about the failure to protect due to a lack of understanding of risk and failure to communicate.

WHAT DO HEALTH AND SOCIAL CARE WORKERS NEED TO KNOW ABOUT CHILD ABUSE?

Practitioners need to know what child abuse is, the nature and prevalence of abuse, how to recognise abuse and how to respond effectively.

WHAT IS CHILD MALTREATMENT?

The abuse and neglect that occurs to children under 18 years of age. 'It includes all types of physical and/or emotional ill-treatment, sexual abuse, neglect, negligence and commercial or other exploitation, which results in actual or potential harm to the child's health, survival, development or dignity in the context of a relationship of responsibility, trust or power. Exposure to intimate partner violence is also sometimes included as a form of child maltreatment' (WHO, 2015).

In the UK in 2018, there were approximately 53,790 children placed on protection plans due to a risk of abuse and neglect; this is an increase of 5.3 per cent (Department of Education, 2018).

FACTORS WHICH INCREASE THE LIKELIHOOD OF ABUSE

There are several factors that are believed to increase the risk to children and make them more vulnerable to abuse, e.g. the age of a child, disability, previous experience of abuse or trauma, low self-esteem and limited opportunities to develop resilience.

CATEGORIES OF ABUSE

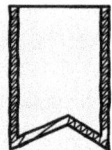

PAUSE FOR THOUGHT 9.1

We have looked at abuse and factors which might increase the likelihood of abuse, but do you know what the different categories of child abuse are?

The HM Government's (2018) *Working Together to Safeguard Children* advises that there are four categories of abuse in relation to child maltreatment. Abuse is broadly defined in terms of:

- Physical abuse
- Emotional abuse
- Neglect
- Sexual abuse

Physical abuse is: unexplained physical injuries, such as burns, bruises, broken bones, bites and head injuries.

Emotional abuse is: 'The persistent emotional maltreatment of a child such as to cause severe and persistent adverse effects on the child's emotional development. It may involve conveying to a child that they are worthless or unloved, inadequate, or valued only insofar as they meet the needs of another person' (HM Government 2018, p. 103).

Neglect is: the persistent failure to meet a child's basic physical and/or emotional needs, likely to result in the serious impairment of the child's health or development. Brandon et al. (2010) highlighted that neglect was apparent in 60 per cent of serious case reviews: 'Practitioners still frequently fail to recognise the severity or underestimate the potential consequences of neglect' (p. 8).

Sexual abuse: 'involves introducing a child who is below the age of consent to take part in activities, which result in the sexual gratification of the perpetrator. This abuse involves the misuse of power and trust and can lead to the grooming and exploitation of vulnerable children' (HM Government, 2018, p. 103).

LEGISLATION PROTECTING AND SAFEGUARDING CHILDREN

The CA 1989 came into force on 14 October 1991, making radical changes in the law relating to children and their families. The Act stipulates that professionals have a duty to act in a child's best interests to ensure that their welfare is the paramount consideration. The Act provides social workers with the legal mandate to protect children who may be at risk of significant harm (Chisnell and Kelly, 2019).

Parts IV and V of the Act provide the legal framework for the protection of children and the legal mandate to intervene to protect a child at risk of significant harm. Section 47 places a duty on the local authority to investigate the circumstances where a child appears to be suffering significant harm or is believed to be at risk of significant harm.

EMERGENCY PROTECTION ORDERS (EPOS)

An EPO can be sought in an emergency, to protect a child who is likely to suffer significant harm. A local authority applying for an EPO must demonstrate in evidence that they have 'reasonable cause to believe that the child is likely to suffer significant harm'.

POLICE PROTECTION S46

Section 46 provides police with powers to remove a child into police protection, as a matter of urgency and without any application to court. This action is short term and can only last up to 72 hours (www.legislation.gov.uk/ukpga/1989).

If a child is in need of longer-term care and protection the Act makes provision for this. A care order is a long-term option and is sought in order to protect children and young people. The local authority (LA) must demonstrate in evidence that 'the child is suffering or likely to suffer significant harm and this is attributable to the care given to the child, or the child is beyond parental control'. If a care order is granted the LA acquires shared parental responsibility with the child's parents.

THE SCOTTISH LEGAL CONTEXT: SAFEGUARDING CHILDREN

The Children (Scotland) Act 1995 is the main piece of legislation in relation to children which introduced specific rights and responsibilities towards children. There are three main principles which underpin the Act:

- The welfare of the child should be paramount.
- No order should be made unless it is essential to do so.
- Children should be given the opportunity to express their views in relation to matters that affect them.

There are a number of similarities between the Children Act 1989 and the Children (Scotland) Act 1995, especially in relation to support for children and families and the provision of emergency protection. The main differences relate to how to make an application for compulsory measures of care and the treatment of young people who are involved in the juvenile justice system.

THEORIES OF HUMAN BEHAVIOUR

Theories help us to try to understand human behaviour and the nature and complexity of relationships. Understanding the aetiology of behaviour should help professionals to recognise abuse and respond more effectively.

Freud developed the psychodynamic perspective which suggested that the unconscious mind influences the development of personality. This theory suggests that if a person has experienced childhood abuse in their childhood this may increase the risk of them displaying inappropriate sexualised behaviour. However, the focus on individual pathology does not take into account other factors that could account for abuse (Corby et al., 2012).

Sociological perspectives suggest that society accepts violence and abuse because of the existence of social problems that have developed because of structural inequality, poverty and social exclusion (Corby et al., 2012).

Learning theories propose that aggression and abusive behaviour may develop as learned conditions as opposed to being a symptom of individual pathology. Social learning theory is most closely associated with Albert Bandura (Bandura et al., 1961). This perspective suggests that aggressive and abusive behaviour can result because of a person's interaction with their social environment rather than individual pathology.

This theory has been used to explain how violent behaviour can be learnt from observing aggressive role models, for example when children who have witnessed domestic violence later also engage in this behaviour, suggesting that a child's behaviour can be influenced by exposure to the misuse of power and aggression. This approach has been criticised because it does not account for the victims of abuse who do not become perpetrators when they are adults (Corby et al., 2012).

A feminist perspective suggests that abuse and violence develop because of patriarchy and the domination of male power over women and children (Parrish, 2014). This perspective also recognises that in many cases the response to abuse and family violence is engendered which can lead to the victim being blamed for a perceived failure to protect their children.

Finklehor (1984) suggests that a more integrated approach as opposed to single-factor theories is required to understand why perpetrators might develop a sexual interest in children. He suggested that if abuse is likely to take place four preconditions would need to be present.

The perpetrator:

1   Will be motivated to sexually abuse (want to);
2   is able to overcome internal inhibitors (guilt conscience);
3   is able to overcome external inhibitors (groom protectors/create opportunity);
4   is able to overcome child's resistance (groom child). (Chisnell and Kelly 2019)

Finkelhor's model has been criticised on the basis that this model illustrates the process of sexual abuse as opposed to understanding why it occurs. There needs to be a more systematic understanding of the factors which can increase risk factors, different offending styles, developmental influences and better clarification of the factors which can increase vulnerability (Ward et al., 2006).

CASE STUDY 9.1   RESPONDING TO RISK

Sarah Michaels is 28 years old and has a long history of both mental health and substance misuse issues. She is a lone parent to Elijah (ten) and Keira (three). Sarah's care of the children is erratic and on occasions they have been reported to have been home alone. Concerns are raised at Keira's nursery as she has been coming into nursery in dirty clothes and appears to be hungry and withdrawn. There are concerns that Keira may not be meeting her developmental milestones and has outstanding immunisation appointments. The school have also noticed a deterioration in Elijah's presentation but when he has been asked if he is OK, he becomes very defensive and is clearly protective of his mother.

Questions

What would be your main areas of concern?

What agencies should you contact to obtain information about the welfare of the children?

What are your duties in relation to the children?

Comments

There appears to be areas of concern, but more information would be required to enable an accurate assessment of risk and needs to be undertaken. Throughout the assessment, it would be vital that practitioners listen to the voice of the children and always keep them at the centre of the assessment process. Although the priority is always to ensure that children are safe, it is also important to identify areas of strength and support which may exist within the family, extended family and community. It is crucial to ensure that communication is effective, with information being recorded and shared appropriately. However, as practitioners who are faced with possible abuse and neglect it is important to remember that when a professional is exposed to increased levels of secondary trauma over time they can experience emotional exhaustion. Effective supervision is a key tool to enable practitioners to develop their emotional resilience.

SAFEGUARDING ADULTS

THE DEVELOPMENT OF ADULT SAFEGUARDING IN THE UK

Like child abuse, awareness of the abuse of adults has evolved in recent decades although this process has been rather later to occur for adults than for children. The development of the welfare state after the Second World War acknowledged state duties towards people in need in UK society and provision for adults with care and support needs often occurred in the context of long stay institutions (Goble, 2011). Awareness of the inhumane nature of many institutionalised regimes grew alongside political priorities to reduce state responsibility for care and led to the development of community-based forms of support. Building on the rights-based approach enshrined in the Human Rights Act 1998, the No Secrets guidance (Department of Health, 2000) provided the first central framework for multi-agency adult protection policies and procedures to prevent and investigate abuse. The Care Standards Act 2000 legislated for regulation and inspection of care services in England, with equivalent organisations in other areas of the UK. While significant changes to regulatory bodies have occurred since then, many of the challenges to improving services have persisted across the different jurisdictions (Campbell, 2017). While there has been a considerable shift towards community-based forms of care, marginalisation of people with care and support needs has often prevailed (Home Office, 2017).

PERSONALISATION AND SAFEGUARDING

The shift towards community-based care has been accompanied by a raft of policies to achieve personalisation, emphasising rights to individual choice, control and self-directed support. Whether such aspirations have yet been achieved in adult social care is contentious, particularly in the context of current budget constraints (Carr and Needham, 2018). Achieving personalisation within safeguarding has been slow to develop with ongoing concerns about managing risk (Stevens et al., 2018). The Making Safeguarding Personal (MSP) initiative in England was developed in 2010 as a response to research which highlighted that safeguarding practice had often focused on processes without seeing people as experts in their own lives. Such restrictive practice has been identified as counter-productive with the potential to further disempower people who have been abused (Lawson et al., 2014). While MSP initially centred around the interventions of local authorities, more recent developments have highlighted the need for person-centred safeguarding responses across partner agencies such as the police, health services and the housing sector (Lawson, 2017a, 2017b, 2017c, 2017d). Research has suggested that where MSP approaches have been successfully developed, there has been a focus on relationship-based work to achieve the outcomes that people themselves want to achieve and that this has can lead to earlier resolution and prevention of further abuse (Cooper et al., 2016). Involving people experiencing abuse in the development of appropriate responses at both individual and policy levels is a key priority for adult safeguarding. There have been significant initiatives in Northern Ireland, for instance, to establish the views of people who have encountered safeguarding and develop user-led approaches (Montgomery et al., 2017).

LEGAL FRAMEWORKS FOR SAFEGUARDING

The Care Act repealed much of the previous legislation relating to the assessment and provision of adult care and support in England and highlights the principles of well-being, independence, prevention, choice and control. It was the first legislation in England to outline adult safeguarding statutory duties for local authorities and partner agencies. Section 42 of the Act requires local authorities to make enquiries or instruct others to do so when adults with care and support needs may be at risk of abuse or neglect. It also includes a statutory requirement for Safeguarding Adults Boards (SABs) with membership from a range of stakeholders. Local authorities are also required to arrange for an independent advocate to represent and support a person if they need help to understand and express their views in a safeguarding enquiry or review (Department of Health, 2018). There have been considerable challenges in relation to achieving effective multi-agency working in safeguarding (Graham et al., 2016) and the require-ments of the Care Act aim to ensure accountability for safeguarding across the range of agencies.

The Care Act emphasises integration of health and social care and requires the agencies involved to streamline approaches and responses in safeguarding (Graham et al., 2016). Research suggests that further clarity around thresholds for safeguarding intervention and scrutiny of local differences in approaches is required (Action on Elder Abuse, 2017).

The approaches advocated by MSP have been enshrined in law through the Care Act. The Care Act guidance suggests that safeguarding needs to be considered in the wider context of the overall well-being of the individual and that all safeguarding work should be underpinned by the six principles for safeguarding which are: empowerment, prevention, proportionality, protection, prevention and accountability (Chisnell and Kelly, 2019).

The Care Act does not give local authorities any new powers to enter a person's property although this was identified as an important additional power by practitioners prior to its incep-tion (Manthorpe et al., 2017). Equivalent legislation in Wales – the Social Services and Well-Being (Wales) Act 2014 – permits Adult Protection and Support Orders to be applied for from a magis-trate to fully investigate where there is risk of abuse (UKQCS, 2014).

In Scotland safeguarding legislation was introduced much earlier through the Adult Support and Protection (Scotland) Act 2007 (ASP). The ASP is based on the following principles:

- that any intervention must provide benefit to the adult;
- that this benefit could not have been reasonably achieved without intervention;
- that any intervention is the least restrictive option to the adult's freedom.

The Act provides a framework to intervene to prevent harm continuing and to promote inter-agency co-operation. Section 35 of the ASP allows for overriding the consent of the adult, with the agreement of a Sheriff, if there appears to be undue pressure being applied to the adult by a suspected perpetrator to withhold their consent (Scottish Government, 2014). While the Care Act reflects many of the principles of the ASP, the ASP goes further in terms of strengthening powers of intervention and the role of state agencies in safeguarding (Chisnell and Kelly, 2019).

MENTAL CAPACITY

Mental capacity relates to the ability of individuals to make decisions and there are legal frame-works in place in each area of the UK to support this. Capacity legislation exists to allow legally valid decisions to be made about finances, welfare or medical treatment where the individual lacks mental capacity. In Scotland this occurs through the Adults with Incapacity (Scotland) Act 2000 (AWIA) and in England and Wales as the Mental Capacity Act 2005 (MCA). The Mental Capacity Act (Northern Ireland) provides similar legislation in Northern Ireland (Wilson, 2017).

Legislation such as the Mental Capacity Act 2005 is highly significant in relation to safeguard-ing as it allows for best-interest decision-making when a person is unable to make a decision themselves and also gives those with capacity the right to make their own decisions. As such it is pivotal in terms of establishing responsibility for decision-making in relation to safeguarding. Section 44 of the MCA also introduced an offence of ill-treatment or neglect of a person lacking capacity (Godefroy, 2015). The principles of the Act include a presumption of capacity of adults, supporting individuals to make decisions and the right to make what others may consider unwise decisions if they have the capacity to do so. Where someone is unable to make a decision, then decisions made for them must be made in their best interest and should be the least restrictive option. Assessment of capacity must always be decision and time specific rather than an over-arching conclusion. The MCA also introduced the Court of Protection which has powers to make declarations about capacity and oversee the legality of decisions (SCIE, 2009).

CATEGORIES OF ABUSE/PREVALENCE

The Care Act defines the different types of adult abuse as:

- **Physical abuse** – including assault, hitting, slapping, pushing, misuse of medication, restraint or inappropriate physical sanctions.
- **Domestic abuse** – including psychological, physical, sexual, financial, emotional abuse or so-called 'honour'-based violence.
- **Sexual abuse** – including rape, indecent exposure, sexual harassment, inappropriate looking or touching, sexual teasing or innuendo, sexual photography, subjection to pornography or witnessing sexual acts, indecent exposure and sexual assault or sexual acts to which the adult has not consented or was pressured into consenting.
- **Psychological abuse** – including emotional abuse, threats of harm or abandonment, deprivation of contact, humiliation, blaming, controlling, intimidation, coercion, harassment, verbal abuse, cyber bullying, isolation or unreasonable and unjustified withdrawal of services or supportive networks.
- **Financial or material abuse** – including theft, fraud, internet scamming, coercion in relation to an adult's financial affairs or arrangements, including in connection with wills, property, inheritance or financial transactions, or the misuse or misappropriation of property, possessions or benefits.
- **Modern slavery** – encompasses slavery, human trafficking, forced labour and domestic servitude. Traffickers and slave masters use whatever means they have at their disposal to coerce, deceive and force individuals into a life of abuse, servitude and inhumane treatment.
- **Discriminatory abuse** – including forms of harassment, slurs or similar treatment; because of race, gender and gender identity, age, disability, sexual orientation or religion.
- **Organisational abuse** – including neglect and poor care practice within an institution or specific care setting such as a hospital or care home, for example, or in relation to care provided in one's own home. This may range from one-off incidents to ongoing ill-treatment. It can be through neglect or poor professional practice as a result of the structure, policies, processes and practices within an organisation.
- **Neglect and acts of omission** – including ignoring medical, emotional or physical care needs, failure to provide access to appropriate health, care and support or educational services, the withholding of the necessities of life, such as medication, adequate nutrition and heating.
- **Self-neglect** – this covers a wide range of behaviour including neglecting to care for one's personal hygiene, health or surroundings and includes behaviour such as hoarding. (Department of Health, 2018)

Many types of abuse are also criminal offences and early involvement of the police is required to establish this. Types of abuse in reality are often overlapping and there can be multiple forms of abuse occurring at the same time. Signs that abuse is occurring can be difficult to detect, may be absent even when abuse is occurring and also some indicators of abuse may have other explanations. It is important that practitioners who come into contact with people with care and support needs are able to recognise potential indicators of abuse.

SERIOUS CASE REVIEWS

Serious Case Reviews (SCRs), or Safeguarding Adults Reviews (SARs), occur when an adult dies or is seriously injured and there are concerns about the conduct of the agencies involved. SCRs have had a significant impact on the development of safeguarding practice and some of these will be examined here.

HATE CRIME

Steven Hoskin was a 38-year-old man with learning disabilities who was tortured and murdered by a group of people in his local community. His death highlighted significant failings in safeguarding systems. The SCR found that there were over 40 missed opportunities for intervention to protect Steven by the range of agencies involved. The SCR found that individual organisations held key information which was not shared with other agencies. Had this information been shared there would have been a much clearer picture of the concerns regarding Steven's situation. The SCR also highlighted concerns around effective assessment of mental capacity and the need to respond effectively to people on the periphery of service involvement who are experiencing marginalisation within communities. Overall the SCR emphasised the need for accountability among all of the agencies who have contact with adults at risk of abuse (Flynn, 2007).

Hate crime against people with learning disabilities continues to be a significant problem although it remains under-reported. The psychological effect on victims and feelings of powerlessness created are cumulative and compounded by services not being equipped to respond adequately (Simmonds et al., 2018). It is important however to acknowledge the strength and resilience of people with learning disabilities or other support needs and avoid assumptions of inherent vulnerability. Simmons argues that the stereotypical assumption of vulnerability can create environments for hate crime to occur.

There are clear parallels between the abuse of people with learning disabilities in communities and other adults with support needs. People with mental health problems are much more likely to be the victims of crime as opposed to perpetrators, despite common media representations (Pettitt et al., 2013). This highlights the challenges that people with support needs face in their relationships with the wider community. There are clear parallels with the exploitation and grooming that can occur in different forms of abuse across the lifespan. Responses to incidents of hate crime can be focused on protecting the individual by restricting their freedom, as opposed to providing access to justice which can create further abuse of rights (Pettitt et al., 2013; Simmonds et al., 2018).

ORGANISATIONAL ABUSE

The abuse of adults with learning disabilities at Winterbourne View assessment and treatment unit has been one of the most high-profile investigations into adult abuse in recent years. Although there were a series of complaints to the Care Quality Commission (CQC) and health professionals, the abuse carried out by staff members continued over several years until BBC's *Panorama* programme exposed this through an undercover reporter in 2011. Six members of staff were ultimately convicted of offences under the Mental Health Act 1983 (as amended by the Mental Health Act 2007) and received custodial sentences. The SCR identified serious failings in relation to the care of patients, physical restraint, unaddressed complaints, staff training and recruitment, and an overall absence of leadership. Wider issues concerned the commissioning of services, lack of consultation with patients and families, no access to advocacy and a failure to respond to whistleblowing by any of the organisations involved, including the CQC (Flynn and Citarella, 2012).

The events at Winterbourne demonstrated that, despite awareness of the negative impact of isolated long-stay institutions over many decades, such environments are still prevalent. Subsequently there was a reform of inspection practices in England and policies to implement alternative community-based services for people with learning disabilities. Despite this there have been ongoing issues with achieving effective oversight and providing suitable alternatives (Brittain, 2016; Care Quality Commission, 2017; Moore, 2017a).

The potential for power imbalances in caring relationships within residential settings is also noteworthy. Features such as dependency, unequal decision-making powers and isolation, can create a climate where individuals are more at risk (Moore, 2017b). The definition of organisational abuse in the Care Act emphasises the fact that abusive cultures of care are not only a feature of large institutions but can also be found in community-based services. On a wider scale, institutional discrimination can also occur in state organisations such as health care or the criminal justice system. Research into the premature deaths of people with learning disabilities has established that inequalities in access and quality of medical treatments is a significant issue (Heslop, et al., 2013).

Negative attitudes and work practices can become entrenched in the culture of any setting with the potential for the actions of those predisposed to harming others to be tolerated or overlooked. These factors can provide warning signs of abuse to practitioners who are in a pivotal position to prevent abuse occurring (Marsland et al., 2015). Good care environments require a culture where people are able to challenge bad practice and speak up about concerns with the standard of care.

DOMESTIC ABUSE

Alongside failure to protect in institutional settings, case reviews have also highlighted significant problems in domestic settings. The SCR into the murder of 81-year-old Mary Russell by her husband found a failure to recognise domestic abuse even though police, social services and health professionals had been alerted to her injuries. Poor communication and deficiencies in multi-agency responses were also identified (Southend Safeguarding Adults Board, 2011). Similarly, the domestic homicide review into the death of Mrs Y, a 79-year-old woman killed by her husband, identified that she was not seen as a potential victim of domestic abuse by the agencies involved and that this was in part due to her age. The review suggested that the death of Mrs Y could not have been predicted but there could have been further investigation of the risks, assessment of domestic abuse indicators and more focus on Mrs Y's views about her relationship with her husband. The panel concluded that there were missed opportunities and that Mrs Y's death could have been prevented if responses that would normally be considered to protect victims of domestic abuse had been put in place. The review recommended setting standards for domestic abuse training across agencies and campaigns to raise public awareness of the domestic abuse of older people (Albiston, 2013).

It is important to consider that domestic abuse is often underpinned by coercive control where abusers threaten and isolate victims in a continuous way with a cumulative impact on the victim. The criminalisation of coercive control in the Serious Crime Act (2015) (legislation.gov.uk) is an important advance in understanding domestic abuse at policy level. The term 'coercive control' has also been included in statutory safeguarding guidance for the Care Act 2014 in England and the Social Services and Well-being (Wales) Act. Research suggests that practitioners working with adults may lack knowledge of specialist domestic abuse services with expertise in situations of coercive control. This can disadvantage groups such as older or disabled people if they are not supported to access services such as the specialist advocacy provided by independent domestic violence advisors (Wydall and Zerk, 2017).

THEORIES AND APPROACHES

It is important to consider adult abuse in the context of wider societal factors. Research into domestic abuse of disabled people suggests that although there is a higher occurrence of abuse of disabled people, particularly women, there are significant barriers to accessing support (LGA/ADASS, 2015). In situations where people are dependent for daily living tasks on an abusive carer there is significant potential for isolation. This is exacerbated by wider societal discrimination and socially constructed perceptions of disabled people which impact on their ability to seek help. People are often reluctant to disclose abuse unless they are asked directly, however, research suggests that professionals rarely ask directly about abuse. People from black and minority ethnic (BME) groups can experience additional barriers to accessing support and leaving abusive circumstances and are more likely to stay in abusive situations for longer before accessing help (Public Health England, 2015). As people need time to build trust, repeated attempts to enquire about abuse when it is safe for the person to disclose may be needed (LGA/ADASS, 2015). The examination of serious case reviews highlighted the impact of socially constructed ideas about older age and how these can impact on recognising the abuse of older people. Practitioners need to be aware of their own and wider societal perceptions of factors such as age, disability and ethnicity, and how these can impact on the experience of abuse and responses. As the proportion of adults with an impairment increases with age (Public Health England, 2015), the dynamics of abuse encountered by disabled people intersects with older people's experiences of ageism and other factors such as race discrimination.

It is particularly relevant here to consider the impact of a medicalised approach to disability and ageing which focuses on the impairments of the individual as opposed to seeing the person in the wider social environment and the barriers that this can create for them (Shakespeare, 2014). A social model of support acknowledges and aims to address marginalisation and is significant in the context of safeguarding adults (Safe Lives, 2017). Awareness of the rights of disabled people to full citizenship and participation in society have been raised over recent years globally and are underpinned by the UN Convention on the Rights of Persons with Disabilities (United Nations, 2006).

While there is a need for awareness of wider societal factors, it is also imperative that practitioners maintain a focus on developing relationships with individuals to build trust for people to disclose abuse. The impact of resource constraints can affect practitioners' capacity to develop effective trusting relationships (Wydall et al., 2018). However, legal mandates to deliver personalised safeguarding and work at a pace which suits the individual are enshrined in frameworks such as the Care Act and wider policies across the UK. These frameworks can provide an impetus for a shift towards relationship-based and value-based practice in safeguarding adults.

The complexity of safeguarding adults lies in the inherent tension between the rights of individuals to self-determination and professional duty of care and protection from harm. This tension requires high levels of effective communication and collaboration with individuals, families and agencies to achieve successful outcomes. Safeguarding is part of a continuum of care and support which has become more of a focus in recent years but is inseparable from wider interventions to meet need. Factors such as addressing social isolation and improving people's social networks are highly significant in preventing abuse as well as enhancing overall well-being (Cook, 2018). The Care Act advocates strengths-based approaches to support which emphasise the need to build on the skills and resources that people have. It is essential in safeguarding adults to acknowledge people as experts in their own lives and build on their personal and social resources to avoid further disempowerment when people have been abused (SCIE, 2015). This, however, must be done in the context of a full assessment of individual needs, risks and challenges which considers the wider inequalities that create barriers for people with care and support needs.

ACTIVITY 9.1

The Care Act suggests that adult safeguarding should comprise six key principles:

- Empowerment
- Protection
- Prevention
- Proportionate responses
- Partnership
- Accountability

Questions

Looking back at the Adult Serious Case Reviews discussed earlier, how would you achieve each of these principles?

Check the end of the chapter for an answer to this activity.

CONCLUSION

This chapter has aimed to provide students of health and social care with a foundational framework of knowledge relating to safeguarding children and adults. Key developments in legislation and policy have been outlined alongside information on the types of abuse and key terms used in safeguarding. Theories, research and approaches which can be applied to inform more effective practice have also been considered.

Key themes that exist within both child and adult safeguarding have been highlighted, such as exploitation, grooming and the misuse of power. The impact of structural factors such as poverty, substance misuse, domestic abuse, mental health, discrimination, marginalisation and isolation in society are also central issues to consider in the context of abuse.

Factors which can achieve more effective practice within safeguarding whatever the age of the individual concerned have been considered. Serious case reviews have consistently highlighted that failures to collaborate and share relevant information lead to serious consequences for people at risk. The principle of effective collaborative working between agencies in safeguarding is central. It is imperative to work together to develop shared knowledge about abuse and ways to safeguard people at risk within our society. Inter-agency training and working practices have a key role in this.

A further essential task is to listen to the voice of the child or adult at risk and ensure that they remain at the centre of safeguarding practice throughout. Advocacy for people who have been disempowered through abuse is also a key element of support. Effective practice should always involve building relationships with families and individuals to encourage a move away from a deficit model towards a strengths-based approach.

Despite the rhetoric of current policies, the prevailing climate of austerity has led to a reduction in public services and a rise in poverty. Current resource constraints potentially narrow the focus of agencies towards safeguarding activity at the expense of wider responses to need. Well-resourced services which allow good practice to flourish and encourage individuals to reflect on their roles and duties are key to achieving positive outcomes in safeguarding and in wider service provision.

GO FURTHER ACTIVITY

In order to develop your knowledge and understanding around aspects of safeguarding policy and the impact on professional practice we would direct the reader to undertake further research around these areas from safeguarding texts and resources available from specialist organisations such as Barnardo's and Age Concern, who campaign to raise awareness of abuse and neglect.

ANSWERS TO CHAPTER 9 ACTIVITIES

——— Activity 9.1: Answers

- Empowerment

Listening to people, provision of advocacy, actively involving people throughout intervention, understanding wider factors which marginalise individuals, relationship-based practice, using preferred methods of communication and settings which the person feels comfortable in, providing clear information throughout.

- Protection

Good multi-agency working and communication, awareness of channels for reporting concerns, understanding of indicators of abuse, appropriate safety planning in a range of contexts, effective use of the law including mental capacity frameworks, providing safe environments for people to disclose abuse.

(Continued)

- Prevention

The removal of isolating environments, establishing support networks, addressing wider needs and rights, raised public awareness of abuse and organisational responsibilities for safeguarding, risk assessment and safety planning.

- Proportionate responses

Seeing the person in wider context and as expert in own lives, focusing on the outcomes they want to achieve, discussion and collaboration with stakeholders on appropriate thresholds for intervention.

- Partnership

Good multi-agency working and communication, seeing the person in wider context and as expert in their own lives, focusing on the outcomes people wish to achieve, relationship-based practice.

- Accountability

Clear understanding of own and other people's roles and responsibilities for safeguarding, risk assessment and safety planning, effective use of the law, collaborative working

FURTHER READING

Bentley, H. et al. (2017). *How Safe Are Our Children? The Most Comprehensive Overview of Child Protection in the UK 2017*. London: NSPCC.

Braye, S. and Preston-Shoot, M. (2017). *Learning from SARs: A Report for the London Safeguarding Adults Board*. London: ADASS.

Cleaver, H., Unell, I. and Aldgate, J. (2011). *Children's Needs – Parenting Capacity. Child Abuse: Parental Mental Illness, Learning Disability, Substance Misuse, and Domestic Violence* (2nd edn). London: The Stationery Office.

Department of Health (2014). *Care and Support: Statutory Guidance Issued under the Care Act 2014*. London: Department of Health.

HM Government (2018). *Working Together to Safeguard Children: A Guide to Inter-agency Working to Safeguard and Promote the Welfare of Children*. London: The Stationery Office.

Local Government Association/ADASS (2015). *Adult Safeguarding and Domestic Abuse: A Guide to Support Practitioners and Managers*. London: Local Government Association. Available at: www.local.gov.uk/publications/-/journal_content/56/10180/3973717/PUBLICATION#sthash.TGS1DVgU.dpuf

Marsland, D., Oakes, P. and White, C. (2015). Abuse in care? A research project to identify early indicators of concern in residential and nursing homes for older people. *Journal of Adult Protection* 17(2), 111–25.

Simmonds, R., Burke, C., Ahearn, E. R. and Kousoulis, A. (2018). *A Life without Fear? A Call for Collective Action against Learning Disability Hate Crime*. London: Mental Health Foundation. Available at: www.mentalhealth.org.uk/publications/life-without-fear

REFERENCES

Action on Elder Abuse (2017). *A Patchwork of Practice*. Available at: www.rbsab.org/ UserFiles/Docs/ Patchwork-of-PracticeDEC2017.pdf

Albiston, K (2013). *Domestic Homicide Review: Executive Summary Mrs Y/2013*. Available at: www. sunderland.gov.uk/media/19435/Domestic-homicide-review-Executive-Summary-Mrs-Y-/pdf/ Domestic_Homicide_Review_Executive_Summary_Mrs_Y.pdf?m=636420329214570000

Bandura, A., Ross, D. and Ross, S. A. (1961). Transmission of aggression through the imitation of aggressive models. *Journal of Abnormal and Social Psychology* 63, 575–582.

Brandon, M., Bailey, S. and Belderson, P. (2010). *Building on the Learning from Serious Case Reviews: A Two-Year Analysis of Child Protection Database Notifications 2007–2009. Research Report*. London: Department for Education.

Brittain, K. (2016) *Time for Change: The Challenge Ahead*. ACEVO. Available at: www.acevo.org.uk/ sites/default/files/ACEVO_report_TCA_final_web.pdf

Campbell, M. (2017). The journey from first inspection to quality standards (1857–2016): are we there yet? *The Journal of Adult Protection* 19(3), 117–129.

Care Quality Commission (2017). *The State of Health Care and Adult Social Care in England 2016/2017*. Available at: www.disabilityrightsuk.org/news/2017/october/care-qualitycommission-state-care-report-2016-17

Carr, S. and Needham, C. (2018). Personalisation: lessons from research. *Community Care Inform* [online]. Available at: https://adults.ccinform.co.uk/research/research-review-personalisationin-adult-social-care-2/

Chisnell, C. and Kelly, C. (2019). *Safeguarding across the Lifespan* (2nd edn). London: Sage.

Cook, S. (2018). Addressing loneliness and social isolation: lessons from research. *Community Care Inform* [online]. Available at: https://adults.ccinform.co.uk/research/addressing-loneliness-andso cial-isolation-lessons-from-research/

Cooper, A., Briggs, M., Lawson, J., Hodson, W. and Wilson, M. (2016). *Making Safeguarding Personal Temperature Check*. London: Association of Directors of Adult Social Services

Corby, B., Shemmings, D. and Wilkins, D. (2012). *Child Abuse: An Evidence Base for Confident Practice* (4th edn). Maidenhead: Open University Press.

Department of Education (2018). *Characteristics of Children in Need: 2017 to 2018*. Available at: https://assets.publishing.service.gov.uk/government/uploads/system/uploads/attachment_data/ file/762527/Characteristics_of_children_in_need_2017-18.pdf

Department of Health (2000). *No Secrets: Guidance on Developing and Implementing Multiagency Policies and Procedures to Protect Vulnerable Adults from Abuse*. London: Department of Health.

Department of Health (2018). *Care and Support: Statutory Guidance Issued under the Care Act 2014*. London: Department of Health.

Finkelhor, D. (1984). *Child Sexual Abuse: New Theory and Research*. New York: Free Press.

Flynn, M. (2007). *The Murder of Steven Hoskin: A Serious Case Review. Executive Summary*. Truro: Cornwall Adult Protection Committee.

Flynn, M. and Citarella, V. (2012). *Winterbourne View Hospital: A Serious Case Review. Executive Summary*. South Gloucestershire Safeguarding Adults Board. Available at: www.hosted.southglos. gov.uk/wv/report.pdf

Goble, C. (2011). Developing user-focused communication skills. In A. Mantell and T. Scragg (eds), *Safeguarding Adults in Social Work* (2nd edn). Exeter: Learning Matters.

Godefroy, S. (2015). *Mental Health and Mental Capacity Law for Social Workers: An Introduction*. London: Sage.

Graham, K., Norrie, C., Stevens, M., Moriarty, J., Manthorpe, J. and Hussein, S. (2016). Models of adult safeguarding in England: a review of the literature. *Journal of Social Work* 16 (1), 22–46.

Heslop, P., Blair, P., Fleming, P., Hoghton, M., Marriott, A. and Russ, L. (2013). *Confidential Inquiry into Premature Deaths of People with Learning Disabilities (CIPOLD) Final Report*. Bristol: Norah Fry Research Centre. Available at: www.bristol.ac.uk/media-library/sites/cipold/migrated/documents/fullfinalreport.pdf

HM Government (2018). *Working Together to Safeguard Children: A Guide to Inter-agency Working to Safeguard and Promote the Welfare of Children*. London: The Stationery Office.

Home Office (2017). *Hate Crime, England and Wales, 2016/17 Aoife O'Neill Statistical Bulletin 17/17*, 17 October. Available at: https://assets.publishing.service.gov.uk/government/uploads/system/uploads/attachment_data/file/652136/hate-crime-1617-hosb1717.pdf

Laming, H. (2003). The Victoria Climbie Inquiry: Report of an Inquiry by Lord Laming. London. The Stationery Office. Available at: www.gov.uk/government/publications/the-victoria-climbie-inquiry-report-of-an-inquiry-by-lord-laming (accessed 23 March 2019).

Lawson, J. (2017a). *Making Safeguarding Personal: What Might 'Good' Look Like for Advocacy?* London: Local Government Association and Association of Directors of Adult Social Services.

Lawson, J. (2017b). *Making Safeguarding Personal: What Might 'Good' Look Like for Health and Social Care Commissioners?* London: Local Government Association and Association of Directors of Adult Social Services.

Lawson, J. (2017c). *Making Safeguarding Personal: What Might 'Good' Look Like for the Police?* London: Local Government Association and Association of Directors of Adult Social Services.

Lawson, J. (2017d). *Making Safeguarding Personal: What Might 'Good' Look Like for Those Working in the Housing Sector?* London: Local Government Association and Association of Directors of Adult Social Services.

Lawson, J., Lewis, S. and Williams, C. (2014). *Making Safeguarding Personal: Guide 2014*. London: Local Government Association.

Local Government Association/ADASS (2015) *Adult Safeguarding and Domestic Abuse: A Guide to Support Practitioners and Managers*. London: Local Government Association. Available at: www.local.gov.uk/publications/-/journal_content/56/10180/3973717/PUBLICATION#sthash. TGS1DVgU.dpuf

Manthorpe, J. et al. (2017). Safeguarding practice in England where access to an adult at risk is obstructed by a third party: findings from a survey. *The Journal of Adult Protection* 19(6), 323–332.

Marsland, D, Oakes, P. and White, C (2015). Abuse in care? A research project to identify early indicators of concern in residential and nursing homes for older people. *Journal of Adult Protection* 17(2), 111–125.

Montgomery, L., Hanlon, D. and Armstrong, C. (2017) 10,000 voices: service users' experiences of adult safeguarding. *The Journal of Adult Protection* 19(5), 236–246.

Moore, S. (2017a). What's in a word? The importance of the concept of 'values' in the prevention of abuse of older people in care homes. *The Journal of Adult Protection* 19(3), 130–145.

Moore, S. (2017b). You can lead a horse to water but you can't make it drink: how effective is staff training in the prevention of abuse of adults? *The Journal of Adult Protection* 19(5), 297–308.

Parrish, M. (2014) *Social Work Perspectives on Human Behaviour* (2nd edn). Oxford: Oxford University Press.

Parton, N. and Williams, S. (2017). The contemporary refocussing of children's services in England. *Journal of Children's Services* 12(2/3), 85–96.

Pettitt, B. et al. (2013) *At Risk, Yet Dismissed: The Criminal Victimisation of People with Mental Health Problems*. London: Victim Support/Mind. Available at: www.mind.org.uk/media/187663/ At-risk-yet-dismissed-report_FINAL_EMBARGOED.pdf

Public Health England (2015). *Disability and Domestic Abuse: Risk, Impacts and Response*. Available at: https://assets.publishing.service.gov.uk/government/uploads/system/uploads/attachment_ data/file/480942/Disability_and_domestic_abuse_topic_overview_FINAL.pdf

Safe Lives (2017). *Disabled Survivors Too: Disabled People and Domestic Abuse*. Available at: http://safelives.org.uk/sites/default/files/resources/Disabled%20Survivors%20Too%20 CORRECTED.pdf

SCIE (2009). SCIE at a glance 5: Mental Capacity Act 2005 at a glance. Available at: www.scie.org.uk/mca/introduction/mental-capacity-act-2005-at-a-glance

SCIE (2015). Care Act guidance on strengths-based approaches. www.scie.org.uk/strengths-based-approaches/guidance

Scottish Government (2014). Adult Support and Protection (Scotland) Act 2007 Code of Practice. Available at: www.gov.scot/publications/adult-support-and-protection-revised-code-of-practice/

Shakespeare, T. (2014). *Disability Rights and Wrongs Revisited* (2nd edn). Abingdon: Routledge.

Sidebotham, P. (2012). What do serious case reviews achieve? *Archives of Disease in Childhood* 97(3), 189–192.

Simmonds, R., Burke, C., Ahearn, E. R. and Kousoulis, A. (2018). *A Life without Fear? A Call for Collective Action against Learning Disability Hate Crime*. London: Mental Health Foundation. Available at: www.mentalhealth.org.uk/publications/life-without-fear

Southend Safeguarding Adults Board (2011). *Mr and Mrs A (Mary Russell) Serious Case Review. Executive Summary*. Southend: Southend SAB.

Stevens, M. et al. (2018) Implementing safeguarding and personalisation in social work: findings from practice. *Journal of Social Work* 18(1), 3–22.

The Children Act 1989. Available at: www.legislation.gov.uk/ukpga/1989/9/contents/enacted (accessed 25 January 2019)

The Children (Scotland) Act 1995. Available at: www.legislation.gov.uk/ukpga/1995/36/contents

UKQCS (2014). Well-being in Wales. Available at: www.ukqcs.co.uk/well-wales/

United Nations (2006). *United Nations Convention on the Rights of Persons with Disabilities*. Geneva: United Nations.

Ward, T., Polachek, D. L. L. and Beech, A. R. (2006). *Theories of Sexual Offending*. Chichester: Wiley.

Wilson, S. (2017). Mental capacity legislation in the UK: systematic review of the experiences of adults lacking capacity and their carers. *BJPsych Bulletin* 41(5), 260–266.

World Health Organization (2015). Child maltreatment. Available at: www.who.int/news-room/fact-sheets/detail/child-maltreatment (accessed 24 November 2018)

Wydall, S., Clarke, A., Williams, J. and Zerk, R. (2018). Domestic abuse and elder abuse in Wales: a tale of two initiatives. *British Journal of Social Work* 48, 962–981.

Wydall, S. and Zerk, R. (2017). Domestic abuse and older people: factors influencing helpseeking. *The Journal of Adult Protection* 19 (5), 247–260.

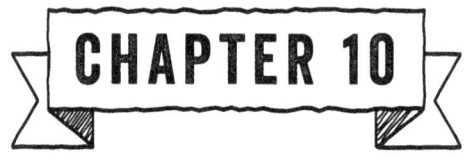

CHAPTER 10

CHILDCARE IN THE UK

Pete King

OVERVIEW

This chapter considers the role of childcare within a health and social care context. The chapter starts with a brief historical account of how childcare has evolved within the United Kingdom (UK) since the Industrial Revolution. The chapter then explains how childcare practice has had to change in relation to the introduction of statutory legislation to reduce child labour and protect children in the nineteenth century to provide the opportunity for mothers to be more active in the workforce in the twentieth and twenty-first centuries. This has led to the growth of childcare provision and the need for the childcare worker to gain professional qualifications to support the health, well-being and development of children in their care. The relationship between the childcare worker and children is considered in respect of attachment theory, and how the role of the childcare worker has an important place within the community, especially with the growth of childcare provision in schools are discussed.

LEARNING OUTCOMES

By the end of this chapter you will be able to:

Explain from both a historical and current perspective the differences and similarities of different childcare provision

Discuss the role of the childcare worker with consideration to attachment theory

Discuss the possible impact of childcare on children's health and well-being

Consider the increase in childcare provision within communities

INTRODUCTION

Let's start with an exercise: defining childcare.

ACTIVITY 10.1

Take one minute and write down as many different environments and contexts where children can be cared for outside of the family home.

The list you have just created may have come from personal experience; you may have memories of using them as a child yourself. In addition, you may have children and they are currently using different childcare facilities. From your list, you may have written:

Pre-schools, playgroups, nursery, childminder, after school clubs, holiday play schemes, residential homes, foster homes, extended family (grandparents, aunts and uncles, etc.), day-care centres, Sunday School, and so on.

For this chapter, childcare is defined by the legislation within the Childcare Act 2006 as 'any form of care for a child … (a) education for a child, and (b) any other supervised activity for a child' (UK Parliament, 2006, p. 10). This does not include formal education within schools, foster care or children living in residential homes. Children in childcare involves a 'contract' between the childcare organisation and the parent/carer where the organisation has responsibility for the care of the child for an agreed period of time. The child is not 'free' to leave the session before they are collected by the parent or carer. The term childcare does not include those environments where there is no 'contract' between parents and play workers working on open access play projects such as play ranging (see King and Sills-Jones, 2018).

The reason, amount of time spent and experience for the child (or young person) will vary between each of the different types of environment. However, for the adult childcare worker, they all have a primary role in the consideration of children's health, development and well-being. Three different types of childcare currently exist include out-of-school provision (after-school clubs and holiday play schemes), day care (including nurseries and childminders) and early education provision (e.g. pre-schools and playgroups).

A BRIEF HISTORY OF CHILDCARE PROVISION IN THE UK

The first recorded nursery provision was in New Lanark, Scotland, set up by the Welsh cotton mill owner Robert Owen in 1816 (Bradburn, 1966). The nursery was set up during the time of the Industrial Revolution in Britain. Owen, a strong believer in social justice (Bradburn, 1966), set up this provision for children under the age of ten where 'the children played freely out of doors, under the supervision of a young woman; sometimes they played inside' (Bradburn, 1966, p. 60) whilst the children's mothers were working in the cotton mill. During this period, children of all ages were employed in the factories and mills until the legislation of the Cotton Mills Act of 1819 (UK Parliament, 2018a) and the Factory Acts of 1833 which stated that no children under the age of nine years could be employed and children under the age of 13 years must have two hours of schooling per day (UK Parliament, 2018b). Now children had 'free time' to fill now not at work, which was increased with the introduction of compulsory education through the Elementary Education Act

1870 (UK Parliament, 1870). This 'free time' worried many of the nineteenth-century social reformers who were concerned about potential anti-social behaviour (Cranwell, 2003). One solution was the formation of organised provision run by adults for children.

From the nineteenth century within the UK, a range of childcare provision was provided organised by churches and schools (Cranwell, 2003). Examples of organised childcare provision set up in London were the formation of two organisations: the Children's Happy Evening Association (CHEA) and the Passmore Edwards Settlement (PES) (Bonel and Lindon, 1996; Cranwell, 2003) which were run in schools and community centres. Childcare provision in children's 'free time', from this early beginning, is still common practice today. After-school clubs, usually running from the end of the school day to up to 6 p.m., provide a space for children to play supervised by childcare workers, as well as holiday play scheme provision. As with the CHEA and PES, schools and community halls are often used.

The roots of early education lie within the Nursery Schools Association (NSA) which formed in 1923 (Jarvis and Liebovitch, 2015). The NSA, developed from the first network of nurseries established during the First World War so women could be employed, was set up by Mary McMillan who was influenced by her belief in Christian socialism and Grace Owen who was influenced by the kindergartens of Friedrich Fröbel (Jarvis and Liebovitch, 2015). Interestingly Fröbel's first kindergarten in Germany was set up later than Robert Owen's first nursery (Bradburn, 1966). The start of public funding for nursery education began with the Education Act 1918 (UK Parliament, 1918) and this enabled the local authority to apply for funding to assist nursery education (West and Noden, 2016). Nursery spaces were not available to all and in 1961, after setting up her own pre-school group, Belle Tutaev orchestrated the first annual meeting of the Pre-School Playgroups Association (PPA) which was to become a 'national body made up of volunteers, (usually parents)' (Faulkner and Coates, 2013, p. 10). The Pre-school Playgroups Association later became Pre-school Learning Alliance in 1995. In 2019, the Pre-school Learning Alliance changed its name to the Early Years Alliance and continues to run pre-school educational provision.

Most often, early education provision (as with after-school clubs) only run for a certain amount of time per day, not the whole day. For some parents, who work or study, they require longer childcare hours, and two popular provisions are day-care nurseries and childminders. Day-care provision often starts at around 8 a.m. and finishes around 6 p.m., enabling parents to work or study, and are run by private (as a business) or voluntary bodies (West and Noden, 2016). There is a national charity organisation which supports day-care providers, the National Day Nurseries Association (NDNA) which was originally formed in 1999. Childminders work from their homes, and their hours of work are flexible to support often looking after their own children, as well as being paid to look after other parents' children. Childminders also have an umbrella organisation with the National Childminding Association, and this was rebranded in 2013 to the Professional Association for Childcare and Early Years (pacey).

The growth of the childcare sector since the first nursery opened by Robert Owen now consists of many different types of provision: nurseries; day care; childminding; after-school clubs and holiday play schemes. Today, childcare provision must adhere to legislation that was not around prior to 1989. This is discussed next.

LEGISLATION AND CHILDCARE

One noticeable difference between childcare practice in the past and the present day was the introduction of the Children Act 1989, and the subsequent legislation of the Care Standards Act 2000 and Childcare Act 2004, which put a regulatory duty on childcare provision applied to all countries in the UK. Part XA of the Childcare Act 1989, Childminding and Day Care for Young

Children, placed for the first time a statutory duty of registration and regulation for any childcare provision that was running for more than two hours a day, more than five days a year, and had children attending under the age of eight years of age. The registration and regulation included the suitability of the premises, the resources and activities being provided and the suitability of the staff in relation to undergoing a police check (now known as a Disclosure and Barring (DBS) check) and any appropriate qualification. The initial role for the regulation and inspection was placed on local authorities. The responsibility of inspection and regulation has now changed and is different between the four UK countries. In England and Wales, childcare provision have had additional legislation with the introduction of both the Children Act 2004 and Childcare Act 2006.

Since the Care Standards Act 2000, registration and inspection of childcare in England is the responsibility for the Office for Standards in Education (Ofsted). Childcare provision in England must comply to The Childcare (General Childcare Register) Regulations 2008, as amended in the Childcare (Welfare and Registration Requirements) (Amendment) Regulations 2014 and be registered on the Childcare Register if the childcare provision has children aged under eight. In Northern Ireland and Wales, registration and inspection for childcare has been raised to 11 years of age, and in Scotland it relates to children up to 16 years of age. In Northern Ireland, under the Children (Northern Ireland) Order 1995, it is the role of the Health and Social Care Trusts for registering and inspecting of childcare (Department for Health, Social Services and Public Safety (DHSSPS), 2012). In Wales, it is the Care Inspectorate for Wales (CIW) formally the Care and Social Services Inspectorate Wales (CSSIW) (Welsh Government, 2016). In Scotland, under The Regulation of Care (Scotland) Act 2001, it is the Scottish Social Services Council (Scottish Government, 2005) that carries out registration and inspection. As well as the increase in legalisation relating to childcare, there has also been an increase in childcare provision.

GROWTH OF CHILDCARE

The 1990s and early 2000 saw an increase in childcare provision (day care, after-school clubs and holiday provision) due to the Labour government's National Childcare Strategy (Department for Education and Employment (DfEE), 1998) which aimed at providing affordable quality childcare so parents (mainly mothers) could get employment, or train to be employed so as to increase family income and reduce childhood poverty (Faulkner and Coates, 2013). This very much reflected Robert Owen's first nursery provision so as to employ the children's mothers in the cotton mills. In Wales, further legislation to tackle poverty was introduced by the Families and Children (Wales) Measures 2010 which included not only childcare, but also the first statutory duty across the UK for children's play.

The increase in both dual and lone parents working resulted in a growth of out-of-school provision (after-school and holiday play schemes) (Smith and Barker, 2000) as well as an increase in day-care nurseries and childminders. The New Opportunities Fund, set up by the Department for Culture, Media and Sport (DCMS), used £220 million from the National Lottery to create 850,000 childcare places through increasing out-of-school provision across the UK (SQW, 2003). In addition, during this time free early years education was made available for 3- and 4-year-olds (Faulkner and Coates, 2013), where under the Childcare Act 2006 (UK Parliament, 2006) any childcare provider (childminder, day care, playgroup) could apply for the funding as long as they have an element of education within the day (West and Noden, 2016). This combination of childcare and education was termed by Betyee Caldwell as 'educare' which has a 'proper blend of education and care' (Caldwell, 1989, p. 266).

The combination of childcare and education, along with health services were integral to the development of SureStart centres (Faulkner and Coates, 2013). SureStart (2003) is linked with the

Childcare Act 2006 and provides integrated services that include both early education and child-care provision (DfE, 2013) with centres located in areas of social deprivation. In Wales, in addition to SureStart, there is another initiative combining early education and childcare for 2–3-year-olds called Flying Start (Welsh Government, 2018). Flying Start, as with SureStart, is targeted provision in areas linked to social deprivation offering other integrated services such as health. Flying Start offers childcare up to two and a half hours a day, five days a week for 39 weeks and can be part of existing childcare provision within a day nursery for example. Although not all parents can access free childcare within SureStart or Flying Start, there is free childcare provision available within the four UK countries, but the number of hours available vary between countries.

In Scotland, children aged 3–4 years have up to 16 hours' free childcare. However, the Children and Young People (Scotland) Act 2014 (Scottish Parliament, 2014) aims for an increase in free early years and childcare provision for 4-year-olds (Care Inspectorate, 2017). In England, there is a universal 15 hours for all children (Jarrett, 2018). A further 15 hours' free childcare is available for eligible children (DfE, 2018a) under the Childcare Act 2016 (UK Parliament, 2016). In Wales, whilst Flying Start childcare provision is only available to children in areas of deprivation, all children are eligible to access up to 10 hours' free part-time Foundation Phase education in registered pre-school or nurseries termed 'Foundation Phase Nursery' (Welsh Government, 2018). Free childcare provision in Wales will increase to 30 hours for working parents (Glover et al., 2018). Northern Ireland currently offers all 3- and 4-year-old children 12½ hours a week (Employers for Childcare, 2018).

Day nurseries cater for children often from 8 a.m. to 6 p.m., which will involve time for children to have food and possibly sleep. Day nurseries need to be large enough to have areas for babies, toddlers (up to 2 years) and for the older children (2–4 years). Childminders work from home, often having to look after their own children at the same time. As with day nurseries, childminders can run from 8 a.m. to 6 p.m., but have a considerably smaller number of children to childcare for. After-school clubs will often run from the end of the school day (3 p.m. to 3.30 p.m.) to up to 6 p.m. Holiday play schemes run in school holidays and can start from as early as 8 p.m. to 6 p.m. A study in England found the use of childcare by parents was highest between 3 p.m. and 5 p.m. (Booth et al., 2013). The number of children any childcare practitioner can look after at a given time is determined by the respective childcare legislation.

PAUSE FOR THOUGHT 10.1

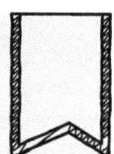

You are a childcare worker working in a nursery during the day with children from 0–4 years of age and then work in an after-school club with children aged 5–11 years attending. What skills and knowledge do you think you need to support children's health and social care in these two different childcare environments?

The skills of the childcare worker will be determined by the nature of the adult themselves, the type of childcare environment, the policies and procedures of the childcare organisation and the legislation (law) that they must adhere to. Another key aspect of the of the Children Act 1989 was for childcare workers to be qualified to demonstrate professional competence working with children, also driven by the Labour government's National Childcare Strategy (Faulkner and Coates, 2013).

THE CHILDCARE WORKER

Although the Childcare Act 2006 states childcare does not include 'any form of health care for a child' (UK Parliament, 2006, p. 10), that is look after children in a medical capacity, the childcare worker does have a duty of care for the well-being of any child being cared for as stated within the Children Act 2004. The childcare worker must have a nationally recognised professional qualification to demonstrate competence to work with children. There are a range of qualifications in early childhood, childcare and playwork which enables people to be employed as a childcare worker. Depending on your role within the childcare organisation, there are different levels of educational attainment. For childcare managers, a level 4 qualification is required (e.g. in Childcare Management) which is the equivalent of the first year of higher education, for supervisors and people in charge of the day to day running a level 3 is required and for childcare workers with no supervisory responsibility a level 2. Level 2 is equivalent to GCSE and level 3 to A Level. A recent study in England on the early years workforce (which includes childcare workers) found the childcare workforce is 'mostly female, low qualified and poorly paid' (Bonetti, 2019, p. 6), which would most probably reflect childcare across the UK.

The childcare worker requires a knowledge of child development, how to resource the childcare environment to stimulate and maintain interest for the children playing there and can plan and deliver play and educational-based tasks and activities to cater for children's physical, emotional, cognitive and social development. The childcare worker, if working in a setting that is linked to early years education will have to have a knowledge of the educational curriculum. The childcare worker will thus play a role in children's health, development and well-being.

CHILDREN'S HEALTH, DEVELOPMENT AND WELL-BEING

The important role of childcare with respect to children's health and development is considered within government legislation and policy, for example the Welsh Early Years and Childcare Plan (Welsh Government, 2013), the Scottish Action Plan (Scottish Government, 2017) and the English Early Years Foundation Phase (Department for Education (DfE), 2017a).

ACTIVITY 10.2

What are the advantages and disadvantages for children attending childcare provision?

Copy out Table 10.1 and use the table to note your answers.

Table 10.1 What are the advantages and disadvantages for children attending childcare provision?

	Childcare	Home
Advantages		
Disadvantages		

Your response to Activity 10.2 may have considered the advantages and disadvantages from the perspective of the child, the adult or both. What does the research evidence indicate? Kamerman (2006) stated that childcare provision, 'Apart from their critical contribution to cognitive stimulation, socialization, child development, and early education, they are an essential service for employed parents' (p. 1). However, there has been some debate around whether children attending childcare provision, particularly from soon after being born, has a negative, positive or no effect at all on children's health, development and well-being.

In America, Baum (2003), using secondary data from the National Longitudinal Survey of Youth (NLSY), analysed children's cognitive development and verbal and maths skills in relation to women returning to work within the first year of having a baby. Baum's (2003) study indicated that 'maternal marketplace work in the child's first year has detrimental total effects on cognitive development' (p. 439) particularly between the child's age of three months to a year. Interestingly, Baum's (2003) analysis found an increase in income (as women go back to work) enhances development. Another American study using the secondary data from the NLSY by James-Burdumy (2005) also indicated that for women who return to work 'there may be some negative effects of maternal employment during the first year of a child's life' (p. 206). This would indicate that maternal leave should be longer to increase children's later development. However, these results from America were not found in Canada. Baker and Milligan's (2010, 2012) analysis of The National Longitudinal Study of Children and Youth (NLSCY) in Canada on women returning to work and children's cognitive and behavioural development found that maternity leave had no negative impact for children at an older age.

In Germany, Sweden and Denmark, policy changes enabled an increase in maternal leave for a positive effect on children's future education attainment (Dustmann and Schönberg, 2011; Liu and Skans, 2010; Rasmussen, 2010). Each of these studies analysing relationships between employment and educational data sets found an increased time with children had no long-term effect on their education outcome. Dustmann and Schönberg's (2011) study in Germany found 'no evidence that the expansions improved children's outcomes' (p. 219), whilst in Sweden Liu and Skans' (2010) analysis found 'the average performance of the children was unaffected by parental leave durations' (p. 31) and Rasmussen's (2010) Danish study found 'at age 15, high school enrolment, or high school grade point average at the age of 21, there does not seem to be an effect' (p. 99). A more recent study in France found children at age 8 who had attended a centre-based childcare provision were less likely to have high levels of emotional symptoms, peer relationship problems or low prosocial behaviours (Gomajee et al., 2018). Similar findings were found in Ireland where children who attended centre-based childcare had better socio-emotional well-being and academic performance at age 9 when compared to children attending other forms of childcare (Byrne and O'Toole, 2015).

As with SureStart across the UK and Flying Start in Wales providing childcare provision in communities of low socio-economic status and deprivation, HeadStart in the United States has been situated within communities since 1965 (Barnett and Hustedt, 2005). Barnett and Hustedt (2005) discuss HeadStart in relation to educational benefits which are sustained over time. However, from a community perspective they state 'In addition, benefits transmitted through parents seem likely to diffuse to siblings, as well' (p.22). However, a study in England looking at educational attainment at ages 5, 7 and 11 with children aged 3 years who attended free childcare found only a small impact at age 5, which by age 11 had disappeared (Blanden et al., 2014).

Research on the benefits of children attending out-of-school childcare outside of the school curriculum (although many out-of-school clubs are run within school premises) is limited. A qualitative study by Barker et al. (2003) on the views of children, parents and staff of the out-of-school clubs found children had space to socialise and make new friendships and the childcare provision contributes to children's self-confidence and social skills. These benefits were also found by Smith's (2010) study in out-of-school provision. They also indicate parents thought the out-of-school care has a positive educational impact for their children, but this did not contribute to children's academic achievement. Another important aspect of out-of-school care identified by Barker et al. (2003) was how it promoted inclusivity with respect to children assessed to have special educational needs (SEN), minority ethnic children and children from deprived areas. As well as deprived areas, out-of-school childcare provision has also had a positive impact for children living in rural locations providing a space for children to meet and play (Smith and Barker, 2001).

Irrespective of the contradictory research evidence in relation to children attending childcare provision, the fact is that the childcare worker will play a role in children's health, development and well-being potentially from a very young age. This was reflected in the Effective Provision of Pre-School Education (EPPE) longitudinal project. The EPPE project aimed to investigate the effectiveness of pre-school education and children's development (Taggart et al., 2013). Although focusing on education provision, the overall results from this longitudinal study indicated 'pre-school experience, compared to none, enhances all-round development in children' (Sylva et al., 2004, p. 1). In addition to children's health and social care, childcare workers can also have a positive contribution to children's well-being with regards to attachment theory (Ainsworth and Bell, 1970; Bowlby, 1969). A brief and concise explanation of Bowlby's (1969) attachment theory is provided by the British Psychological Society (2007):

> 'Attachment theory suggests that infants are biologically predisposed to form attachment relationships from which they can experience security and comfort …. The attachment figure provides a secure base for the child. The child seeks this security when feeling threatened and uses the base as a platform for exploring and learning when the threat is reduced' (p. 2).

When a child feels threatened and scared, they will instantly migrate to the adult (in the first instance the mother or father) with whom they have formed a strong attachment (see Harlow and Zimmermann, 1959 experiments with isolated monkeys). In childcare provision, it is possible children will form attachments with childcare workers. Howes and Hamilton's (1992) study looked at attachment over a three-year period where the infant stayed with the same teacher (childcare worker) up to the age of 4 years. Their study found that where there was consistency between children and the same teacher, 'the child, teacher relationships were as stable as maternal relationships' (Howes and Hamilton, 1992, p. 871).

Another study by Howes and Smith (1995) on the child–caregiver relationship identified three profile types of difficult, avoiding and secure. The secure child–caregiver relationship was one where 'caregivers were more involved with the children in the secure profile than they were with the children in the avoiding or difficult profiles' (Howes and Smith, 1995, p. 59). This secure profile was reflected in Clasien et al.'s (2008) observational study of children and caregivers where 'higher frequencies of positive caregiving were associated with more security in the child–caregiver attachment relationship' (p. 466). These studies indicate the important role the childcare worker has in developing important attachments with children, and in particular supporting children's social development, as well as their health and well-being where the childcare worker, within the childcare environment, provides that secure base, an important role parents have.

THE INCREASING ROLE OF CHILDCARE IN THE COMMUNITY

The main drive of the National Childcare Strategy (DfEE, 1998) was to get adults, particularly mothers, back into the workforce, education or training and a recent study found parents still use childcare provision for both economic reasons (to work or look for work) or potential economic benefit (to study) (DfE, 2017b). With the increase in childcare provision over the last 20 years and the increased free childcare availability to 3- and 4-year-old children, the role of the childcare worker within the community has become just as important as that of teachers in schools. This is reflected where UK schools provide the space for most childcare provision to run (Butler and Rutter, 2016) and a survey of 1,000 parents in England, nearly 60 per cent had used childcare provision within a six-month period (Booth et al., 2013), this figure rising to 66 per cent in 2017 (DfE, 2017b).

The growth in childcare has seen in England 80,000 providers offering 2.8 million registered childcare places (DfE, 2018a) where 430,500 early years and childcare staff are employed (DfE, 2018b). In Wales, there are around 4,012 childcare providers, (including Welsh Medium provision run by Mudiad Meithrin) (Iorwerth, 2017) employing around 23,300 childcare workers (Welsh Government, 2017) offering up to 84,000 childcare places (Welsh Government, 2016). In Scotland, there are 9,726 childcare services providing 196,440 places (Care Inspectorate, 2017) where in 2010 there were 26,010 employed childcare workers (Scottish Government, 2010). In Northern Ireland, it was estimated in 2013 there were around 58,913 childcare places (Equality Commission, 2013). What is evident is childcare provision and the childcare worker have an important role in communities, ranging from the targeted provision with SureStart and Flying Start, day-care provision, out-of-school care provision to childminders. Robert Owen's first childcare provision was part of his philosophy 'aimed at making New Lanark a well-governed community based on his ideals' (Gordon, 1994, p. 280) of social and educational values that should be accessed by all. The National Childcare Strategy (DfEE, 1998) enabled adults to access education and training through the increase in childcare provision. However, this was based more on economic values, rather than the social values which Owen believed in (Gordon, 1994).

The evaluation of the New Opportunities Fund Out-of-school Childcare programme found parents felt they had a better work–life balance which had a positive effect on home life (SQW, 2003), which indicates a benefit more related to a community aspect. The important role of childcare within the community has been acknowledged in other countries. For example, in Australia, the early childcare workers support the community as 'they are creators of new and potentially more effective strategies for creating truly supportive provisions for families and children' (Black, 2004, p. 328). In Malawi, care for children aged between 3 and 5 years has provided both pre-primary school learning and care for orphans and other vulnerable children (Munthali et al., 2014). With the increasing childcare still expanding across the UK, for the Health and Social Care student this can offer an opportunity to work with children across a range of settings in diverse communities.

ACTIVITY 10.3

Go back to the table you created in Activity 10.2. After reading the sections around the research evidence, the role of the childcare worker and growth of childcare provision within communities, what would you keep, add or change?

CONCLUSION

This chapter has discussed the role childcare workers have in respect of health and social care, from the historical background where the first nursery set up by Robert Owen was to address social needs, to the varied childcare provision currently available throughout the United Kingdom. Childcare provision is heavily regulated since the publication of the Children Act 1989 and subsequent legislation in England, Wales, Scotland and Northern Ireland. Although the research evidence is contradictory with respect to the benefits of childcare, childcare provision requires qualified and professionally competent staff who have an important role in supporting children's health, development and well-being within their communities.

GO FURTHER ACTIVITY

What are the different types of childcare provision available where you live? See if you can find out how many playgroups, day-care centres and after-school clubs there are. One tip, many local authorities have Family Information Centres which may have the information you need.

FURTHER READING

Booth, C., Kostadintcheva, K., Knox, A. and Bram, A. (2013). Parents' views and experiences of childcare. Available at https://assets.publishing.service.gov.uk/government/uploads/system/uploads/attachment_data/file/212589/DFE-RR266.pdf.

Bretherton, I. (1992). The origins of attachment theory: John Bowlby and Mary Ainsworth. *Developmental Psychology* 28, 759–775.

Cranwell, K. (2003). Towards playwork: an historical introduction to children's out-of-school play organizations in London (1860–1940). In F. Brown (ed.), *Playwork Theory and Practice* (pp. 32–48). Maidenhead: Open University Press.

Faulkner, D. and Coates, E. A. (2013). Early childhood policy and practice in England: twenty years of change. *International Journal of Early Years Education* 21(2/3), 244–263.

Felfe, C. and Lalive, R. (2012). *Early Child Care and Child Development: For Whom it Works and Why*. Discussion Paper No. 7100. Available at: http://ftp.iza.org/dp7100.pdf.

Jarvis, P. and Liebovitch, B. (2015). British nurseries, head and heart: McMillan, Owen and the genesis of the education/care dichotomy. *Women's History Review* 24(6), 917–937.

REFERENCES

Ainsworth, M. D. S. and Bell, S. M. (1970). Attachment, exploration, and separation: Illustrated by the behavior of one-year-olds in a strange situation. *Child Development* 41, 49–67.

Baker, M. and Milligan, K. (2010). Evidence from maternity leave expansions of the impact of maternal care on early child development. *Journal of Human Resources* 45, 1–32.

Baker, M. and Milligan, K. (2012). Maternity leave and children's cognitive and behavioural development. NBER working paper, NBER.

Barker, J., Smith, F., Morrow, V., Weller, S., Hey, V. and Harwin, J. (2003). *The Impact of Out-of-school Care: A Qualitative Study Examining the Views of Children, Families and Playworkers.* Nottingham: Department for Education and Skills.

Barnett, W. S. and Hustedt, J. T. (2005). Head Start's lasting benefits. *Infants & Young Children* 18(1), 16–24.

Baum II, C. L. (2003). Does early maternal employment harm child development? An analysis of the potential benefits of leave taking. *Journal of Labor Economics* 21(2), 409–448.

Black, A. (2004). Investing in early childhood: creating a community of care for children and families. In E. McWilliam, S. Danby and J. Knight (eds), *Performing Educational Research: Theories, Methods and Practices* (pp. 319–330). Flaxton: Post Pressed.

Blanden, J., Del Bono, E., Hansen, K., McNally, S. and Rabe, B. (2014). The impact of free early education for 3 year olds in England. Available at: www.ifs.org.uk/uploads/publications/docs/MISOC%20Childcare%20briefing%20paper.pdf.

Bonel, P. and Lindon, J. (1996). *Good Practice in Playwork*. Cheltenham: Stanley Thornes (Publishers) Ltd.

Bonetti, S. (2019). *The Early Years Workforce in England: A Comparative Analysis Using the Labour Force Survey*. Available at: https://epi.org.uk/wp-content/uploads/2019/01/The-early-years-workforce-in-England_EPI.pdf.

Booth, C., Kostadintcheva, K., Knox, A. and Bram, A. (2013). *Parents' Views and Experiences of Childcare: Research Report*. Available at https://assets.publishing.service.gov.uk/government/uploads/system/uploads/attachment_data/file/212589/DFE-RR266.pdf.

Bowlby J. (1969). *Attachment. Attachment and Loss: Vol. 1*. New York: Basic Books.

Bradburn, E. (1966). Britain's first nursery infant school. *The Elementary School Journal* 67(2), 57-63

Butler, A. and Rutter, J. (2016). Joseph Roundtree Foundation Programme Paper: An anti-poverty strategy for the UK: creating an anti-poverty childcare system. Available at: www.activematters.org/uploads/pdfs/anti_pov_childcare_full.pdf.

Byrne, D. and O'Toole, C. (2015). *The Influence of Childcare Arrangements on Child Wellbeing from Infancy to Middle Childhood: Technical Report*. Túsla in association with Maynooth University.

Caldwell, B. M. (1989). All-day kindergarten – assumptions, precautions, and overgeneralizations. *Early Childhood Research Quarterly* 4, 261–266.

Care Inspectorate (2017). Scotland's early learning and childcare – an initial overview of the expansion of provision during 2014/15: Implementing Parts 6, 7 and 8 of the Children and Young People (Scotland) Act (2014). Dundee: Care Inspectorate.

Clasien De Schipper, J., Tavecchio, L. W. C. and Van IJzendoorn, M. H. (2008). Children's attachment relationships with day care caregivers: associations with positive caregiving and the child's temperament. *Social Development* 17(3), 454–470.

Cranwell, K. (2003) Towards playwork: an historical introduction to children's out-of-school play organizations in London (1860–1940). In F. Brown (ed.), *Playwork Theory and Practice* (pp. 32–48). Maidenhead: Open University Press.

Department for Education and Employment (DfEE) (1998). *Meeting the Childcare Challenge*. Green Paper. London: HMSO.

Department for Education (2013). Sure Start children's centres statutory guidance: for local authorities, commissioners of local health services and Jobcentre Plus. Available at: https://assets.publishing.service.gov.uk/government/uploads/system/uploads/attachment_data/file/678913/childrens_centre_stat_guidance_april-2013.pdf

Department for Education (2017a). *Statutory Framework for the Early Years Foundation Stage: Setting the Standards for Learning, Development and Care for Children from Birth to Five*. London: Department for Education.

Department for Education (2017b). *Childcare and Early Years Survey of Parents in England*. Available at: https://assets.publishing.service.gov.uk/government/uploads/system/uploads/attachment_data/file/669857/SFR73_2017_Text.pdf

Department for Education (2018a). *Early Education and Childcare: Operational Guidance*. London: Department for Education.

Department for Education (2018b). *Survey of Childcare and Early Years Providers: Main Summary, England*, 2018. Available at: https://assets.publishing.service.gov.uk/government/uploads/system/uploads/attachment_data/file/752919/Survey_of_Childcare_and_Early_Years_Providers_2018_Main_Summary3.pdf

Department for Health, Social Services and Public Safety (2012). *Childminding and Day Care for Children Aged Under 12: Minimum Standards*. Available at: http://childcarepartnerships.hscni.net/wp-content/uploads/2017/04/Minimum-Standards-2012.pdf

Dustmann, C. and Schönberg, U. (2011). Expansions in maternity leave coverage and children's long-term outcomes. *American Economic Journal: Applied Economics* 2011 4(3), 190–224.

Edexcel (2006) *NVQ Guidance for Candidates*. Available at https://qualifications.pearson.com/content/dam/pdf/NVQ-and-competence-based-qualifications/2010/Teaching-and-learning-materials/NVQ-guidance-for-candidates.pdf

Employers in Childcare (2018). *Free Pre-school Places*. Available at www.employersforchildcare.org/app/uploads/2016/10/Free-Preschool-Places.pdf

Equality Commission (2013). *Childcare: Maximising the Economic Participation of Women*. Available at: www.equalityni.org/ECNI/media/ECNI/Publications/Delivering%20Equality/MaximisingChildcareMainReport2013.pdf

Faculty for Children and Young People, Division of Clinical Psychology, British Psychological Society (2007). Briefing Paper No.2: Attachment theory into practice. Available at: www1.bps.org.uk/system/files/Public%20files/DCP/cat-378.pdf

Faulkner, D. and Coates, E. A. (2013). Early childhood policy and practice in England: twenty years of change. *International Journal of Early Years Education* 21(2/3), 244–263.

Glover, A., Harries, S., Lane, J. and Lewis, S. (2018). *Evaluation of the Early Implementation of the Childcare Offer for Wales*. Cardiff: Welsh Government.

Gomajee, R., El-Khoury, F., Côté, S., van der Waerden, J., Pryor, L. and Melchior, M. (2018). Early childcare type predicts children's emotional and behavioural trajectories into middle childhood. Data from the EDEN mother–child cohort study. *Epidemiol Community Health* 72, 1033–1043.

Gordon, P. (1994). Robert Owen (1771–1858). *PROSPECTS* 24(1/2), 279–296.

Harlow, H. F. and Zimmermann, R. R. (1959). Affectional responses in infant monkeys: orphaned baby monkeys develop a strong and persistent attachment to inanimate surrogate mothers. *Science* 130(3373), 421–432.

Howes, C. and Hamilton, C. E. (1992). Children's relationships with child care teachers: stability and concordance with parental attachments. *Child Development* 63(4), 867–878.

Howes, C. and Smith, E. W. (1995). Children and their child care caregivers: profiles of relationships. *Social Development* 4, 44–61.

Iorwerth, H. (2017). *Briefing Note: Welsh Medium Childcare and Early Years Education Provision*. Cardiff: Welsh Language Commissioner.

James-Burdumy, S. (2005). The Effect of Maternal Labor Force Participation on Child Development. *Journal of Labor Economics*, 23(1), 177211.

Jarrett, T. (2018). Childcare: '30 hours' of free childcare – eligibility, access codes and charges (England). Available at:file:///C:/Users/Dr%20Pete%20King/Downloads/CBP-8051.pdf

Jarvis, P. and Liebovitch, B. (2015). British nurseries, head and heart: McMillan, Owen and the genesis of the education/care dichotomy. *Women's History Review* 24(6), 917–937.

Kamerman, S. B. (2006). Background paper prepared for the Education for All Global Monitoring Report 2007 Strong foundations: early childhood care and education: A global history of early childhood education and care. Available at www.ecdgroup.com/docs/lib_003972023.pdf

King, P. and Sills-Jones, P. (2018). Children's use of public spaces and the role of the adult – a comparison of play ranging in the UK, and the leikkipuisto (Play Parks) in Finland. *International Journal of Play* 7(1), 27–40.

Liu, Q. and Skans, O. N. (2010). The duration of paid parental leave and children's scholastic performance. *The B.E. Journal of Economic Analysis & Policy* 10(1), Article 3.

Munthali, A. C., Mvula, P. M. and Silo, L. (2014). Early childhood development: the role of community based childcare centres in Malawi. *SpringerPlus* 3(305), 1–10.

National Assembly for Wales Children, Young People and Education Committee (2018). Flying Start: Outreach. Available at: www.assembly.wales/laid%20documents/cr-ld11425/cr-ld11425-e.pdf

Rasmussen, A. W. (2010). Increasing the length of parents' birth-related leave: the effect on children's long-term educational outcomes. *Labour Economics* 17, 91–100.

Scottish Government (2005). National Care Standards early education and childcare up to the age of 16. Available at: www2.gov.scot/resource/doc/37432/0010250.pdf.

Scottish Government (2010). Pre-School and Childcare Statistics 2010. Available at: www2.gov.scot/Resource/Doc/326162/0105080.pdf

Scottish Government (2017). *A Blueprint for 2020: The Expansion of Early Learning and Childcare in Scotland 2017–18 Action Plan*. Edinburgh: Scottish Government.

Scottish Parliament (2014). Children and Young People (Scotland) Act 2014. Available at: www.legislation.gov.uk/asp/2014/8/pdfs/asp_20140008_en.pdf

Smith, H. H. (2010). Children's empowerment, play and informal learning in two after school club provision. Unpublished doctoral dissertation, Middlesex University.

Smith, F. and Barker, J. (2000). Contested spaces: children's experiences of out-of-school care in England and Wales. *Childhood* 7(3), 315–333.

Smith, F. and Barker, J. (2001). Commodifying the Countryside: The Impact of Out-of-School Care on Rural Landscapes of Children's Play. *Area* 33(2), 169–176.

SQW (2003). *Evaluation of the Out-of-school Childcare Initiative: Final Report*. Cambridge: SQW Limited.

SureStart (2003). *Full Day Care: National Standards for Under 8s Day Care and Childminding*. Nottingham: Department for Education and Skills.

Sylva, K., Melhuish, E., Sammons, P., Siraj-Blatchford, I. and Taggart, B. (2004). The Effective Provision of Pre-School Education (EPPE) Project: Findings from Pre-school to end of Key Stage1. http://dera.ioe.ac.uk/8543/7/SSU-SF-2004-01.pdf

Taggart, B., Sammons, P., Sylva, K., Melhuish, E., Siraj-Blatchford, I., Elliot, K. and Walker-Hal, K. (2013). The Effective Provision of Pre-School Education [EPPE] Project: A Longitudinal Study funded by the DfEE (1997–2003). Available at: www.ucl.ac.uk/ioe/research/pdf/Ratios_in_Pre-School_Settings_DfEE.pdf

UK Parliament (1870). Early Elementary Education Act 1870. Available at: www.educationengland.org.uk/documents/acts/1870-elementary-education-act.pdf

UK Parliament (1918). Education Act 1918. Available at: www.parliament.uk/about/living-heritage/transformingsociety/parliament-and-the-first-world-war/legislation-and-acts-of-war/education-act-1918

UK Parliament (1989). Children Act 1989. Available at: www.legislation.gov.uk/ukpga/1989/41/contents

UK Parliament (2000). Care Standards Act 2000. Available at: www.legislation.gov.uk/ukpga/2000/14/pdfs/ukpga_20000014_en.pdf

UK Parliament (2004). Children Act 2004. Available at: www.legislation.gov.uk/ukpga/2004/31/pdfs/ukpga_20040031_en.pdf

UK Parliament (2006). Children Act 2006. Available at: www.legislation.gov.uk/ukpga/2006/21/pdfs/ukpga_20060021_en.pdf

UK Parliament (2016). Childcare Act 2016. Available at: www.legislation.gov.uk/ukpga/2016/5/pdfs/ukpga_20160005_en.pdf

UK Parliament (2018a). Living Heritage Reforming Society in the 19th century: early factory legislation, Available at: www.parliament.uk/about/living-heritage/transformingsociety/livinglearning/19thcentury/overview/earlyfactorylegislation/

UK Parliament (2018b). Living Heritage Reforming Society in the 19th century: the 1833 Factory Act. Available at: www.parliament.uk/about/living-heritage/transformingsociety/livinglearning/19thcentury/overview/factoryact/

Welsh Government (2013). *Building a Brighter Future: Early Years and Childcare Plan*. Cardiff: Welsh Government.

Welsh Government (2016). National Minimum Standards for Regulated Childcare for children up to the age of 12 years. Available at: https://careinspectorate.wales/sites/default/files/2018-01/160411regchildcareen.pdf

Welsh Government (2017). *Childcare, Play and Early Years Workforce Plan*. Cardiff: Welsh Government.

Welsh Government (2018). *Foundation Phase Nursery: A Guide for Parents and Carers*. Cardiff: Welsh Government.

West, A. and Noden, P. (2016). Public funding of early years education in England: an historical perspective. Clare Market Papers, 21. London School of Economics and Political Science, Department of Social Policy, London.

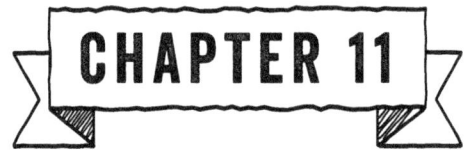

CHAPTER 11

HEALTH PROMOTION AND HEALTH PSYCHOLOGY

*Michelle Anderson and
Llewellyn Morgan*

OVERVIEW

Diseases of lifestyle (otherwise known as non-communicable diseases) are a major challenge facing the National Health Service (NHS). The cost of poor lifestyle choices and resulting disease has been estimated to cost the NHS £7 out of every £10 spent (Musgrove, 2017). The link between behaviours and the subsequent development of chronic disease is irrefutable. Therefore, promoting healthy behaviour and positive behaviour change within the population has become a vital undertaking and is a responsibility of every professional working within the field of health. This is, however, a complex and multifaceted task, which draws upon the skills of those working in not only health care but also the wider public sector. The development of interventions such as Making Every Contact Count (MECC) has meant that all workers who encounter the public can be trained to provide positive health messages and direct the public towards sources of help. Although seemingly simplistic, these interventions are based upon various theories, models and approaches to behavioural ideation, intention and change.

LEARNING OUTCOMES

By the end of this chapter you will be able to:

- Identify the scale and effects of lifestyle choices on health
- Discuss health promotion in the context of behaviour change
- Examine the underpinning theory supporting interventions like MECC
- Discuss behavioural change through approaches such as motivational interviewing and cognitive behavioural therapy
- Discuss and apply these theories to a variety of common lifestyle issues such as smoking, physical activity, substance abuse and healthy eating

INTRODUCTION

Public Health England (2016) identified the cost to the NHS of lifestyle choices at approximately £11 billion per year in England alone. This could be seen as a rather conservative estimate with the true cost being 70 per cent of the overall NHS annual budget nationally (Musgrove, 2017). The media regularly sensationalise and vilify those they deem to be responsible – smokers, drinkers, 'couch potatoes' and drug users – when in reality we all do things that are seen as unhealthy in varying degrees.

The personal costs of chronic and long-term conditions are often overlooked. It is these costs that increase the overall burden on services with effects felt in all sectors of health, social care and the wider public sector. Additionally, the contributors to these behaviours are often discounted or seen as not important. A further consideration must also be given in relation to the social determinants of health such as housing, employment status and education as examples, as these have an impact when addressing health and lifestyle factors during health behavioural change interventions (Green et al., 2018). They are, however, fundamental to the behaviours seen and these aspects must be acknowledged when trying to address health-related behaviour, as they may well influence how successful the change is viewed or implemented.

Health promotion, under the umbrella of public health, has been charged with developing new and innovative ways of delivering evidence-based approaches to address health and lifestyle behaviours. Many of these draw upon theories and models that come from a psychological perspective. Within this chapter some of the various theories that underpin health promotion and behaviour change will be explored.

THE SCALE AND EFFECTS OF LIFESTYLE CHOICES ON HEALTH

There are strong links between behaviours and subsequent disease development, yet people continue to carry out health-damaging behaviours. So surely if people are told the consequences of their behaviours they will stop? Isn't it easy not to smoke, drink, take more exercise and eat well? The answer, unfortunately, is no. Behaviours result from complex conscious and unconscious decisions influenced by numerous factors. These will be discussed later in the chapter. Ayers and De Visser (2018) further suggest where and who the information comes from may also have an impact on an individual's willingness or ability to change. This can be linked to the psychological concepts of the locus of control and theory of self-efficacy which will be explained later in this chapter.

Marmot (2010) identifies that health inequalities will have an effect on people's lifestyle and health choices and can contribute to the impact of non-communicable diseases (NCDs). Furthermore, Marmot (2010) also suggests that health inequalities are those factors which are preventable but arise from the unequal differences in the distribution of resources within society. This can impact on an individual's ability to prevent illness or access treatment when illness occurs, and this is evident in the presenting behaviours of the population which are affected by health inequality. The World Health Organization give a stark warning about NCDs. The WHO (2017) state that non-communicable diseases kill 41 million people each year, equivalent to 71 per cent of all deaths globally. The main types of NCDs identified are cardiovascular diseases, respiratory diseases, diabetes and cancers. What is more concerning is that these deaths are mostly preventable and are attributed to four main behaviours – tobacco use, physical inactivity, the harmful use of alcohol and unhealthy diets all increase the risk of dying from an NCD (WHO, 2017).

In the UK rates of these behaviours remain worryingly high. In Wales smoking rates have dropped, though are still at approximately 19 per cent of the population (Welsh Government, 2018) overall, but there are huge regional variations often related to social class. People living in Rhondda Cynon Taf, which is an area that is identified as having lower social class/socio-economic conditions, are seven times more likely to smoke than those living in the more affluent county of Powys. This is replicated over the entire United Kingdom and demonstrates the effect of deprivation upon health-related behaviours.

Obesity is rarely out of the news and its links with physical activity and diet make concerning reading especially in relation to young people. In England in 2016–2017, there were 617,000 hospital admissions where obesity proved a factor, which was an 18 per cent increase from 2015/2016 (NHS Digital, 2018a). Furthermore, 26 per cent of adults are classified as obese (NHS Digital, 2018a). From a gender perspective, 40 per cent of men were deemed to be overweight (27 per cent were classified as obese) and 31 per cent of women were classified as overweight (30 per cent were classified as obese) (NHS Digital, 2018b).

In addition, one in ten children in school reception classes, and one in five children in school year six were classified as being obese (NHS Digital, 2018a). 'Children in most deprived areas are twice as likely to be obese than children in least deprived areas' (Health and Social Care Information Service, 2016, p. 2). There are also contrasts between England and Wales in terms of childhood obesity. Current statistics in Wales for reception-aged children (those aged between 4 and 5 years old) indicate that 27.1 per cent of children in Wales are overweight or obese, compared to 22.6 per cent in England with those children living in Wales at significantly more risk of being obese if they live in areas of high social deprivation (Public Health Wales, 2018).

Within Wales there are also stark contrasts in terms of how obesity presents. For example, the highest prevalence is in Merthyr Tydfil (recognised as an area with a high prevalence of social deprivation) with 17.5 per cent of children obese which is more than double when compared to 7.8 per cent of children presenting as obese in the Vale of Glamorgan – an area with low levels of social deprivation (Public Health Wales, 2018). This potentially means we are 'storing up' significant health risks in the future for people living in socially deprived areas. This means that if this does not change then there is a risk that they will go on to develop some form of related NCD.

The proportion of adolescent boys who met the weekly physical activity guidelines of 60 minutes per day fell from 28 per cent in 2008, to less than 20 per cent in 2018 (Public Health Wales, 2019). The proportion of girls who met the weekly physical activity guidelines fell from 19 per cent in 2008 to less than 10 per cent in 2018 (Public Health Wales, 2019). For adults in Wales, 54 per cent of adults undertake the recommended 150 minutes of physical activity per week; however, the rate for females is lower than that of males across all ages (Public Health Wales, 2019). Worryingly, the percentage of adults meeting physical activity guidelines is 15 per cent higher in the least deprived areas compared with the most deprived areas.

In relation to diet within the UK, the percentage eating five or more portions of fruit or vegetables a day was 26 per cent for England, 20 per cent for Scotland and 32 per cent for Wales (NHS Digital, 2018a). Again, there is a strong link with social deprivation where rates were poorer still. This is strongly supported in Obesity in Wales (Public Health Wales, 2019) which found one in ten Welsh residents reported that they could not always afford to eat a balanced diet and one in twenty often worried that they would run out of food before having enough money to buy more.

However, given the current financial climate, this can make it a challenging area to address in practice. The guidelines provided by the NHS in relation to healthy eating could also fuel these opinions because they could be viewed as difficult or impossible to achieve for some individuals, because of what they consider to be the increased cost of eating healthily, which they may not be able to afford to do so. Individuals may also need to access the increasing number of food banks in order to feed themselves and their families, and often the food parcels provided do not provide for what could be considered a healthy diet when compared to NHS guidelines around this. This then requires health professionals to adapt how they approach giving advice around healthy eating using approaches outlined with Making Every Contact Count (discussed later in this chapter), thus tailoring advice to individual need.

Alcohol consumption rates have also shown a concerning increase. In 2015/16 there were 41,161 alcohol-related inpatient hospital admissions in Scotland. This equates to 6.4 per cent of all hospital admissions with men being twice as likely as women to be admitted to hospital (NHS Health Scotland, 2018). An inequality gap for alcohol-related admissions between those living in the most and least deprived parts of Scotland was again seen. Conversely, around one in five adults in Wales report to drink above guidelines, with higher rates in the less deprived areas and this is attributed predominately to occupational stressors (Public Health Wales, 2019).

All of the above factors have resulted in an increase in lifestyle-related conditions, which has had, and will continue to have, a massive impact on health care provision and services as well as societal and personal impact.

HEALTH PROMOTION AND BEHAVIOUR CHANGE

Promoting health is a complex multifaceted task. Health is dependent not only on individual choices about how we live our lives but is also affected by numerous other variables such as social, demographic as well as psychological factors. It would appear that by encouraging individuals to simply live a healthier lifestyle then many of the NCDs we currently see would disappear. However, for an individual to make any change it is necessary to go through a complex psychological process which is affected by internal and external factors, and may be mitigated by their motivation to make any form of behavioural change, which complicates matters further.

Health education has always been a mainstay of health promotion and involves a mix of behavioural advice and risk communication, which aimed to elicit positive behaviour change. In psychology, this is described as a social cognitive approach, which assumes that behavioural choices are a reflection of how people see and view the world (Upton and Thirlaway, 2016). Any decisions related to an individual changing their behaviour involves, at a fundamental level, a cost–benefit analysis. So, an obese patient may see the cost involved in eating a healthy diet as not eating high-calorie fat-rich foods which are enjoyable versus the benefit of being slimmer and healthier, but this is over-simplistic. There are numerous other variables that will affect that decision, and as a result a number of models of change have been developed based around the cost–benefit model, which expands on this basic principle.

The following section aims to discuss some of these models of change and to develop theoretically focused strategies when working with individuals and their families, which are based on the five key approaches to health promotion.

APPROACHES TO PROMOTING HEALTH

Naidoo and Wills (2016) identify five main approaches that can be taken when promoting health with individuals, families, communities and populations:

- Medical
- Behavioural

- Educational
- Empowerment
- Social change

Each of these approaches has differing aims and methods, which will be discussed further.

MEDICAL

As the name suggests this approach is based around the traditional medical model prevalent in health services and aims to reduce mortality and premature morbidity. Its aim is the prevention of disease at three differing levels:

1   Primary – preventing onset of a disease state through risk education – immunisation, encouraging healthy lifestyles.
2   Secondary – preventing disease progression through early identification – screening for diseases such as cancer where it is still deemed to be treatable.
3   Tertiary – preventing an illness reoccurring or reducing further disability or improving quality of life – palliation, rehabilitation.

The medical approach is expert-led, often instigated because of epidemiological data. It has been used throughout public health and has seen large gains in population and individual health through immunisation and screening however the shortcomings of this approach must be recognised in that it ignores the socio-economic determinants of health and can be deemed as victim blaming when those who do not uptake the services offered become ill.

BEHAVIOURAL

The behaviour change approach is perhaps the most widely used health promotion method which aims to encourage individuals to adopt healthy behaviours. It assumes that by providing information individuals will choose to change their lifestyles but, as with the medical approach, does not take into account the effect of socio-economic factors and the influence they will have on behaviour. This approach can be used with individuals (making changes in diet) or through mass media (stop smoking campaigns).

EDUCATIONAL

The educational approach is sometimes confused with the behaviour change approach because of the provision of information. However, its aim is not to elicit change in behaviour but instead to provide the individual with knowledge, so they can then make a voluntary choice about their health. This approach works through the provision of knowledge and information which in turn aids individuals to develop the skills necessary to make informed decisions about their health and health-related choices. This approach again ignores the socio-economic determinants of health, and the psychological complexities of decision-making, which will be further discussed later in this chapter.

EMPOWERMENT

This approach aims to work with individuals and communities to enable them to identify and meet their own perceived needs. The role of the health promoter within this approach differs to the previous three approaches outlined in that they act as a facilitator only, withdrawing as the change grows and develops. Unlike the previous approaches discussed the empowerment approach can be seen to be proactive and allows recognition of socio-economic factors that may affect the individual or community. The empowerment approach can be used very successfully. However, it must be recognised that the issues identified are those perceived as important to the patient and this process cannot be influenced by the health care practitioner.

SOCIAL CHANGE

Also known as radical health promotion, the social change approach aims to bring change in the physical, social and economic environment to promote health. At times, this may require a legislative change to enact, such as no smoking bans in enclosed public places and seat-belt use in cars. Although this approach is often seen as beyond the remit of the health professional there are times when it will be utilised, for example provision of health profiles, research and lobbying through professional organisations. This approach can also be used within organisations, for example healthy eating in a staff canteen.

All of the above approaches have advantages and disadvantages. When used in combination they are usually more successful.

ACTIVITY 11.1

Try to answer the following questions:

- What are the pros and cons of each approach?
- What areas of health promotion could these approaches be applied to?
- What media campaigns using these approaches are you aware of?

Check the end of the chapter for an answer to this activity.

HEALTH PSYCHOLOGY: AN INTRODUCTION

Naidoo and Wills (2016: 322) define health psychology as 'a discipline that seeks to understand the psychological and behavioural processes in health, illness, and healthcare'. In other words, it seeks to study how people perceive the effects of health or ill-health and its impact upon them, and how they negotiate their way through the health care system as part of addressing this. Alongside this is how individuals perceive the impact of a health-related diagnosis and its effects upon their social functioning, and whether they feel able to deal with this appropriately or whether they believe they are not able to deal with, or cope with, this.

Bandura (1994) defined this coping concept further and termed it self-efficacy. Thus, a person with a notion of high self-efficacy has a stronger internal belief that they are able to cope with a condition due to various personal factors such as a positive support network of family and friends, a well-paid secure job, a good level of education, and so on. Whereas a person with a notion of low self-efficacy has a weaker internal belief that they will be able to cope with the condition, and thus are less likely to believe that they can. This also may be due to various factors which can influence this such as social isolation, lack of support network, poor access to health care, lack of transport, and so on. The term self-efficacy can be viewed as a continuum with individuals moving up and down this (i.e. from low to high, or high to low) at different stages based on individual perceptions and circumstances. Thus, it is a dynamic concept as opposed to a static one. As shown in the above description individual views related to the social determinants of health also can influence this individual self-efficacy concept to a greater or lesser extent, dependent on individual resilience and their perceptions of being in control of the situation that they find themselves in (Prestwich et al., 2018).

If we apply this notion of self-efficacy to health behaviour change those who view themselves as having strong internal motivation to change would be considered to have high self-efficacy, and are therefore more likely to make and adapt to that change, because they see themselves as capable of making and sustaining the change. Whereas those who are being told to change lack motivation to change (i.e. they say they want to make a change, but demonstrate no inclination to change), or who lack the appropriate support to instigate that change would be considered to have low self-efficacy and thus are less likely to make that change (Prestwich et al., 2018), as they may not feel in control. Consequently, they may not feel capable of making the change even if appropriate support and facilitation is provided (Corcoran, 2013).

Therefore, for health practitioners working with people interested in undertaking any form of health behaviour change, due consideration needs to be given regarding the individual's motivation for that change. This can be linked into various health-promotion models which will be discussed later in this chapter. Furthermore, assessment of readiness or willingness to change has to be undertaken in conjunction with the person seeking to make the change, so that appropriate support can be provided to assist them with this (Green et al., 2018; Prestwich, et al., 2018). Support will vary depending on the needs of the individual and potentially may need to be provided over a long-term period, in order to successfully achieve the planned change. This may well impact on individual notions of self-efficacy, which in turn may impact on the success of the health behaviour change, and this must be considered and planned for, as part of this change process (Prestwich, et al., 2018).

Tools or techniques such as Making Every Contact Count or Motivational Interviewing may assist here in empowering individuals to successfully make the relevant health changes. Through utilising these tools it may allow a person to change their perception of not being in control of the change to one of being in control as a result of being empowered to do so, which in turn may well affect their individual self-efficacy. As can be seen this is potentially a cyclical process and can predict where a person sees themselves on the self-efficacy continuum, and may also give some underlying prediction of how motivated they are to successfully make and sustain a behavioural change.

MAKING EVERY CONTACT COUNT (MECC)

Making Every Contact Count (Public Health Wales, 2017) provides a web-based learning resource for anyone who has contact with members of the general public. The tool provides information about how to make the most of the opportunities to help people lead healthier lives. This tool is based around the principles of brief intervention which relates to available face-to-face time with patients as opposed to any particular theory. Within MECC the conversation you have with the person is the intervention. It does not need to be long or involved and usually is less than five minutes in duration. The main aim of brief intervention is concentration upon the change needed underpinned by the following principles:

1   Educating about risks of current behaviour.
2   Emphasis of patient's responsibility towards their health.
3   Provision of advice about making a change.
4   Exploring strategies and methods for changing.
5   Action planning in collaboration with the patient.

Another method is Motivational Interviewing (Rollnick and Miller, 2012) which draws on the principles of cognitive behavioural therapy used within mental health and aims to:

1   Build an empathetic relationship with the patient about the health issue and need to change.
2   Advantages and disadvantages of the change for the individual are discussed.
3   Resistance to change is seen as a normal part of the process.
4   Support autonomy in changing the behaviour.

The goal of this method is one of empowerment of the patient and allows them to identify their own strategies and goals to achieve. Within motivational interviewing the health professional acts as a facilitator to enable the person to come up with their own solutions, in order to plan a potentially successful change (Prestwich et al., 2018).

MODELS OF BEHAVIOUR CHANGE

There are numerous models that aim to explain the many complexities of behaviour change and how people move to healthier behaviours. Many come from the fields of health psychology or learning theory. While it is beyond the remit of this chapter to fully explore them all, the key models will be outlined that explain intention to change and the actual change process.

Understanding why people behave in a particular way is central to planning health-promotion interventions. Factors that can inhibit or encourage the intervention must be taken into account to enable the practitioner to fully support the individual. No one will make a change to their behaviour in isolation. There are both internal and external factors which will affect decisions such as education, culture, family, environment, income and peer pressure (Anderson, 2015). In addition to this, as discussed above, individual notions of self-efficacy also add an additional layer of complexity to the change process and this also may be mitigated by the above factors as described by Anderson (2015).

A number of theories have been developed to try to explain the different factors that will affect individual health-related behaviours. These theories suggest that an individual's behaviour is determined by their attitude towards that behaviour. For example, an individual may smoke despite thinking that it is an unhealthy behaviour or eat an extra helping of food even though they are trying to decrease their weight. Attitudes are developed from two parts – cognitive (knowledge and information) and affective (feelings and emotions). Attitudes to behaviour are influenced by beliefs held towards that action or intention. For example, a smoker may believe that smoking helps to calm them but if the person is then encouraged to believe that smoking is a stimulant their belief may alter. This view of beliefs is identified in a relatively simplistic model known as knowledge-attitudes-beliefs (KAB) which views a change in behaviour as a result of information alone. The giving of information only, as seen in numerous early health campaigns, has proven to be ineffective and does not automatically lead to behaviour change (Naidoo and Wills, 2016).

Other factors that influence behaviour include values, which are developed through socialisation and are an emotional belief and drives, which are described as strong motivating factors. The term drive can be used to describe addictions or factors such as hunger.

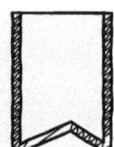

PAUSE FOR THOUGHT 11.1

Try to think of a behaviour you have which is perceived as not being healthy. For example, you may not exercise regularly, not eat enough fruit or vegetables or smoke.

Write down the internal and external factors that may contribute to or influence this behaviour.

Check the end of the chapter for an answer to this activity.

HEALTH PSYCHOLOGY THEORIES AND MODELS

These theories come from cognition models, social cognition models and empowerment models, all of which must be considered when helping a person to change behaviour.

HEALTH BELIEF MODEL (BECKER, 1974, 1988; JANZ AND BECKER, 1984)

This is perhaps the most widely recognised model that shows how beliefs affect decision-making. These beliefs in turn will affect the feasibility of the individual changing their behaviour, and in many ways this takes the form of a cost/benefit analysis. When considering, for example, attending a screening appointment or making a health-related behaviour change, the individual will consider their perceived susceptibility to and severity of a disease against the costs and benefits of undertaking or altering behaviour. Often this model is used to predict protective health behaviour and compliance with medical advice.

Ayers and De Visser (2018: 117) identify that the health belief model is 'the only model that explicitly recognises the importance of the cues to action that will prompt people to change'. This indicates an acknowledgement that other external factors will influence how a person will view the planned change. Corcoran (2013) and Ayers and De Visser (2018) also suggest that the health education messages must be presented in the right way to have an impact upon the individual in order for them to potentially view the health harming behaviour as a risk. Thus by doing so will mean that the individual then views the threat to the health and how susceptible they are to this threat in order to make the change.

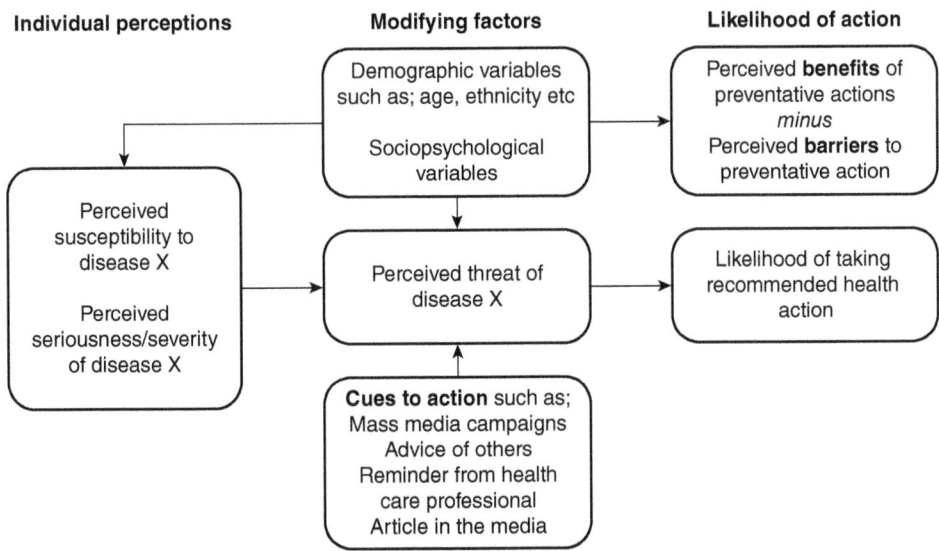

Figure 11.1 Health belief model (Becker, 1974) modified from Janz and Becker (1984)

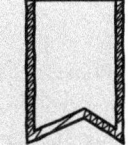

PAUSE FOR THOUGHT 11.2

Think about a health-related behaviour you intend to undertake and try to apply the HBM to it. For example, you may have a screening appointment to attend, have joined a gym to get fitter or stopped smoking. What factors will help or hinder you to achieve this?

THEORIES OF REASONED ACTION AND PLANNED BEHAVIOUR (AJZEN AND FISHBEIN, 2005)

This theory suggests that individual behaviour is a result of two factors, attitudes and subjective norms. These are influenced by beliefs, motivation and personal evaluations. These two factors combine to form a behavioural intention. Ajzen and Fishbein (2005) acknowledge that behavioural intention is not always consistent and may be affected by the stability of their beliefs and the effect of social norms. For example, a group of friends may go out on a weekend and one has decided not to drink alcohol; however, pressure is exerted to join in and drink alcohol. Not wanting to be perceived as a killjoy or outsider the person may then drink.

THE HEALTH LOCUS OF CONTROL THEORY (ROTTER, 1954)

Locus of control relates to an individual's perception of control over events. The theory suggests that those with a strong internal locus of control are more likely to change their

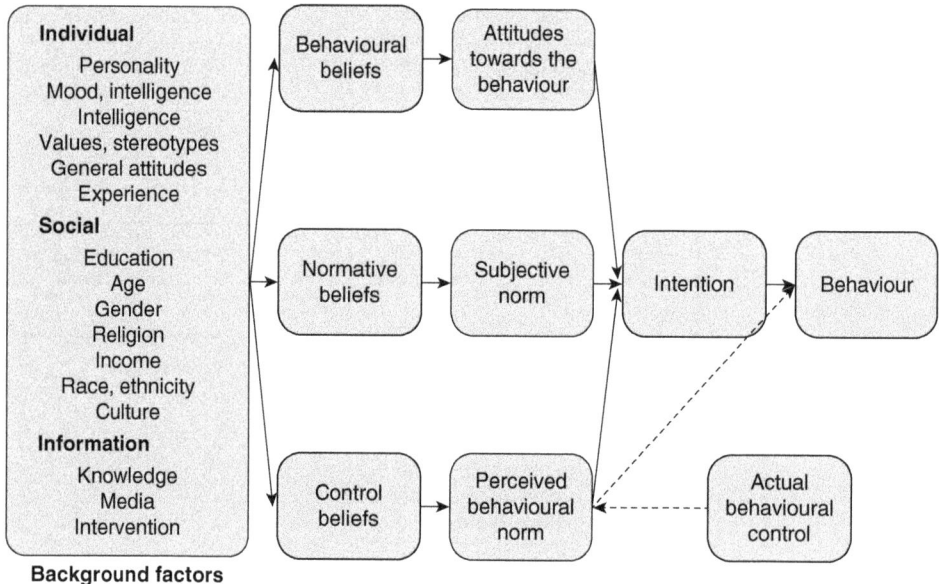

Figure 11.2 Visual representation of the theory of reasoned action and planned behaviour (Azjen and Fishbein, 2005)

behaviour than those with an external locus of control. Wallston and Wallston (1981) suggest that beliefs about health control fall into three categories: internal – the extent to which the individual believes that they are responsible for their health; powerful others – the extent to which the individual believes that other people such as health professionals are responsible; and chance – the extent to which individuals believe that things happen to them by fate or luck rather than because of what they choose to do. This has some links to Bandura's (1994) self-efficacy concept as discussed above.

STAGES OF CHANGE (PROCHASKA AND DICLEMENTE, 1986)

A model of behaviour change which, the authors state, incorporates all of the theories above is the transtheoretical stages of change model (Prochaska and DiClemente, 1986). This model is used to explain how an individual moves from having no intention of making a change towards adopting behaviour that will maintain good health. This model draws on different theories of health psychology around a core construct of cyclical change. Strategies based on this model can be successful for changing a range of behaviours such as alcohol and drug abuse, smoking, exercise and weight control. The key to this model is one of a revolving door as usually an individual would go round more than once before permanent change is maintained (Corcoran, 2013; Prestwich, et al., 2018). The authors of the model suggest that the goal of the health professional when working with patients is not to get them through the whole change cycle but instead is to move them on from one stage to the other.

This model represents the stages that people go through where at first they may not consider changing their health behaviour (pre-contemplation), then start to think about it (contemplation). The next stage is to get ready for change (preparation) followed by starting to

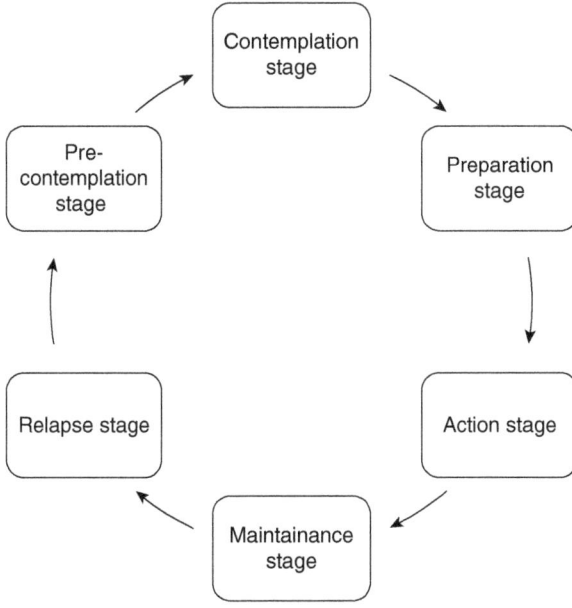

Figure 11.3   Diagram of 'stages of change' model from Prochaska and DiClemente (1984)

make the change (action). The final stage is either maintenance of the change or relapse back to the pre-contemplation stage. At any stage within this process an individual can relapse and go back to old behaviours. Stop Smoking Wales report that people commonly go around this change cycle four to five times before they may stop smoking. Progressing through each stage is not easy but is possible with motivation and help back onto the cycle after relapse.

Table 11.1 provides an outline of each stage a person will go through when changing behaviour and provides the health professional with methods for helping them move on from one stage to the next.

Table 11.1   Stages of changing behaviour

Stage of Change	Process	Moving On
Pre-contemplation	Not aware of the need for change or has no interest in changing their health-related behaviour	Peer support/pressure
		Professional advice
		Effects upon current health
		Role model
Contemplation	Starting to realise that there may be a need to change. Expressing some interest in change	Discussion of costs/benefits
		Ways of making the change discussed
		Assess confidence level
		Reflect on past experiences
		Others who have been successful

(Continued)

Table 11.1   (Continued)

Stage of Change	Process	Moving On
Preparation	Actively seeks information and support May be planning when the change will happen	Provide information such as leaflets, support groups, books, websites Set SMART goals Set a start date Discuss potential barriers and ways to overcome Identify facilitators
Action	The change begins – this may be viewed as a trial period or may be approached with enthusiasm	Keep a diary of thoughts, feelings, barriers and facilitators Review progress regularly Praise success
Maintenance	The new health behaviour has been established – on average six months is considered the time that the behaviour has changed with small chance of relapse	Review coping strategies Acknowledge that everyone has set backs and ways of dealing with them Reviewing progress Rewards Ask them to help/speak with other people in their old situation
Relapse	The patient does not like the change, lacks motivation, feels pressured Finds certain situations difficult Does not feel supported	Reinforce that relapse is not the end of the process Review the goals and adjust if needed Self-monitoring Revisit earlier stages

Source: Prochaska and DiCemente (1984) and Improving Health and Changing Behaviour (DOH, 2008).

SOME CRITICISMS OF THE PRESENTED MODELS

Various authors have provided criticism regarding the above presented modules (see Corcoran, 2013 and Prestwich et al., 2018 as examples of this). The reasoning for the critism is that these theoretical models do not take into account spontaneity of behavioural change, or explain why some people continue to demonstrate health-risk behaviours even though they have said they wish to make the change. Alongside this they fail to account other extraneous factors that can influence behaviour such as the social determinants of health. For example, young people engage in unprotected sexual activity even though they have actively sought advice around the use of appropriate contraception to prevent unplanned pregnancy or sexually transmitted infections, with acknowledged high rates of these in socially deprived areas. The models only appear to account for planned and thought-out changes.

Furthermore some consideration has to be given to the fact that these models are also based on Western theories of health and illness so may not be suitable to use with people from differing cultures and ideologies. There may also be some concerns related to using some of these models to approach health-promotion practice with what are considered traditionally hard to reach groups and may need to be adapted to their circumstances in order to be effective (Corcoran, 2013).

In relation to the Prochaska and Diclemente (1984) model described above, in some cases people assume that they are on a different stage of the cycle to that where they realistically are. Furthermore the stages can appear arbitrary rather than clearly delineated and distinct. Prestwich et al. (2018) suggest that some of the stages could be combined to allow the model to be more flexibly applied to individual circumstances.

Corcoran (2013: 13) suggests that 'other approaches should be integrated alongside theoretical models such as social marketing and technology-based behavioural change models'. This is beyond the scope of this chapter to explore fully here, and we would direct the reader to the book edited by Nova Corcoran in the further reading section for further exploration of these issues. Therefore it must be acknowledged that a 'one size fits all' approach may not be successful and health practitioners may need to select differing aspects of individual models and combine them into a tailor-made approach in order to help approach successful health behaviour change interventions (Green, et al., 2018; Naidoo and Wills, 2016).

ACTIVITY 11.2

Having read this chapter please try to answer the following questions in order to test your knowledge:

1   What are the key lifestyle factors that influence people's health?
2   How does the principle of self-efficacy affect people's ability to make a health
     behaviour change?
3   Describe and apply the 'stages of change' model to a person who is looking to stop
     smoking

Check the end of the chapter for an answer to this activity.

CONCLUSION

This chapter has looked at a number of key areas related to the theme of health promotion and health psychology. It has identified that this is a complex and multifaceted area of health and social care practice that requires an understanding of a number of differing things. It has identified that a 'one size fits all approach' is not always suitable and that health promotion needs to be tailored to individual needs. It requires consideration of individual capabilities and willingness to change, alongside the impact upon individuals of the social determinants of health which may predict the success of a health behaviour change intervention.

This chapter has also explored the impact on individuals related to factors of non-communicable diseases. It has identified that this is further impacted on by areas of deprivation in which people live, and that people living in socially deprived areas are at greater risk of developing health concerns as a result of various lifestyle factors which include smoking, alcohol use, and lack of exercise that can potentially impact on developing obesity. It has also demonstrated that there are distinct differences in obesity presentation between England and Wales.

This chapter has also discussed the impact of some aspects of health psychology related to the theories of self-efficacy and the locus of control, and applied this to the field of health-promotion practice. It has discussed the various approaches to health-promotion practice, including some tools (e.g. MECC) to help promote health behaviour change.

Finally, the chapter has discussed some of the various health-promotion models available to support practice and has provided some commentary around the criticisms of their use in isolation. It has identified that in some cases these models only consider planned changes and do not account for spontaneity, alongside difficulty in their use with what are considered traditionally hard-to-reach groups.

As can be seen the field of health promotion is a complex area of practice and this chapter has tried to demonstrate and explain that complexity. It has provided information on how to use this information to support people considering making a positive health behaviour change.

ANSWERS TO CHAPTER 11 ACTIVITIES

———— Activity 11.1: Answers

1   What are the pros and cons of each approach?

- Medical: Based on lots of available data which is collected routinely so it can identify trends in behaviour. It has led to large campaigns such as immunisation programmes and the public are aware of them. However, it often adopts a 'victim blaming' approach where the ill-health is the result of the behaviour undertaken by the individual so they are at fault. Also, it fails to take account of the effect of various social determinants of health upon the individual.
- Behavioural: It assumes individuals will make a behavioural change if they are provided with lots of information. It is a traditional approach used in practice. However, it also fails to take into account the impact of the various social determinants of health.
- Educational: This has close links with the behavioural approach, and is often confused with the behavioural change approach. However, the difference is that through education it is hoped that individuals will change their behaviours voluntarily. Furthermore, one of the additional considerations it fails to take into account are the psychological complexities of people's willingness or motivation to make a change. Nor does it take into account the impact of the social determinants of health.
- Empowerment: This model takes into account the effects of the social determinants of health and works with individuals and communities to identify the areas they wish to change. In this approach the health-promotion practitioner acts as a facilitator to support the change process. One of the challenges of this is that the individual not the facilitator has to identify the area to change and the facilitator must not present their own views.

- Social Change: This is a difficult area for individual health-promotion practitioners and often this area is one where direct intervention is not possible, as it will often require legislative change in order to promote social change. However, individual practitioners can be influential in policy change through lobbying those in political power to make the necessary changes to enact this.

2   What areas of health promotion could these approaches be applied to?

There are various areas that these approaches could be applied to; for example healthy eating campaigns, reducing alcohol intake, uptake of various screening services, immunisation uptake and promoting mental health.

3   What media campaigns using these approaches are you aware of?

- Seasonal drink drive campaigns
- Cervical screening
- Breast screening (mammography)
- Various immunisation campaigns

——— Pause for Thought 11.1: Answers

Facts that may help you to take action: peer support, personal experience, experience of others, media messages, health benefits, reminders from others, internal locus of control, sense of achievement, professional advice/support, role model, confidence.

Factors that may hinder action: negative experience, poor role models, lack of time/money, lack of support, enjoying current behaviour, external locus of control, lack of knowledge, lack of skills.

——— Activity 11.2: Answers

1   What are the key lifestyle factors that influence people's health?

Lack of exercise, smoking, diet and obesity, social deprivation, alcohol use, housing. In fact, any of the social determinants of health will affect individual lifestyle factors which, as shown in the introductory section of the chapter, can lead to a number of health conditions developing.

2   How does the principle of self-efficacy affect people's ability to make a health behaviour change?

The principle of self-efficacy describes the individual characteristics associated with the view of being able or willing to make the change to improve their health. It also relates to the view of how successful the individual thinks that they will be in making that change. It is a continuum and can vary for individuals based on any number of factors, and can

(Continued)

be influenced by previous successes or failures in similar areas of experience. Thus, for individuals with high self-efficacy they will be internally motivated to succeed in making a change and will feel they are able to do so. Whereas a person with low self-efficacy may lack the motivation to change or believe that they are unlikely to be able to do this change successfully. This may in turn require the health-promotion practitioner to provide additional support to the individual in order to successfully achieve the change. It must also be acknowledged that even when support is provided in this case the person may still be unwilling or unlikely to make a change.

3 Describe and apply the 'stages of change' model to a person who is looking to stop smoking.

- Pre-contemplation (haven't thought about making a change): At this stage the person hasn't really thought about the effect of smoking upon their health and are thus unlikely or unwilling to change this behaviour because they do not see a need to do so.
- Contemplation (considering making the change): Something in their life has triggered them to think about making a change; for example, they may be getting breathless, coughing or have had a relative develop complications from smoking. Thus, they will be seeking out how to make that change, where they go for information and support. They may be looking into smoking cessation aids to help.
- Preparation (getting ready to make a change): At this stage the person may be cutting down the amount of cigarettes they are smoking. They may be looking at joining a support group, or speaking to individuals who are ex-smokers. They may continue to seek advice and start 'collecting' nicotine replacement therapy devices to 'trial' them to see what suits, or works for them before they actively look to stop smoking.
- Action (making the change: At this stage the person 'takes the plunge' to stop smoking and either attempts to stop completely without any form of nicotine replacement therapy, or uses these items to help them with the cravings associated with stopping smoking. They may also be looking at building rewards into their actions to mark their success and to reinforce sustaining the change.
- Maintenance/relapse (behaviour change sustained more than six months, but realising the potential for going back to old habits based on differing factors): At this stage the person has now likely stopped smoking and has begun to 'wean' themselves off of the devices that have helped them quit. They will have begun to notice the health benefits from stopping smoking. Also during this period something may 'trigger' them and a relapse ensues where the person starts smoking again. During this stage it is important to recognise that relapse is a common aspect, and they should be encouraged not to view this as a failure. Instead they should be supported to explore why this relapse occurred and work out a strategy to prevent it happening again in the future.

FURTHER READING

In order to develop your knowledge around the various aspects of health promotion we would suggest the reader undertakes some additional reading around relevant topics such as smoking cessation (linked with Activity 11.2 above), healthy eating, sexual health, immunisation uptake, or any other topic which interests you, and reflect upon how this is addressed in the practice setting. This will enable you to identify the relevant steps that are required when working with individuals in addressing these behaviours, using health-promotion approaches, models and theories.

Corcoran, N. (ed.) (2013). *Communicating Health: Strategies for Health Promotion* (2nd edn). London: SAGE. This very useful book looks at the various ways in which health promotion can be applied in the context of today's media and how this can be used to develop health-promotion campaigns to target various audiences.

Prestwich, A., Kenworth, J. and Conner, M. (2018). *Health Behavior Change: Theories, Methods and Interventions*. Abingdon: Routledge. This textbook examines the various theories of health promotion, the relevant research and the application of this to health-promotion contexts. This enables the reader to develop a deeper understanding of the challenges associated with health behaviour change.

REFERENCES

Ajzen, L. and Fishbein, M. (2005). The influence of attitudes on behaviour. In D. Albarracin, B. T. Johnson and M. P. Zanna (eds), *The Handbook of Attitudes*. Mahwah, NJ: Erlbaum.

Anderson, M. (2015). Public Health and Health Promotion. In T. D. Barton and D. Allan (eds), *Advanced Nursing Practice: Changing Healthcare in a Changing World*. London: Palgrave.

Ayers, S. and De Visser, R. (2018). *Psychology for Medicine & Healthcare* (2nd edn). London: SAGE.

Bandura, A. (1994). Self-efficacy. In V. S. Ramachaudran (ed.), *Encyclopedia of Human Behavior* (Vol 4: 71–81). New York: Academic Press. (Reprinted in H. Friedman [ed.], *Encyclopedia of Mental Health*. San Diego, CA: Academic Press, 1998.)

Becker, M. H. (1974). *The Health Belief Model and Personal Health Behaviour*. Thorofare, NJ: Slack.

Corcoran, N. (2013) Theories and models. In N. Corcoran (ed.), *Communicating Health: Strategies for Health Promotion* (2nd edn, pp. 5–28). London: SAGE.

Green, J., Tones, K., Cross, R. and Woodall, J. (2018). *Health Promotion Planning & Strategies* (4th edn). London: SAGE.

Health and Social Care Information Service (2016). *Statistics on Obesity, Physical Activity and Diet – England, 2016*. England: ONS.

Janz, N. K. and Becker, M. H. (1984). The health belief model: a decade later. *Health Education and Behaviour* 11(1), 1–47.

Marmot, M. (2010). *Fair Society, Healthy Lives: The Marmot Review*. Available at: www.parliament.uk/documents/fair-society-healthy-lives-full-report.pdf (accessed on 21 May 2019).

Musgrove, J. (2017). *The NHS and the Funding of Lifestyle Diseases*. Available at: https://prezi.com/-jpt_u0nrrag/the-nhs-and-the-funding-of-lifestyle-diseases/

Naidoo, J. and Wills, J. (2016). *Foundations for Health Promotion* (4th edn). Oxford: Elsevier.

NHS Digital (2018a). *Statistics on Obesity, Physical Activity and Diet*. Available at: https://files.digital.nhs.uk/publication/0/0/obes-phys-acti-diet-eng-2018-rep.pdf (accessed on 12 February 2019).

NHS Digital (2018b). *Health Survey for England – Summary of Key Findings*. Available at: https://files.digital.nhs.uk/5B/B1297D/HSE%20report%20summary.pdf (accessed on 12 February 2019).

NHS Health Scotland (2018). *Hospital Admissions, Deaths and Overall Burden of Disease Attributable to Alcohol Consumption in Scotland*. Edinburgh: NHS Health Scotland.

Prestwich, A., Kenworthy, J. and Conner, M. (2018). *Health Behavior Change: Theories, Methods and Interventions*. Abingdon: Routledge.

Prochaska, J. O., and DiClemente, C. C. (1984). *The Transtheoretical Approach: Towards a Systematic Eclectic Framework*. Dow Jones Irwin: Harnewood.

Prochaska, J. O. and DiClemente, C. C. (1986). Towards a comprehensive model of change. In W.R. Miller and N. Heather (eds), *Treating Addictive Behaviours: Processes of Change*. New York: Plenum.

Public Health England (2016). Illnesses associated with lifestyle cost the NHS £11 billion. Available at: www.bbc.co.uk/news/health-37451773

Public Health Wales (2017). *Making Every Contact Count*. Available at: www.wales.nhs.uk/sitesplus/888/page/65550

Public Health Wales (2018). *Child Measurement Programme for Wales 2016/17*. Cardiff: Public Health Wales NHS Trust.

Public Health Wales (2019). *Obesity in Wales*. Cardiff: Public Health Wales NHS Trust.

Rollnick, S. and Miller, W. R. (2012) *Motivational Interviewing* (3rd edn). New York: Guilford Press.

Rosenstock, I.M., Strecher, V.J. & Becker, M.H (1988) Social Learning Theory and the health belief model. *Health Education Quarterly* 15(2) pp.175–183.

Rotter, J. B. (1954). *Social Learning and Clinical Psychology*. Englewood Cliffs, NJ: Prentice Hall.

Upton, D. and Thirlaway, K. (2016). *Promoting Healthy Behaviour: A Practical Guide* (2nd edn). Abingdon: Routledge.

Wallston, K. A. and Wallston, B. S. (1981). *Health Locus of Control Scales*. Available at: http://citeseerx.ist.psu.edu/viewdoc/download;jsessionid=8312F478460697B764B776BCB24E95B3?doi=10.1.1.467.6716&rep=rep1&type=pdf

Welsh Government (2018). *National Survey for Wales 2017–18: Population Health – Lifestyle*. Available at: https://gov.wales/docs/statistics/2018/180627-national-survey-2017-18-population-health-lifestyle-en.pdf

World Health Organization (2017). *Noncommunicable Diseases*. Geneva: WHO.

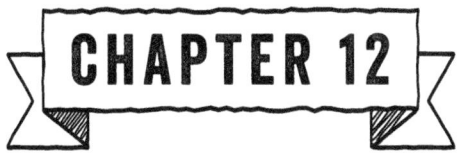

CHILDREN'S RIGHTS AND PARTICIPATION

Tracey Maegusuku-Hewett and Pete King

OVERVIEW

This chapter seeks to explore and provide health and social care students with an overview of children's rights and participation. This will be achieved by setting out the historical context of the evolution of children's rights, and locating this in the current legislative and policy context of the UK's devolved nations. There will be an overview of the purpose and underlying principles of the United Nations Convention on the Rights of the Child 1989 (UNCRC) and a subsequent focus on children's rights to participation. There will be some unpicking of the concept of participation and various models that help to understand it as well as activities and case examples of children's right to participation in play and rights to participation in the decision-making process. The chapter will provide insight into factors that hinder or promote children's participation in these contexts and give students further sources of reading and resources on this topic.

LEARNING OUTCOMES

By the end of this chapter you will have:

- An awareness of the historical and political context of children's rights in the UK
- Reflected on the extent to which children are afforded human rights and considered ways in which health and social care professionals can support children to exercise their rights to protection, participation and provision
- Become familiar with different levels of child participation ranging from non-participation to children and young people as full and active participants

INTRODUCTION

Health and social care professionals often intervene in the lives of children and young people, whether to protect them from harm, or in the provision of services such as emergency health, palliative care, social work services to children and families in need, etc. Sometimes when engaging with families there are complex and competing rights at stake, however in all our work with families, UK legislation asserts that the welfare of the child is paramount. Likewise, the United Nations

Convention on the Rights of the Child 1989 (referred to hereafter as the UNCRC) advocates 'the best interests of the child shall be a primary consideration' (Article 3). In more recent years, in recognition of children's rights, there has been a shift towards rights-based and child-centred health and social care practice in which practitioners need to possess the necessary skills and knowledge to champion children's enjoyment of their rights and enable their participation in matters that are important to them or when decisions may impact on their lives. Concepts such as 'children's rights' and 'participation' are variously defined, understood and operationalised (Lundy et al., 2012), yet the UNCRC, Article 54 imposes a duty upon state parties to systematically improve knowledge of the UNCRC and promote an affirmative child rights culture. In this chapter, we introduce you to the main principles of the UNCRC which apply to all children in all aspects of their lives. This will provide you with the grounding to help you on your trajectory of becoming a rights-based student and practitioner. Before we embark on this chapter, you are encouraged to complete the following activity, thinking about the questions posed. These questions form the basis of this chapter and will aid your reflection and learning.

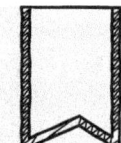

PAUSE FOR THOUGHT 12.1

As an adult, make a list of all the rights you think you have. Look at your list and then think how many of these rights do children have. Did you have these rights as a child? Do children now have these rights? If children have rights, how can adults who work with children support these rights?

A BRIEF HISTORY AND BACKGROUND TO CHILDREN'S RIGHTS IN THE UK

Historically, children's rights have not been explicit (or even desirable from an adult perspective). In earlier times, children were seen as the legal and moral property of their parents or as an extension of their parents (Archard and Macleod, 2002). Pre- industrialisation, children as young as six were expected to contribute to society, deemed to be young adults. Child labour was widespread and legitimised by a society that did not ascribe children any legal status or rights (Kosher et al., 2016).

The Industrial Revolution signalled a shift in the conceptualisation of childhood helped by legislation which abolished child labour and established the universal provision of education in the late nineteenth and early twentieth centuries. Children during this period were perceived as 'becoming adults', thus children's rights manifested in terms of their protection and access to certain provisions with greater dependence upon parents, and the state (Kosher et al., 2016). There was a noticeably increased role of philanthropists and the state in child and family matters to promote children's health and development through the establishment of the NHS and through social welfare institutions that sought to protect children from harm, and to provide support for children in need. (Some interventions we now deem to have been well intentioned but causing children harm, such as the various child migration schemes – see Independent Inquiry Child

Sexual Abuse, 2018). Meanwhile on an international stage, and following the First World War, Eglantyne Jebb (Founder of Save the Children International) was instrumental in the League of Nations' adoption of the Declaration of Geneva of Children's Rights 1924; a declaration containing five Articles that asserted provisions and protections to children (see Humanium, 2019, for the text of the Declaration).

By the second half of the twentieth century, thinking on rights had begun to expand to encapsulate children as 'being' (children and not becoming adults), as well as children's right to self-determination, expression and participation (Kosher et al., 2016); though this was a protracted process. Most prominently, the aftermath of the Second World War saw the creation of the United Nations and significant Declarations such as the 1948 Declaration of Human Rights and the UN Declaration of the Rights of the Child in 1959. Both of these international treaties mirrored earlier rights principles of protection and provision, but the latter treaty was expanded upon by Poland in 1978, with the aim of making a more comprehensive legally binding convention. In its early format and a year later, with the International Year of the Child, the UN Committee for Human Rights established a working group that would progress the draft convention over a further ten years of negotiation and re-drafting to become the United Nations Convention on the Rights of the Child in 1989 (Sandberg, 2014).

THE UNCRC

The UNCRC set a precedence for ratifying nation states to treat children as the subject of human rights and to confer civil, social, political, economic and cultural rights specifically to children owing to their unique status as children and human beings in their own right. The convention has since been the foundation upon which three further protocols were developed. For example, of importance to hearing the voice of the child, the Optional Protocol to the Convention on the Rights of the Child on a Communications Procedure (UN, 2011) enables a child to complain against alleged rights violations directly to the UN Committee. (At the time of writing, the UK has not ratified this protocol.)

In total there are 54 Articles of the UNCRC, 13 of which advocate how governments and adults need to embrace and implement the rights of children and Article 1 defines a child as being below the age of 18 years. A common way to understand and categorise the remaining Articles is to refer to the 'three Ps': rights that relate to children's **p**rotection, **p**articipation and **p**rovision.

ACTIVITY 12.1

To explore the UNCRC and the full wording of the 54 Articles please refer to the further reading section. Below you will find a summary list of Articles that relate to children's protection, participation and provision.

Consider and categorise each one as being a protection right, a participation right or a provision right. You may find that some rights are more clearly aligned with a particular category, whereas others seem to be a bit more ambiguous or open to interpretation.

Check the end of the chapter for an answer to this activity.

ARTICLES

Article 2: Access to rights without discrimination

Article 3: Best interests of the child

Article 5: Rights and responsibilities of families to bring up children

Article 6: Right to life, survival and development

Article 7: The right from birth to a name, nationality and knowledge of, and where possible to be cared for by their parents

Article 8: Governments should respect children's right to identity, including nationality, name and family relations

Article 9: Right to be brought up by family and to have contact with both parents unless not in the child's best interests

Article 10 : A right to move between countries for family contact

Article 11: Not to be taken out of their own country illegally

Article 12: Participation – a right to a say in decisions about them

Article 13: A right to information about them and to share their information

Article 14: A right to belief and practice of religion/faith

Article 15: A right to association with other people and organisations

Article 16: Right to privacy

Article 17: Right to reliable, understandable information from the mass media

Article 18: Both parents are responsible for the upbringing of the child. Governments should provide services to support them

Article 19: Right to protection from harm, abuse and neglect at home

Article 20: Children looked after by others should have their religion, culture and language respected

Article 21: The child's best interests are central to adoption or when children are taken outside of their country to live

Article 22: Children who enter a country seeking refuge should have the same rights as other children born in that country

Article 23: Disabled children should have special care and support to enable them to live as independently as possible

Article 24: Right to good-quality health care and clean water, nutrition and environment

Article 25: Children looked after by the state should have their situation reviewed regularly

Article 26: Governments should provide resources for families in need

Article 27: Right to a sufficient standard of living to meet physical and mental needs

Article 28: Right to an education

Article 29: Education should develop children's full potential

Article 30: A right to learn and use the language and customs of their families

Article 31: A right to relax and play and join in activities

Article 32: Governments should protect children from work that is dangerous, or harmful to health and education

Article 33: Governments should protect children from dangerous drugs

Article 34: Governments should protect children from abuse

Article 35: Governments should make sure children are not abducted or sold

Article 36: Children should be protected from any activity harmful to their development

Article 37: Children who break the law should not be treated cruelly; they should not be imprisoned with adults and have a right to contact with their families

Article 38: Governments should not allow children to be conscribed into the military; children in war zones should be afforded special protection

Article 39: Abused and neglected children should receive special support to help

Article 40: Children accused of committing an offence should be afforded legal help; prison sentences should only be used for the most serious crimes

Article 41: If the laws of a country protect children better than the Articles of The UNCRC, then the laws of the country should be referred to

RATIFICATION OF THE UNCRC

The UK signed the convention on 19 April 1990 and ratified it on 16 December 1991. The UNCRC 1989 has now been ratified by 196 nation states across the globe; the USA is the only country to sign but not ratify the convention. Ratification refers to a state's agreement to be bound by the convention; it is legally binding in international law. Though this does not mean that ratifying states necessarily abide by it. That said, at the least the United Nations Committee of the Rights of the Child works as an 'accountability committee' to monitor, report and bench mark ratifying nations' commitment to children's UNCRC rights. The UN Committee makes recommendations to all ratifying states, though these are not legally binding. States respond to such recommendations and essentially interpret and implement the convention to varying degrees. Individual nations may place a 'reservation' on a particular Article, which has the effect of the state reserving the right to use their sovereign rule.

AN EXAMPLE OF A RESERVATION ON A *PROTECTION* RIGHT

A UK example can be found with Article 22, which relates to all children subject to immigration control, guaranteeing asylum-seeking children's rights and protection. However, upon ratifying the UNCRC in 1991, the UK government entered a general reservation 'as regards the entry, stay in and departure from the UK of children who are subject to immigration control'. The government's position was that 'the reservation is necessary to maintain effective immigration control' (Baroness Scotland of Asthal, 2004). Consequently, asylum-seeking children may have been placed in detention, and were denied access to certain other rights (Joint Committee on Human Rights, 2005). The UK government eventually withdrew the reservation in September 2008 and by 2010 had committed to alternatives to detention.

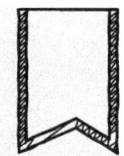

PAUSE FOR THOUGHT 12.2

With the above example of asylum-seeking children in the UK, how might detention have impacted on children and their families? What other UNCRC rights would have been infringed as a consequence.

THE UNCRC AND UK NATIONS

Whilst the UK has ratified the UNCRC, there is some divergence in how Wales, Scotland, Northern Ireland and England interpret and integrate the convention into policy, practice and, to some extent, law. Upon devolution in 1999, Wales formally adopted the UNCRC in 2003 and was the first nation in Europe to introduce legislation specifically concerned with children's rights and the UNCRC via the auspices of the Rights of Children and Young Persons' (Wales) Measure 2011. The crux of the Measure obliges all Ministers to give *due regard* to the UNCRC 1989 in all law and policy-making (Williams, 2013). Scotland followed suit in 2014 with the Children and Young People (Scotland) Act requiring ministers to '*keep under consideration* whether there are any steps which they could take which would or might secure better or further effect in Scotland of the UNCRC requirements' (section 1). Neither Northern Ireland nor England have taken this legislative pathway. Instead, in Northern Ireland the emphasis is upon children and young people's well-being. To this end, the Children's Services Co-operation (Northern Ireland) Act 2015 places an obligation on certain public authorities to co-operate in order to improve the well-being of children and young people. When determining what well-being means, authorities are to *have regard* to the Articles of the UNCRC. The Act also provides powers for ministers to initiate a Children and Young Person's Strategy for the purposes of implementing well-being. (At the time of writing this was in the final stages of consultation.) Finally, in England, there is no specific children's rights legislation, nor is there a 'due regard duty'. In fact, the government rejected the need to incorporate the 'due regard duty' into its most recent and prominent child welfare legislation, the Children and Social Work Act 2017 (Rosa et al., 2019). The Committee on the Rights of the Child has frequently requested the UNCRC be incorporated into UK law; however, the language of the UNCRC has been argued by ministers as being too aspirational and difficult to integrate into domestic law, whilst it is argued that children's rights are protected by other existing laws such as the Equality Act 2010, Children Act 1998, albeit not explicitly articulated as children's rights (Fortin, 2009). This seemingly less than enthusiastic and inadequate stance towards the rights of children contrasts with the UK government's incorporation of the European Convention on Human Rights (also known as ECHR 1950) which was integrated into UK domestic law via the Human Rights Act 1998. Children may well be afforded rights through this mechanism; however, as Baroness Hale of Richmond states, 'there is virtually nothing in the ECHR about children' (cited in Fortin, 2009, p. 50).

THE EXTENT TO WHICH CHILDREN'S RIGHTS ARE REALISED IN THE UK

Aside from the variable approach to implementation of the UNCRC across UK nations, it is fair to say there has been a significant ideological and policy shift on children, childhood and rights in the twenty-first-century UK. This amounts to positive changes brought about by greater commitment to children, with some notable examples including the Welsh government's initiative to adopt a play policy, the Northern Ireland and Scottish governments' guardianship scheme for unaccompanied asylum-seeking children, the England cross-government care leavers' strategy and charter (UNCRC, 2016). Other rights advances may have been brought about by legislation; for example, all UK nations have established a Children Commissioner. The Commissioners' remit varies across each nation; for example, in Scotland the Commissioner has the power to investigate children's allegations of mistreatment, whilst other roles may include scrutinising policy and legislation and the impact on children, gathering evidence, presenting concerns and making recommendations. The fundamental aim is to champion the rights and best interests of children and young people. Where matters are non-devolved such as immigration and youth justice, then the England-based commissioner represents each nation. However, there are concerns about this approach, as well as the variance in remit and the level of autonomy that Commissioners may or may not have (Joint Children Commissioners, 2015; UN Committee Rights of the Child (UNCRC), 2016). Finally, other rights may have been won as a result of jurisprudence, or case law. For example, see *Child's Rights Alliance for England v. Secretary of State for the Home Office* [2012] EWHC 8 (Admin) which relates to staff restraint of young people in secure training units.

Notwithstanding these strides, children across the UK experience a variable quality of life, well-being and protection, participation and provision. For example, in Northern Ireland, the NI Committee on Human Rights were seriously concerned that paramilitary organisations continue to direct shootings and other violence at children (NICHR, 2015), whilst in Scotland the age of criminal responsibility is just age eight. In Wales, despite an increase in demand for early intervention mental health provision, the evidence suggests availability to be limited; similarly in England, children with mental health needs are being placed on adult wards due to a lack of bed capacity. Looking at the UK as a whole, for example, concerns relate to the levels of obesity amongst children, lower numbers of breast feeding, the impact of air pollution on child health, the increase in homeless families, residual welfare provision and austerity, increasing child poverty with fuel and food insecurity, and increased use of food banks (UNCRC, 2016).

FORECASTING THE FUTURE OF CHILDREN'S RIGHTS IN THE UK

Whilst at the time of writing the UK is in a state of Brexit uncertainty, it would be foolish not to acknowledge the potential impact of our exit from the European Union (EU) on the rights and well-being of children and young people. This is a significant issue that has the commitment and campaigning momentum of a collective of child rights organisations across all four nations. In their collaborative report (see Children's Legal Centre, 2017), they strongly advocate the need to facilitate the inclusion of children and young people's views on Brexit and beyond. They also see crucial issues relating to child poverty, safeguarding, cross-border family contact, children living in Northern and the Republic of Ireland, and EU national children and settlement status. There is also trepidation for the potential dilution of children's rights during the transposition of EU and

UK law and the exclusion of EU mechanisms such as the EU Charter of Fundamental Freedoms as prescribed in the EU Withdrawal Act 2018 (Rosa et al., 2019). This is coupled with the current UK government signalling their desire to repeal the Human Rights Act 1998 post-Brexit (House of Lords, 2019). Potentially in the future, then, children may suffer if there are diminished rights and enforcement mechanisms; this could certainly be their reality whilst the UNCRC remains unincorporated into UK law.

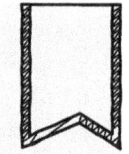

PAUSE FOR THOUGHT 12.3

At the time of reading this chapter, reflect on the UK's position in the EU. Are there any specific children's rights matters that have arisen and are reported on that you know of? How do these compare to the crucial issues highlighted above?

WHY SHOULD THOSE WORKING IN HEALTH AND SOCIAL CARE FACILITATE CHILDREN'S VOICE AND PARTICIPATION?

In Chapter 9 you will have been introduced to child and adult safeguarding and to the historical context of safeguarding policy and practice which emerged in the wake of a number of high-profile child abuse deaths, some of whom were discussed: Maria Colwell (1973), Jasmine Beckford (1984), Victoria Climbié (2000), Peter Connolly (Baby Peter) (2007). More recently there have been revelations of long-standing child sexual exploitation of girls in Rochdale, Rotherham and Oxford. These grab the public attention, causing outrage and criticism of the role played by police, education, health and social care practitioners who may have engaged (sometimes on numerous occasions) with children in these pernicious circumstances (Ferguson, 2017).

In their conclusion, Kelly and Chisnell (Chapter 9) see it as essential to listen to the voice of the child and keep them at the centre of any safeguarding context. This is reinforced by the evidence base and well-publicised child death cases which have all failed to ensure children and young people are given proper opportunity and support to have their voices heard (Bedford, 2015; Ferguson, 2017; Jay, 2014; Munro, 2011). Ferguson (2017) describes children in these contexts as 'invisible'. He questions, 'how is it possible for practitioners to be in the same room as children and not engage with them in ways that reveal their experiences' (p. 1009). The UN Committee (2016) noted:

> Many children feel that they are not listened to by their social workers, reviewing officers, paid carers, judges, personnel working with children in conflict with the law or other professionals in matters affecting them, including in family proceedings (p. 6).

This, of course, is a compelling rationale for health and social care professionals to ensure they enable children's participation and voice and to listen fully and meaningfully to children in their care, particularly in safeguarding contexts. Meanwhile on a daily level, all nations of the UK can be seen to aspire to a greater commitment to children's participation in matters affecting them, be this in relation to them being cared for by the state as looked after children, gaining views on changes to school curriculum and activities, asking children about their play and fun, health and development, or how to make the local neighbourhood more youth and environmentally friendly and so on.

As a future health and social care practitioner you are encouraged to take a child-centred rights-based approach; after all, the UN Committee (2016) made recommendations to 'ensure that children are not only heard but also listened to and their views given due weight by all professionals working with children'.

CONSULTATION AND *PARTICIPATION* WITH CHILDREN

What do we mean by participation? The UN Committee on the Rights of the Child's (2009) General Comment on the child's right to be heard considers the meaning of participation: 'to describe ongoing processes, which include information-sharing and dialogue between children and adults based on mutual respect, and in which children can learn how their views and those of adults are taken into account and shape the outcome of such processes' (p. 3).

Skivenes and Strandbu (2006) identify four aspects key for children's consultation and participation where children have the opportunity to form opinions; express their viewpoints; have their arguments taken seriously; and be informed after a decision.

ACTIVITY 12.2

What factors do you need to consider when obtaining children's views? Write down a list of all the factors you need to consider when consulting with children.

Check the end of the chapter for an answer to this activity.

When consulting with and participating with children, we have to consider their age and stage of development. For example, according to Piaget (1953) children go through four stages of cognitive development: sensorimotor (birth to 2 years); preoperational (2 to 7 years); concrete operational (7 to 11 years); and formal operational (12 years onwards). Obviously, consultation and participation with a 16-year-old girl will differ when compared to a 5-year-old boy as, according to Piaget, the 16-year-old girl will make logical choices, whereas the 5-year-old boy may still only think egocentrically, that is from their own perspective only.

The second point relates to typical and atypical development. Consulting with a 12-year-old boy with typical development (that is adjudged to meet standardised developmental norms) would be different with a 12-year-old boy with a learning impairment or Down's syndrome. All children's views are needed and valid, but you must consider ability and disability, in addition to a child's age and stage of development, as there may be additional challenges involved where 'adequate preparation, commitment, resources, flexibility and skilled, trained facilitators are required' (Franklin and Sloper, 2009).

The third aspect of context is needed; that is the specific area that children are being consulted about. Children's participation exists within areas of disability (Franklin and Sloper, 2009), mental health (LeFrancois, 2009), health care (Moore and Kirk, 2010), schools (Johnny, 2006) and child protection (Cossar et al., 2016). This is obviously not a definitive list (see if you can find other contexts where children have been consulted and have participated in). Other contextual factors to be considered could be cultural, socio-economic or access.

The final aspect is in relation to power. Children will often see adults as figures of authority and control and it is important that consultation and participation is on a voluntary basis; that is children are nor forced or coerced to take part.

ACTIVITY 12.3

You want to find out children's views on their local park. What methods could you use within consultation and participation taking into account the four aspects discussed earlier:

1   Children aged 5–7 years old in primary schools?
2   Young people in secondary school?
3   A local charity who support disabled children in the local area?

You may have thought of more creative ways for younger children to participate (e.g. use of drawings), whereas for older children more 'formal' dialogue such as a focus group may be used. For disabled children, a mixture of both techniques may be needed, often with the support of specialist workers. Useful resources for consulting and participating include for pre-school and primary-aged children the publication 'Listening to young children: the Mosaic approach' (Clark and Moss, 2001), for secondary school aged children is the publication 'Empowering children and young people' (Treseder, 1997) and for disabled children 'The Disabled Child's Participation Rights' (Callus and Farrugia, 2016).

To have a dialogue to obtain children's views on a particular subject or concept, we as adults have to consult with children. As stated by Skivenes and Strandbu (2006), 'Consideration must be given to the ways in which states (Governments) and adults view children and gain a proper understanding of their opinions, as well as ways in which adults can facilitate their participation' (p. 11). In addition, how adults interpret children's views are of equal importance where 'there is always a danger that these interpretations are wrong. Errors are particularly likely when children are concerned, as their language skills and social and cognitive maturity vary considerably' (Skivenes and Standbu, 2006, p. 15). One framework for adults to consult with children was developed by Hart (1992) and refined by Treseder (1997).

A FRAMEWORK FOR CONSULTATION AND PARTICIPATION

Hart (1992) introduced a model for consultation and participation based on the concept of a 'ladder'. The 'ladder of participation' consists of eight rungs, where the first three rungs are considered as non-participatory and rungs four to eight as participatory. A brief outline of the eight rungs are (Hart, 1992):

- **Rung 1**: Manipulation is where children are being used for an adult agenda or outcome. An example of this could be where children are with adults protesting with placards against the closure of a school where children have no idea or inclination of being involved.
- **Rung 2**: Decoration is where children are involved in an adult agenda to promote a cause, for example a national event such as a state visit, where children are dressed up and paraded.
- **Rung 3**: Tokenism is where children's views and opinions are sought, but are often 'muted' to meeting an adult agenda; for example a local government office obtaining children's views but being used as a 'tick box exercise' so adults can say children have been consulted, but do not provide any feedback to the children, and the views are not followed up or acted upon.

Although from an adult perspective this may appear to be consultation and participation, in reality it is not. Children often will not participate voluntarily in relation to rungs one to three. It is not until rung four, which Hart (1992) calls 'genuine participation' (p. 11), does it take place:

- **Rung 4**: Assigned but informed. This is where Hart (1992) explains, 'children understand the intentions of the project … know who made the decisions concerning their involvement and why … have a meaningful (rather than 'decorative') role … and volunteer for the project after the project was made clear to them' (p. 11).
- **Rung 5**: Consulted and informed is a project which is 'designed and run by adults, but children understand the process and their opinions are treated seriously' where children act as 'consultants' (Hart, 1992, p. 12).
- **Rung 6**: Adult initiated, shared decisions with children. Hart (1992) explains this is 'true participation because, though the projects at this level are initiated by adults, the decision making is shared with the young people' (p. 12).
- **Rung 7**: Child initiated and directed.
- **Rung 8**: Child-initiated, shared decisions with adults is where children have more control, where at rung eight the adults really are taking on a supportive role.

Treseder (1997) adapted Hart's (1992) rungs four to eight, not as 'hierarchy' (p. 7) as the 'ladder of participation' suggests, but more as 'degrees of participation' (p. 7) moving away from a 'hierarchy' to a 'circular layout' which takes into account that a particular way of consultation and participation (e.g. rung seven, 'child initiated and directed') may not be suitable for, say, four-year-old children starting primary schools, whereas rung four ('assigned and informed') would be more appropriate. The key aspect is to get to know the children you are working with to gauge the best method for consultation and participation.

An example of where consultation and participation has taken place is briefly discussed within the context of playwork.

CONSULTATION AND PARTICIPATION IN PLAYWORK: A BRIEF EXAMPLE OF A *PROVISION* RIGHT

Playwork is defined as 'a highly skilled profession that enriches and enhances provision for children's play. It takes place where adults support children's play but it is not driven by prescribed education or care outcomes' (SkillsActive, 2010, p. 3). The adult, or more correctly the play-worker, works with school-aged children (Russell, 2006) in the primary school age group (4–11 years); however, it is not uncommon for children as young as 3 years and as old as 17 years in a variety of settings that include adventure playground, after-school club provision and holiday play schemes (Russell, 2006) and in more recent times within children's local parks and open spaces (King and Sills-Jones, 2018). Since the UK government ratified the UNCRC in 1991, playwork prac-tice has been the vehicle to promote and implement Article 31 of the UNCRC – children's right to play (King and Newstead, 2017). This has involved extensive consultation and participation with children, considering both Article 12 (children's right to have a view) and Article 13 (children's right of freedom of expression) as well as Article 31 and reflecting the primary role of the play-worker to support children's play. To support children's play, this can only be achieved if children are consulted and participate in all aspects of the play environment: the space, the activities and even the rules (Save the Children, 1996; Shier, 1995); that is to 'work exclusively with the child's agenda' (Wragg, 2011, p. 71). Consultation and participation with children has been pivotal in the development of playwork during the 1990s where today, nearly 20 years later, the playwork-ers' role is not only to support children's play, but act as advocates for children's right to play (Playwork Principles Scrutiny Group (PPSG), 2005).

ACTIVITY 12.4

Using the internet, explore some potential participation tools that can be used to engage children and young people.

CONCLUSION

Finally, the chapter has outlined the development of children's rights and by association, the changing conceptualisation of children and childhood. The UNCRC has been a prominent catalyst in modern-day child-centred and rights-based policy and provision, though as outlined the extent of UK nations' interpretation and explicit commitment to the UNCRC is variable. This in turn man-ifests in inequity across nations of children's quality of life and enjoyment of rights, with some devolved nations seemingly more progressive in their endeavours to afford children their civil, political, social, economic and cultural rights.

We have implored you to consider your professional accountability to children you will work with as a health and social care professional. We've exemplified some past high-profile child deaths and child sexual exploitation cases where evidence points to the misgivings of profes-sionals from all disciplines in the protection, provision of services and meaningful participation of children. We caution that this is not to blame individual practitioners, but rather to be pre-pared that there are myriad factors that come into play in the complexity of some encounters with children and families, often the potential for competing rights and needs, as well as more systemic failings.

As a health and social care worker it is your obligation to familiarise yourself with the UNCRC, to learn about legislation where rights are implicit or explicit, in the nation where you practise.

It is your obligation to find out your organisation's ethos towards children and to secure children's best interests. Of the upmost importance, and as advocated here, it is imperative that you take the time to develop your active listening skills, to explore different participatory tools, and to provide meaningful opportunity for the children in your care to have the support and trust to communicate their views and opinions about their lives, what matters to them, and to be given a genuine voice in decisions that impact on them.

GO FURTHER ACTIVITY

Consider which health or social care professional discipline you may like to work in in your future career, post-graduation.

- What might be your role in relation to children and young people?
- How might taking a rights-based approach present opportunities and challenges?
- What skills might you need to develop now in order to enable children's active participation in this context?

ANSWERS TO CHAPTER 12 ACTIVITIES

——— Activity 12.1: Answers

Table 12.1   Children's UNCRC rights to **P**rotection, **P**articipation and **P**rovision.

Protection	Participation	Provision
Article 3: best interests of the child	**Article 12**: participation – a right to a say in decisions about them	**Article 2**: access to rights without discrimination
Article 6: right to life, survival and development.	**Article 13:** a right to information about them and to share their information	**Article 5:** rights and responsibilities of families to bring up children
Article 7: the right from birth to a name, nationality and knowledge of, and where possible to be cared for by their parents	**Article 15:** a right to association with other people and organisations	**Article 10:** right to move between countries for family contact

(Continued)

Table 12.1 (Continued)

Protection	Participation	Provision
Article 8: governments should respect children's right to identity, including nationality, name and family relations.	Article 25: children looked after by the state should have their situation reviewed regularly	Article 14: a right to belief and practice of religion/ faith
Article 9: right to be brought up by family and to have contact with both parents unless not in the child's best interests.		Article 18: both parents are responsible for the upbringing of the child. Governments should provide services to support them
Article 11: not to be taken out of their own country illegally		Article 20: children looked after by others should have their religion, culture and language respected.
Article 16: right to privacy		Article 21: the child's best interests are central to adoption or when children are taken outside of their country to live
Article 17: right to reliable, understandable information from the mass media		Article 22: children who enter a county seeking refuge should have the same rights as other children born in that country.
Article 19: right to protection from harm, abuse and neglect at home		Article 23: disabled children should have special care and support to enable them to live as independently as possible
Article 32: governments should protect children from work that is dangerous, or harmful to health and education		Article 24: right to good-quality health care and clean water, nutrition, and environment.
Article 33: governments should protect children from dangerous drugs		Article 26: governments should provide resources for families in need.
Article 34: governments should protect children from abuse		Article 27: right to a sufficient standard of living to meet physical and mental needs.
Article 35: governments should make sure children are not abducted or sold		Article 28: right to an education

Protection	Participation	Provision
Article 36: children should be protected from any activity harmful to their development		**Article 29:** education should develop children's full potential
Article 37: children who break the law should not be treated cruelly. They should not be imprisoned with adults and have a right to contact with their families.		**Article 30:** a right to learn and use the language and customs of their families
Article 38: governments should not allow children to be conscripted into the military. Children in war zones should be afforded special protection		**Article 31:** a right to relax and play and join in activities
Article 41: if the laws of a country protect children better than the Articles of the UNCRC, then the laws of the country should be referred to		**Article 39:** abused and neglected children should receive special support to help
		Article 40: children accused of committing an offence should be afforded legal help. Prison sentences should only be used for most serious crimes.

———— Activity 12.2: Answers

From your list, the following should be considered:

- Age and stage of development of children
- Ability and disability of the children
- Power relationship between adults and children
- Context of the consultation

FURTHER READING

Children's Views on their Well-Being:

Watch this short video for a glimpse of how children and young people perceive child well-being in the UK: https://youtu.be/QATU67eFlDE (2 minutes 18 seconds)

Or if you want more details, read this summary:

UNICEF (2013). *The Well-being of Children: How Does the UK Score?* UNICEF: Retrieved at:

https://downloads.unicef.org.uk/wp-content/uploads/2013/04/ReportCard11_CYP.pdf?_ga=
2.213316371.605874803.1560875218-2132505281.1560875218

UNCRC

Please click on the link to read the full text of the UNCRC:

www.unicef.org.uk/wp-content/uploads/2010/05/UNCRC_united_nations_convention_on_the_
rights_of_the_child.pdf

Or for a summary version:

www.unicef.org.uk/wp-content/uploads/2010/05/UNCRC_summary–1.pdf

Children's Participation

Morrison, F. (2016). *Social Workers' Communication with Children and Young People in Practice*, IRISS.
Retrieved at: www.iriss.org.uk/sites/default/files/insights-34.pdf

Tisdall, E. K. M, Davis, J. and Gallagher, M. (2008). Reflecting upon children and young people's participation in the UK. *International Journal of Children's Rights* 16(3), 343–354.

REFERENCES

Archard, D. and Macleod, C. (eds) (2002). *The Moral and Political Status of Children*. Oxford: Oxford
University Press.

Baroness Scotland of Asthal (2004). *United Nations Convention on the Rights of the Child*. Hansard
Written Answers 2nd November, House of Lords, vol. 656. [online]. Cited at: https://hansard.
parliament.uk/Lords/2004-02-02/debates/ed170684-ad8c-4619-8704-9edeef8075f0/
UnConventionOnTheRightsOfTheChild

Bedford, A. (2015). *Serious Case Review into Child Sexual Exploitation in Oxfordshire: from the experiences of Children A, B, C, D, E, and F*. Oxfordshire Safeguarding Children Board. Cited at: www.oscb.
org.uk/wp-content/uploads/SCR-into-CSE-in-Oxfordshire-FINAL-FOR-WEBSITE.pdf

Callus, A.-M. and Farrugia, R. (2016). *The Disabled Child's Participation Rights*. London: Routledge.

Children's Legal Centre (2017). *Making Brexit Work for Children: The Impact of Brexit on Children and
Young People*. CLC. Cited at: www.childrenslegalcentre.com/wp-content/uploads/2017/08/Brexit_
Discussio--n_Paper_FINAL.pdf

Children and Social Work Act (2017), ch. 16. England and Wales.

Children and Young People (Scotland) Act (2014), asp.8. Scotland.

Children's Services Cooperation (Northern Ireland) Act (2015), ch. 10. Northern Ireland.

Clark, A. and Moss, P. (2001). *Listening to Young Children: The Mosaic Approach*. London: National
Children's Bureau for the Joseph Rowntree Foundation.

Cossar, J., Brandon, M. and Jordan, P. (2016). 'You've got to trust her and she's got to trust you': children's
views on participation in the child protection system. *Child and Family Social Work* 21(1), 103–112.

Ferguson, H. (2017). How children become invisible in child protection work: findings from research
into day-to-day social work practice. *British Journal of Social Work* 47(4), 1007–1023.

Fortin, J. (2009). *Children's Rights and the Developing Law* (3rd edn). Cambridge: Cambridge University
Press.

Franklin, A. and Sloper, P. (2009). Supporting the participation of disabled children and young people in
decision-making. *Children & Society*, 3–15.

Hart, R. (1992). *Children's Participation: From Tokenism to Citizenship*. UNICEF International Child Development Centre. Cited at: www.unicef-irc.org/publications/100-childrens-participation-from-tokenism-to-citizenship.html.

House of Lords (2019). *Human Rights Act Is Not Safe After Brexit*. Cited at: www.parliament.uk/business/lords/media-centre/house-of-lords-media-notices/2019/january-2019/human-rights-act-is-not-safe-after-brexit/

Humanium (2019). *Geneva Declaration of the Rights of the Child 1924 – Text*. Available at: www.humanium.org/en/text-2/

Independent Inquiry Child Sexual Abuse (2018). *Child Migration Programmes. Investigation Report March 2018*. Available at: www.iicsa.org.uk/key-documents/4265/view/child-migration-programmes-investigation-report-march-2018.pdf

Jay, A. (2014). *Independent Inquiry into Child Sexual Exploitation in Rotherham, 1997–2013*. Rotherham MBC. Available at: www.rotherham.gov.uk/downloads/file/1407/independent_inquiry_cse_in_rotherham

Johnny, L. (2006). Reconceptualising childhood: children's rights and youth participation in schools. *International Education Journal* 7(1), 17–25.

Joint Children Commissioners UK (2015). *Report of the UK Children's Commissioners UN Committee on the Rights of the Child Examination of the Fifth Periodic Report of the United Kingdom of Great Britain and Northern Ireland*. Available at: www.childcomwales.org.uk/uploads/publications/61.pdf/

Joint Committee on Human Rights (2005). *Reservation to the UNCRC: Immigration and Nationality*. 17th Report. UK Parliament: https://publications.parliament.uk/pa/jt200405/jtselect/jtrights/99/9907.htm#a13

King, P. and Newstead, S. (eds) (2017). *Researching Play from a Playwork Perspective*. London: Routledge.

King, P. and Sills-Jones, P. (2018). Children's use of public spaces and the role of the adult – a comparison of play ranging in the UK, and the leikkipuisto (Play Parks) in Finland. *International Journal of Play* 7(1), 27–40.

Kosher, H., Ben-Ariah, A. and Hendelsman, Y. (2016). *Child's Rights and Social Work*. Cham Switzerland: Springer.

LeFrancois, B. A. (2007). Children's participation rights: voicing opinions in inpatient care. *Child and Adolescent Mental Health* 12(2), 94–97.

Lundy, L., Kilkelly, U., Byrne, B. and Kang, J. (2012). *The UN Convention on the Rights of the Child: a Study of Legal Implementation in 12 Countries*. UNICEF UK. Cited at: www.qub.ac.uk/research-centres/CentreforChildrensRights/filestore/Fileupload,368351,en.pdf

Moore, L. and Kirk, S. (2010). A literature review of children's and young people's participation in decisions relating to health care. *Journal of Clinical Nursing* 19(15), 2215–2225.

Munro, E. (2011). *Munro Review of Child Protection: Final Report: A Child-Centred System*. London: Department for Education.

Northern Ireland Human Rights Commission (2015). *Submission to the UN Committee on the Rights of the Child on the United Kingdom's Fifth Periodic Report on Compliance with the UN Convention on the Rights of the Child*. Cited at: https://tbinternet.ohchr.org/Treaties/CRC/Shared%20Documents/GBR/INT_CRC_IFN_GBR_21222_E.pdf

Piaget, J. (1953). *The Origin of Intelligence in the Child*. London: Routledge.

Playwork Principles Scrutiny Group (PPSG) (2005). *The Playwork Principles*. Available at www.playwales.org.uk/login/uploaded/documents/Playwork%20Principles/playwork%20principles.pdf.

Rights of Young Persons (Wales) Measure (2011). Nawm 2. Wales.

Rosa, G., King, L., Stephens, M. and Smith, L. (2019). *The State of Children's Rights in England*. Children's Rights Alliance England. Cited at: www.crae.org.uk/media/126982/B2_CRAE_GMI_2018_WEB.pdf

Russell, W. (2006). 'Playwork', In T. Bruce (ed.), *Early Childhood a Guide for Students*. London: Sage.

Sandberg, K. (2014). *25 Years of the UNCRC. The Genesis and Spirit of the Convention on the Rights of the Child*. UNICEF. Cited at: www.unicef.org/crc/files/03_CRC_25_Years_Sandberg.pdf

Save the Children (1996). *Children's Participation Pack: A Practical Guide for Playworkers*. London: Save the Children and Kirklees Metropolitan Council.

Shier, H. (1995). *Article 31 Action Pack: Children's Rights and Children's Play – Resources for Action to Implement Article 31 of the United Nations Convention on the Rights of the Child*. Birmingham: PlayTrain.

SkillsActive (2010). *SkillsActive UK Play and Playwork Education and Skills Strategy 2011–2016*. Cited at: www.skillsactive.com/PDF/sectors/PDF_28_-skillsactive_Playwork_Strategy_2011-2016.pdf.

Skivenes, M. and Strandbu, A. (2006). A child perspective and children's participation. *Children, Youth and Environments* 16(2), 10–27.

Treseder, P. (1997) *Empowering Children and Young People*. London: Save the Children.

United Nations (UN) (1948). *Declaration of Human Rights*. Geneva: UN.

United Nations (UN) (1959). *Declaration of the Rights on the Child*. Geneva: UN.

United Nations (UN) (1989). *Convention on the Rights of the Child*. Geneva: UN.

United Nations (UN) (2011). *Optional Protocol to the Convention on the Rights of the Child on the Application of Communications*. Available at: https://treaties.un.org/doc/source/signature/2012/CTC_4-11d.pdf

United Nations (UN) Committee on the Rights of the Child (2009) *General Comment Number 12: The Child's Right to Be Heard*. Cited at: www2.ohchr.org/english/bodies/crc/docs/AdvanceVersions/CRC-C-GC-12.pdf.

United Nations (UN) Committee on the Rights of the Child (2016). *Concluding Observations on the Fifth Periodic Report of the United Kingdom of Great Britain and Northern Ireland*. Cited at: http://tbinternet.ohchr.org/Treaties/CRC/Shared%20Documents/GBR/CRC_C_GBR_CO_5_24195_E.docx

Williams, J. (ed.) (2013). *The UNCRC in Wales*. Cardiff: University of Wales Press.

Wragg, M. (2011). The child's right to play: rhetoric or reality? In P. Jones and G. Walker (eds), *Children's Rights in Practice*. London: SAGE.

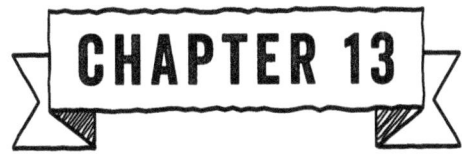

CHAPTER 13

WORKING WITH PERSONS EXPERIENCING MENTAL DISORDER

MENTAL HEALTH CONDITIONS

Keith Bradley-Adams

OVERVIEW

Mental illness is the leading cause of disability in the Western world. It is accountable for more absences from work and education than any other cause and is a major financial burden for health services. One of the surprising facts about mental illness is the difficulty many who have not experienced mental ill-health, or do not know someone with mental ill-health (although we probably all know people with mental ill-health, even if we are not aware of those persons' issues), have in differentiating between the terms mental illness and mental health. This is bizarre as when we take away the word mental most adults can differentiate between health and illness.

LEARNING OUTCOMES

By the end of this chapter you will be able to:

- Define mental disorder
- Differentiate between mental health and mental illness
- Recognise how mental disorder may interfere with mood, thinking and understanding
- Describe commonly occurring conditions
- Identify barriers to mental health care

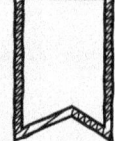

PAUSE FOR THOUGHT 13.1

Try asking family, friends or colleagues if anyone has ever had mental health, most will say no. Once you have read this chapter you will be able to point out to them that they probably all have had long periods of mental health but that some may also have experienced periods of mental illness.

Check the end of the chapter for an answer to this activity.

DEFINING MENTAL DISORDER

Before we can discuss the health and social care needs of people experiencing mental disorder it is necessary first to define what mental disorder is. The World Health Organization (2014) describe mental health as a state of well-being in which every individual realises his or her own potential, can cope with the normal stresses of life, can work productively and fruitfully, and is able to make a contribution to her or his community. Mental disorder therefore is a period of poor mental health where a person is unable to achieve these ideals. This eudemonic view of mental health and well-being is common in literature, particularly nursing texts, and forms the basis for much nursing care although Westerhof and Keyes (2010) suggest that taking a eudemonic stance is not holistic, as it is seeing only part of the picture, and that for a true interpretation of a person's mental health you must also consider hedonic elements such as their individual beliefs about their mood and perceived well-being.

Mental health, or well-being, includes not only psychological health but emotional health and social well-being too. When well we are able to regulate our emotions and behaviours; form and maintain relationships; act independently and autonomously; solve problems; and manage stress. When ill these skills are diminished or absent. Historically mental disorders were divided into two categories, neurosis and psychosis (Bradley-Adams, 2012). Psychotic conditions refer to those conditions where perception and cognition are altered and are now more commonly referred to as 'serious mental illness' and include conditions such as schizophrenia, bipolar affective disorder, and so on. Neurotic conditions are now referred to as 'common mental health problems' and include those conditions such as anxiety or depression where 'normal' emotional responses become exaggerated or absent (Bradley-Adams, 2012). The UK Adult Psychiatric Morbidity Survey (McManus et al., 2016) reports that 17.5 per cent of adults in the UK will have experienced a common mental health problem in the last week whilst 2 per cent will have experienced a serious mental illness (SMI). The report also states that for adults 25 per cent will have experienced a mental disorder in the last 12 months, whilst for persons under the age of 16, 10 per cent will have experienced a disorder during this timescale.

Although the term 'mental illness' is widely used it is more appropriate to adopt the term mental disorder. Both the International Classification of Diseases, 11th edition (ICD-11) and the US Diagnostic and Statistical Manual of Mental Disorders, 5th edition (DSM-5) adopt this term. The term 'illness' was employed in the UK when the 1983 Mental Health Act was introduced but by 2007, when the act was amended, the term had been superseded by disorder. Section 1(2) of this act states, 'In this Act "mental disorder" means any disorder or disability of the mind; and "mentally disordered" shall be construed accordingly'. Mental disorder is the leading cause of absence from work and/or education in the Western world (Vos et al., 2013; Whiteford et al., 2013) with the most common condition attributing to absence being major depression.

WHAT IS MENTAL HEALTH AND WHAT IS MENTAL DISORDER?

One of the confounding factors in diagnosing mental disorder is recognising when someone is ill and that the signs and symptoms are not just their usual behaviours. Ellerby (2015) suggests that eccentric behaviours (literally behaviours 'off-centre') are not in themselves an indication of mental disorder, arguing that eccentricity is often a 'lifestyle choice' whilst mental disorder is something the sufferer has no choice in. The UK has many persons who may be considered eccentric as they live a life of their choice, elements of which are removed from conventional 'norms', but we would not normally consider these persons who celebrate the freedom of personal expression to be mentally ill. Tucker (2015) describes many 'Great British Eccentrics' who lived (or live) lives which are very different to the common 'norms' although it is unclear how Tucker defines eccentricity as many of the behaviours described share similarity with symptoms of mental disorders.

O'Connell (2017) suggests that the eccentric straddles the void between a formal diagnosis of mental disorder and the assumption of conventional 'wellness'. Eccentrics may be unusual in their behaviour, their quirks and their beliefs but this is an indication of their uniqueness and not of insanity she argues. This is in keeping with, though not fully supportive of, the anti-psychiatry movement of the 1960s and 1970s which argued that insanity is a medical construct and should not be used to describe symptoms that are essentially a set of social concepts.

Formal diagnosis can also be confused by the necessity to differentiate between appropriate adaptation to change and episodes of ill health. For example grief is a normal and natural experience and one would be expected to experience a period of unhappiness following the death of a loved one or the end of a relationship and should not therefore be diagnosed as depressed when feelings and behaviours are in keeping with societal norms. Similarly when a person receives joyous news a period of profound happiness should not be identified as evidence of mania.

Roper (2000) describes a set of 'activities of daily living' (ADL) which are the basic actions adults can usually undertake independently when well. These activities include mostly physical and social needs (such as maintaining nutrition, having adequate rest, establishing and maintaining relationships, etc.) where if a person's ability to undertake the ADL independently is compromised we would usually accept that this is an indication of a health and/or social care need. Periods of poor mental health can severely inhibit a person's ability to manage their ADL and it is the absence of the capability to undertake ADL that is commonly accepted as indication of mental disorder.

We all exhibit symptoms of mental illness from time to time but do not necessarily consider ourselves to be ill. For example many of us talk to ourselves, but would not say we have psychosis; many of us get out of bed to check we did lock the back door or turn the kettle off, but we do not say we have obsessive compulsive disorder; and of course many more of us use substances in a way that breaches national guidelines, but we do not say we have a substance misuse issue.

What, then, are the criteria for describing someone as being mentally ill? Clinicians rely on diagnostic tools and guidelines such as the International Classification of Diseases, 11th revision (ICD-11, World Health Organization, 2018) or the Diagnostic and Statistical Manual of Mental Disorders, 5th edition (DSM 5, American Psychological Association, 2013).

These international diagnostic guidelines have two main advantages. Firstly, they enable clinicians to diagnose with some degree of confidence by employing a set of carefully described symptoms sharing a common aetiology. Secondly, they allow international comparison to occur i.e. that clinicians in the UK can compare research data with that from any other country in the world and be sure they are comparing like for like (Steel et al., 2014). These are both important paradigms as they enable international consensus on signs, symptoms, occurrence and aetiology to take place. However, Rogers and Pilgrim (2014) argue that diagnosis is a system of 'labelling' clients and that there is a danger of clinicians focusing on the disorder rather than the individual.

HOW MAY MENTAL DISORDER INTERFERE WITH MOOD, THINKING AND UNDERSTANDING?

As we all experience some symptoms of mental disorder from time to time diagnosis focuses on an individual's ability to live the life they want to live. This may not mean that we are able to 'self-actualise' (Goldstein, 1939; Maslow, 1943; Rogers, 1951) but rather that we are able to undertake the activities we would wish to undertake without being prevented from doing so by symptoms of a mental disorder. It is when we lose the ability to undertake the activities of daily living that we become ill. Mental disorder can have a global effect on the individual experiencing ill health; that is to say they effect the ABC of mental health – A, affect, ; B, behaviour, C, cognition.

Affect is the term used in psychological medicine to describe mood, feelings or emotions (Miller-Keane and O'Toole, 2003). Schnall (2011) reports that whilst most definitions do describe affect as comprising emotions and mood there is no common consensus on what mood actually is, arguing that it appears to be a subjective construct influenced by the researchers' methodology. However most authors do link affect, mood and emotion together when describing symptoms of mental well-being and of mental disorder and it could be argued that the best person to describe mood is the individual themselves. Many mental illnesses will cause mood disturbances which may involve severely suppressing mood, elevating mood, or fluctuations from high to low mood, such as bipolar affective disorder. Where a person is unable to regulate their mood or emotions they would be considered to be experiencing a mental disorder.

Behaviour refers to how we as humans interact with environments, situations and with others (Starr and Taggart, 2009). Reber (1995) asserts that psychologists have spent many years attempting to define behaviour and proposes a brief summary of these findings – behaviour is a measurable response. That is, we can measure how individuals respond to stimuli and the differences in these responses are what we term behaviour. Where an individual displays behaviours out of keeping with others or with their own common behaviours we may consider them to be experiencing a disorder. For example, a person with a phobia may avoid certain situations or settings; a person with post-traumatic stress disorder may be hyper-vigilant and respond to loud noises, etc. in a manner out of keeping with others; persons experiencing schizophrenia may exhibit bizarre behaviours if experiencing positive symptoms or may appear apathetic and withdrawn if experiencing negative symptoms, etc.

Cognition has been described as the internal processes through which humans make sense of the environment around them and select appropriate actions and responses (Eysenck and Keane, 2013). The ability to reason or to think clearly and logically may become impaired in many conditions. Although perhaps the most obvious illnesses where cognition becomes impaired are the dementias (where memory, ability to calculate, perception, etc. may become altered) these symptoms could be present in many other disorders including depression, psychosis or substance misuse.

Where an individual has experienced changes to one or more of their ABC which result in a reduced ability to undertake the activities of daily living and to lead the independent life of their choice then they would be considered to no longer be mentally well and thus to be experiencing mental disorder. When assessing a person's mental status using the ABC approach the clinician must take account of the person's age, culture, and so on, as these may influence the validity of their beliefs. For example, a child of five would probably believe in Santa Claus; however, you would be surprised if an adult held this belief. Similarly many African cultures have strong beliefs in witchcraft which you would not expect most Europeans to believe (Radford, 2010). Mansel and Bradley-Adams (2017) have devised a mnemonic 'I AM A STAR' for undertaking mental status examinations in which the clinician is able to carry out a holistic assessment of the client (see Table 13.1).

Table 13.1 I AM A STAR Mental Status Examinations

I	Introduce Yourself	Hello my name is (#hellomynameis.org.uk)
A	Appearance & Behaviour	Appearance Body build – Under/overweight. Clothing – Appropriate to age, season, clean, casually dressed, dishevelled, colours. Hygiene and grooming – Odour, clean/dirty, unkempt, meticulous. Behaviour Facial expression – Sad, happy, excited, elated, worried. Eye contact – No eye contact, fleeting, appropriate. Compulsions
M	Movement & Gait	Foot tapping, hand wringing, nail-biting, tics, chewing. Agitated. Difficulty rising from the chair, balance. Awkward, clumsy, agile, falling easily. Gait (manner of walking) – Brisk, shuffling, normal.
A	Affect & Mood	Affect – Lively, flat, normal, superficial. Mood – Tearful, sad, appropriate, hopelessness, depressed, anxious, elated. Both mood and affect can be described as euthymic (normal), labile (rapidly changing from one mood state to another), euphoric (excessively happy). Congruous/incongruous – Some depressed service users look depressed; however, others who are depressed appear euthymic. Approach to you – Open, warm, guarded, friendly, suspicious.
S	Speech	Rapid, slow, slurred, clear, monotonous, dramatic, talkative, hesitant, mumbling, incoherent. Responds only to questions, scant, mute, repetitive. Pressure of speech-seen in mania, rapid changing topics.

(Continued)

Table 13.1 (Conitnued)

I	Introduce Yourself	Hello my name is (#hellomynameis.org.uk)
T	Thought Pattern	Coherent, incoherent, confused, vague.
		Excited.
		Relevant, irrelevant.
		Difficult to follow thought process.
		Suicidal ideations – BEGIN RISK ASSESSMENT.
		Hallucinations – sensations experienced by the service user without external stimuli (e.g. auditory, visual, olfactory, gustatory, tactile).
		Delusions – Persistent false beliefs (e.g. persecution).
		Flight of ideas – in mania, pressure of speech, rapid changing topics.
		Paranoid ideations.
		Compulsions.
		Obsessions – unwanted thoughts.
		Grandiose – unrealistic exaggeration of own importance.
		Somatic – misinterpretation of physical symptoms.
		Phobias.
		Preoccupation.
A	Attention & Concentration	Easily distracted, poor concentration, memory.
		Orientated to time, place and person (full name, current location, date and time).
		Impulsive behaviour.
		Unrealistic decisions.
		Complete denial.
		Level of consciousness – Respond when spoken to in a normal/loud voice.
R	Respond & Record.	Pass on information if you have concerns, share information as appropriate and within confidentiality guidelines (e.g. with Medic/CRHT).
		Document your findings.

Source: Mansel and Bradley-Adams (2017).

This tool includes the advice to ensure that assessment includes subjective elements – real life experiences as interpreted and reported by the client, and objective assessment from the clinician's observations. This is important as what the client says is not always congruent with what the clinician sees (Mansel and Bradley-Adams, 2017) as many persons will, consciously or subconsciously, misreport symptoms and behaviours and clinicians will interpret findings in their own unique way (Aboraya et al., 2006) although Cella et al. (2010) report a good level of accuracy in self-reporting of symptoms where a specific tool is employed. Labelling of persons as 'mad' or 'bad' was common in mental health care in the last century but this outdated approach is no longer acceptable; even terms such as 'them' and 'us' can be seen as labelling (Tew, 2005).

One of the challenges in diagnosing symptoms as being psychological in origin is the need to first exclude any possible somatic (physical or biological) causes. For example neoplasms, or tumours, in the brain can affect the organs functionality and can mimic the symptoms of other disorders such as in peduncular hallucinosis, where persons with a tumour in the mid-brain may develop vivid hallucinations (Geddes et al., 2016). Persons with concussion can present with symptoms of confusion and memory loss which may appear similar to dementia (Coppel, 2014) whilst persons who have taken psychoactive substances, including alcohol, can present with a range of features which may be confused with other disorders including dementia, depression and psychosis (Bradley-Adams, 2012). Engel (1977) first proposed the biopsychosocial model which suggests that causes of mental illness are not dependent on a single paradigm but rather the interaction between a number of factors in the biological, psychological and sociological domains. Engel observed that whilst many psychiatric patients share common social history in that they had experienced childhood abuse, been brought up in poverty, and had low levels of education, and so on, these were not necessarily determinants of poor mental health. Persons brought up with similar life experiences did not develop psychiatric conditions and, conversely, some persons brought up in relevant affluence did. Similarly whilst some changes in the brain (e.g. chemical imbalance) of persons with some conditions can be observed other persons can exhibit the same symptoms without any changes to the brain and persons with apparent changes may not exhibit symptoms.

Engel's work laid the foundations for a more holistic approach to diagnosis and treatment. In contemporary psychiatry it is uncommon to attribute a person's presentation to a single cause. More importantly the interventions offered to individuals experiencing mental disorder will include biological, psychological and sociological elements. As no one member of the multi-disciplinary and inter-disciplinary team will have the skills and knowledge to address needs or deficits in all of these areas a team approach to care and treatment is vital. Persons experiencing mental illness are likely to come into contact with a range of health and social care professionals and possibly the criminal justice system during the course of their disorder therefore.

COMMONLY OCCURRING DISORDERS

The common cold is, as its name rather conveniently suggests, the most common disease on the planet. However, when we begin to look at other common conditions they are dominated by mental illness, particularly those disorders known under the umbrella term of 'common mental health problems' including, anxiety and depression. Steel et al. (2014) report that in a global survey of mental disorder they found that almost a fifth of the world's adults reported experiencing a mental disorder in the previous 12 months, whilst a third reported experiencing a mental disorder at some point in their lifetime. There are some variations in these figures when gender is taken into account with female respondents being twice as likely as males to experience disorders of mood whilst males are three times more likely to experience substance misuse (Steel et al., 2014).

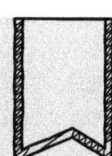

PAUSE FOR THOUGHT 13.2

Why may this be the case? What is it about females that make them apparently more likely to experience commonly occurring conditions? What is it about men that makes them more likely to use substances in an unhealthy way?

Check the end of the chapter for an answer to this activity.

It is highly likely that the incidence of mental disorder in males is similar to the incidence in females (Smith et al., 2018) but that the reported incidence is lower due to under-reporting and the absence of a formal diagnosis. Women are twice as likely as men to seek support for psychological symptoms (Singleton and Lewis, 2003) whilst it is also recognised that men will report psychological symptoms as somatic (physical) symptoms such as sleep disturbance, lower back pain, reduced appetite, etc. (Walsh, 2009). Bradley-Adams (2012) suggests that limited-self disclosure is more common in men and that they are less likely to firstly identify issues as being psychological in origin; and secondly less likely to seek help. A scenario typified by the 'big boys don't cry' attitude of previous generations. Seidler et al. (2016) support this view asserting that masculine gender norms prevent men from seeking help and suggesting that male suicide rates (75 per cent of all suicides are male) are a clear indication that male depression rates must be comparable to female rates.

Some of the conditions which are prevalent in the UK are described below. The list includes both serious mental illnesses and commonly occurring conditions. Although there are many conditions that could be discussed here discussion is limited to those conditions which either due to severity of symptoms or commonality of occurrence are those that health and care professionals are more likely to encounter.

ANXIETY

Anxiety is a common and 'normal' response to a range of life events including exams, meeting new people, starting a new job, and so on. For some people this response becomes exaggerated and becomes an anxiety disorder. Anxiety disorder is the most common of all mental disorders with an estimated 16 per cent of the population experiencing anxiety at any given time (Walters et al., 2012). Anxiety disorder is a maladaptive response to stimuli known as 'stressors' or situations that can induce stress.

Although humans have a natural physiological and emotional response mechanism to stress, known as the 'fight or flight response' (Cannon, 1929), this should be a short-lived response which does not result in long-term harm. In anxiety disorders this response appears heightened and will reduce the individual's ability to undertake activities of daily living. Anxiety may be termed as 'general anxiety disorder', a free-floating set of behaviours not linked to a single stimulus; or where linked to single stimulus as a 'phobia'. Anxiety can be severely disabling and can prevent an individual from participating in work, education, social activities, and so on.

Although anxiety may be a symptom of mental disorder there may also be occasions when anxiety may in fact be of benefit. Selye (1974) describes the concept of eustress (or good stress) where for some individuals the pressure of, for example, a watching audience or a looming deadline is necessary in order for them to motivate themselves to perform to the best of their ability. Without this motivation the individual is unable to give their best. This is commonly seen in students who do not begin their essay until a day or two prior to submission and cannot understand why their peers spend weeks undertaking research!

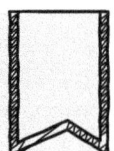

PAUSE FOR THOUGHT 13.3

Think about the last time you felt anxious. How did it feel? What were the emotional/psychological/mental changes you noticed? What were the physical changes? Anxiety is characterised by fear, restlessness, shortness of breath, tightness in the chest, etc. It is sometimes difficult to tell (without appropriate diagnostic equipment) if a person with these symptoms is having a panic attack or a heart attack.

Check the end of the chapter for an answer to this activity.

DEPRESSION

Depression is a period of low mood, extreme sadness and anhedonia (WHO, 2018). Although more commonly reported in women, one in four women compared to one in ten men (Singleton and Lewis, 2003), it is believed incidence rates in both genders are broadly comparable. Estimates suggest that about 60–70 per cent of adults will experience a period of intense unhappiness and/or low mood at some point in their lives and that for most persons experiencing these changes a diagnosis of depression may be appropriate.

Typical symptoms include: anhedonia (an inability to enjoy simple pleasures); gloomy or pessimistic outlook; sleep disturbances; decreased libido; and asociality. Symptoms may vary between genders, however, with the Royal College of Psychiatrists (2015) reporting that certain symptoms are more prevalent in male patients including: irritability; sudden anger; increased loss of control; greater risk-taking; and aggression. This is of concern as suicide is often linked to depression and these traits predispose males to suicidality which, as discussed above, is three times more common in men.

The WHO have described three levels of depression depending on the number of symptoms and their severity (i.e. the impact of symptoms on the individual's activity to undertake the ADL). Depression is classified as either mild, moderate or severe. Persons with mild depression will have less profound symptomology and would normally begin to recover within two to three weeks of receiving treatment/support; in moderate depression symptoms will be more debilitating and would last for at least two weeks; in severe depression the range and intensity of symptoms is greater and can last for many weeks or even months. Severe depression is a life-changing condition which will impact on the individual's ability to work, study, socialise etc. There is also an increased risk of suicide during periods of severe depression.

SCHIZOPHRENIA

Schizophrenia is a severe and enduring mental illness which affects about 1 per cent of the population (Rethink Mental Illness, 2017). Although there is no conclusive evidence to suggest the causes of schizophrenia many theories have been proposed including changes to the physiology of the brain or to levels of certain chemicals in the brain. Although some of these theories are quite credible it is also true to suggest that whilst for some persons with schizophrenia changes are evident it is also true that for many others with schizophrenia there are no changes present and that some persons who appear to have these somatic markers do not have schizophrenia. One thing we do know is that whilst 1 per cent of the general population are likely to develop schizophrenia this risk is significantly increased when a close family member has schizophrenia where the occurrence increases to 15 per cent. The evidence is unclear as to whether this is a genetic risk factor (nature) or if this is a result of family and societal influences (nurture).

The disorder is characterised by alterations to perception and thought processes. As these changes can occur in other conditions and also as a result of substance use it is necessary to undertake careful assessment of the individual before making a diagnosis. Formal diagnosis is usually confirmed where two or more symptoms are present in the absence of any relevant somatic influence. Symptoms are divided into 'positive symptoms' (things the disorder adds to the person's premorbid state) and 'negative symptoms' (things the disorder takes away). The main positive symptoms are hallucinations and delusions. Hallucinations are the perception of stimuli which are not present. They can occur in any modality (visual, auditory, tactile, gustatory and olfactory) although hearing voices is the most common symptom (Bradley-Adams, 2012). Delusions are a false, fixed belief which cannot be changed (e.g. I am the Queen of England). Negative symptoms are often referred to as 'the four As': avolition; anhedonia; asociality/ autism; alogia.

Avolition is described as a lack of motivation. Persons experiencing avolition have extreme difficulty in making decisions and in motivating themselves to engage in any activities; they also appear withdrawn and inactive. Anhedonia is an inability to experience pleasure, characterised by 'flat affect' or a mood that changes little irrespective of stimulus, persons with anhedonia may appear sullen and uncaring. Asociality or autism is a reduction in the ability to develop social relationships and to engage with others; persons often appear solitary and to express a limited range of emotions. Alogia is described as poverty of speech, where a person says very little and will rarely initiate conversations.

BIPOLAR AFFECTIVE DISORDER

Bipolar affective disorder (BAD) used to be referred to as 'manic depression'; however, as it is recognised that the disorder is a mood disorder the term 'affective disorder' is more appropriate. The bipolar element refers to mood swings which can be at absolute extremes, i.e. from pole to pole. As both titles suggest the disorder is characterised by experiencing symptoms of depression and symptoms of mania. Mania refers to episodes of increased excitability, hyper-arousal and over-activity (MIND, 2013). Persons who are manic, or hypomanic, will be extremely talkative, experience flight of ideas, be physically active and may become frustrated with persons moving at a slower pace (Bradley-Adams, 2012).

A diagnosis of BAD may be made therefore if a person experiences 'highs' or 'lows' and if in between their mood is only slightly lowered or slightly elevated from their premorbid baseline. Where a cycle develops of recurring highs and lows this is referred to as 'Bipolar 1' whilst if a person experiences frequent highs but does not experience significant lows the diagnosis would be 'bipolar 2' (MIND, 2013). If the predominant mood is low with periods of 'normality' in between the individual is more likely to be diagnosed with 'unipolar depression'. Whilst for a true diagnosis of BAD to be made a person must experience mood swings where in at least one direction the change is marked, an alternative diagnosis of cyclothymia may be made where the individual experiences periods of low and high moods without excessive change in both directions, although change in one direction may be greater (WHO, 2018).

DEMENTIA

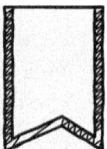

PAUSE FOR THOUGHT 13.4

What do you think of when you hear the term 'dementia'? What sort of behaviours do you associate with the term? Who may experience dementia? Is it just part of the normal ageing process?

Check the end of the chapter for an answer to this activity.

Dementia is an umbrella term given to over 100 different organic brain disorders; that is disorders where the organ of the brain has undergone change which results in the illness. The World Health Organization (2018) define organic brain disorders as, 'A range of mental disorders grouped together on the basis of their having in common a demonstrable aetiology in cerebral disease, brain injury or other insult leading to cerebral dysfunction'. Organic brain disorders include conditions where the changes are passing or transient, such as intoxication or delirium, and conditions where the changes are permanent, such as dementias. The diagnostic criteria for an organic disorder being classed as dementia are that the symptoms or condition are present for at least six months without improvement. If treated promptly and appropriately it is expected that recovery rates for individuals experiencing acute organic brain disorders are 75 per cent i.e. that 75 per cent of persons are expected to recover within the first three weeks; 20 per cent will recover within three months; 5 per cent will become chronic or die.

The most common cause of dementia in the world is Alzheimer's disease (Alzheimer's Association, 2015; Alzheimer's Society, 2018). Dementia is typified by the changes you would yourself experience if you have a transient organic brain condition, such as being drunk (i.e. changes to perception, understanding, mood, language, etc.). Persons with dementia experience these changes for a period of six months or longer without remission or recovery and, typically, the condition will worsen over time. The main risk factor in developing Alzheimer's disease is old age; the longer you live the more likely you are to develop the condition. However Alzheimer's disease is not a normal part of the ageing process as although the incidence increases over time the incidence in persons over the age of 80 is still a fifth so 80 per cent of persons who are 80 and above do not have dementia. Indeed the most common mental disorder in persons aged over 80 is depression which will affect at least 25 per cent of older persons (Bradley-Adams, 2012).

ADDICTIONS AND APPETITIVE BEHAVIOUR

The World Health Organization (2010) describe addiction as becoming dependent on a substance to the extent that its use becomes uncontrolled and harmful. Under this definition a person may become addicted to a substance but not to a behaviour. The WHO offer the alternative description of 'appetitive behaviours' for those behaviours persons have an appetite to engage in, even if the behaviour is harmful. Under these criteria an individual could, for example, be addicted to nicotine, alcohol or heroin but not addicted to gambling, sex, or exercise. The WHO defend this interpretation by arguing that when persons engage in 'risky' activities they produce chemicals (neuro-transmitters and hormones including dopamine, cortisol, adrenaline, etc.) that make the activity pleasurable and that if an addiction occurs then it is to these chemicals and not to the behaviour which caused their levels to rise (Barry et al., 2009). Under this model one risky activity can be replaced by another with the same effect; for example, a person with an appetite for gambling could switch to exercise instead.

However, in 2018 the WHO revised this guidance and in the latest version of the International Classification of Diseases (ICD-11) gambling is now recognised as a mental disorder. This is probably more to do with the real harm that excessive, uncontrolled gambling can have on an individual and their family rather than a change in the basic belief of the need to experience chemical addiction for a behaviour to be deemed dependent. This is an interesting development which may in time change our views on addiction to include other behaviours such as gaming, texting or even tattooing. There is already evidence which suggests that engagement in appetitive behaviours may lead to other disorders including anxiety and depression (Demirci et al., 2015).

Although much of the focus on addictions is on class 1 drugs (as defined under the Misuse of Drugs Act 1971) the most commonly abused chemicals are caffeine, alcohol, nicotine and prescription drugs. This focus on illicit drugs may be counterintuitive given that some illicit drugs may be less harmful than their legitimate contemporaries (e.g. cannabis) and the ease of access to legitimate substances which may actually be more harmful when used long term (e.g. alcohol and nicotine) (Lachenmeier and Rehm, 2015).

Another confounding factor in substance use is that even low or moderate use may increase other risks. Grossman and Markowitz (2002) found that teenagers and adolescents are more likely to engage in unprotected sexual intercourse, with all the inherent risks, when drinking even moderately. Baskin-Sommers and Sommers (2006) support this view and in fact go further suggesting that other risky encounters such as having group sex with multiple partners is more likely when substances are involved. The risks increase if more than one substance is involved and there is also an increased risk of being the victim of non-consensual sexual activity and assault (Baskin-Sommers and Sommers, 2006).

Shinew and Parry (2005) found that college students' use of alcohol, nicotine, ecstasy and cannabis is higher than in persons of similar ages not in higher education. This contradicts the lay perception of substance use as being more common in persons not in employment or education. Shinew and Parry (2005) also found that substance use is an infrequent activity linked to events such as attendance at clubs or raves rather than a daily event for many young people which again counters the image many lay persons have of drug users. These findings are no surprise to most health professionals, however, and it is because of this picture of young professionals using drugs infrequently that the lay image of an 'addict' is not shared by mental health professionals.

EATING DISORDERS

There are three main eating disorders – anorexia nervosa, bulimia nervosa and compulsive overeating (Bradley-Adams, 2012). Anorexia nervosa (AN) may occur in both males and females irrespective of age, gender, sexuality, orientation, etc. although it is most commonly identified in young females (Zipfel et al., 2015). AN is not just about managing weight; it is a serious mental disorder which has a very high mortality rate (Westmoreland et al., 2016). Suicide is one of the most prevalent risks in AN (Chesney et al., 2014) and AN is believed to carry the highest risk of suicide in all mental disorders (Preti et al., 2011). Lay persons generally refer to AN as 'anorexia' which is wrong as it suggests that it is a physical disorder rather than a psychological disorder; it is only through widening public understanding of this serious mental disorder as a mental disorder that sufferers can access appropriate treatment. Anorexia is a physical illness, such as oral cancer or a stroke, which prevent a person from eating.

Anorexia is a physical illness, such as oral cancer or a stroke, which prevent a person from eating. Anorexia Nervosa is a psychological condition where the sufferer has altered body perception and other delusional beliefs in relation to diet (Treasure and Alexander, 2013). These delusional beliefs include a refusal to accept that the behaviour is harmful and a denial of the individual's emaciation (Mountjoy et al., 2014). Other explanations for the disorder include feelings of low self-worth as a driver to starvation and an avoidance of reaching sexual maturity (Treasure and Alexander, 2013). AN is extremely difficult to manage and is life threatening; it has the highest death rate of all psychiatric disorders (Kaye, 2008).

Bulimia Nervosa (BN) is characterised by periods of binge eating and periods of purging (induced vomiting or diarrhoea) in an attempt to retain or reduce weight (Berg et al., 2013).

Mortality rates are estimated at 1–8 per cent with most studies suggesting a rate of around 2.5 per cent (Keel and Brown, 2010). Waxman (2009) suggests that although there are many similarities in eating disorders persons with BN differ from those with AN as they are more likely to exhibit impulsive behaviours, typically binge eating. However, Waxman (2009) also asserts that other impulsive behaviours such as self-harm and suicide are prevalent in binge-eaters.

Compulsive overeating disorder (COD), sometimes referred to as *binge eating disorder* (BED), is a disorder where the individual is compelled to eat vast amounts of, typically, unhealthy foods (Barry et al., 2009). As with BN there is a compulsion to eat even where the person knows the behaviour is unhealthy. Many studies suggest that BED is the most common of all eating disorders and is a significant contributor to the worldwide obesity epidemic (Guerdjikova et al., 2017).

BARRIERS TO MENTAL HEALTH CARE

Persons experiencing mental disorder often face the additional challenge of dealing with the stigma of being labelled 'mentally ill' (Clement et al., 2015; Corrigan et al., 2014; Corrigan and Wassel, 2008). This stigma can be socially disabling, preventing individuals from accessing the opportunities available to others. Stigma also affects the rates at which persons choose to seek help, engage with services and follow care and treatment plans (Corrigan et al., 2014). Alongside the stigmatisation from wider society many persons with mental disorder also stigmatise themselves. This increases the likelihood of not seeking help or adhering to treatment regimens and is seen as a key factor in relapse, particularly for those persons who will not take their medication as this is seen as a clear indication of their having a mental disorder (Kao et al., 2017).

Students are seen as particularly susceptible to self-stigma, and the resultant non-engagement (Eisenberg et al., 2009). This may be surprising on the one hand as students are by definition well educated and intelligent although it should be borne in mind that they are also young people trying to fit in with a new group of peers and would not wish to stand out for what they may perceive as 'wrong' reasons. There is also evidence to suggest that males are more prone to self-stigmatisation than females and that men who see themselves as weak are less likely to engage with services (Judd et al., 2008).

Livingston and Boyd (2010) undertook a systematic review of literature on the subject of self-stigmatisation and concluded that this 'insidious social force' is a determinant of the development of mental disorder and that for those persons diagnosed with, or experiencing, mental disorder self-stigma is a perpetuating force which prevents recovery. Crucially they determined that self-stigmatisation robs the individual of hope.

CONCLUSION

In this chapter we have looked at definitions of mental disorder/illness and become familiar with how to identify persons who are mentally well and persons whose mental health may be compromised. Through accessing diagnostic criteria such as DSM-5 and ICD-10 we are able to understand the changes to affect, behaviour and cognition which may be present in certain conditions and to recognise serious mental illness and commonly occurring conditions. We have also considered the assessment process of these conditions and some of the barriers to providing health care.

GO FURTHER ACTIVITY

At the beginning of the chapter, we discussed the question, 'Have you ever had mental ill-health?' If you were asked this now how would you respond? You should be able to differentiate between mental health and mental illness, and recognise signs and symptoms of some conditions. Importantly you should also be aware that although some of these conditions may be limiting they should not become the primary focus of your life. In the next chapter we will discuss concepts of recovery and see how it is possible to live with mental illness.

Check the end of the chapter for an answer to this activity.

ANSWERS TO CHAPTER 13 ACTIVITIES

—— Pause for Thought 13.1: Answers

This activity requires you to reflect on your own thoughts and experiences and to recognise the difference between mental health and mental illness.

—— Pause for Thought 13.2: Answers

This may relate to psychosocial conditions. Males may report mental health issue less frequently than females, perhaps due to perceived stigma. Males may also have greater difficulty in recognising and labelling emotions, a condition called alexithymia which is more common in males than females.

—— Pause for Thought 13.3: Answers

Anxiety is characterised by a range of physical (somatic) and psychological symptoms which can make diagnosis difficult. The fear and panic felt can be exacerbated by the perceived physical symptoms e.g. fear of sudden death.

—— Pause for Thought 13.4: Answers

You may associate the following when you think about dementia: loss of memory, difficulty in performing familiar tasks, and problems with keeping track of things. Typically, dementia is associated with older persons (2% of persons aged of 66-70 suffer from dementia, rising to 20% of persons aged 80 or more). It is not part of the normal ageing process and is regarded a brain disease rather than normal age associated memory impairment.

——— **Go Further Activity: Answers**

This activity requires you to reflect on your own thoughts and experiences.

REFERENCES

Aboraya, A., Rankin, E., France, C., El-Missiry, A. and John, C. (2006). The reliability of psychiatric diagnosis revisited: the clinician's guide to improve the reliability of psychiatric diagnosis. *Psychiatry (Edgmont)* 3(1), 41–50.

Alzheimer's Association (2015). Alzheimer's disease facts and figures. *Alzheimer's & Dementia: The Journal of the Alzheimer's Association* 11(3), 332.

Alzheimer's Society (2018) Alzheimer's disease. Available at: www.alzheimers.org.uk/about-dementia/types-dementia/alzheimers-disease (accessed 25 July 2018)

American Psychological Association (2013). *Diagnostic and Statistical Manual of Mental Disorders*, 5th edition (DSM 5). New York: APA.

Barry, D., Clarke, M. and Petry, N. M. (2009). Obesity and its relationship to addictions: is overeating a form of addictive behavior? *The American Journal on Addictions* 18(6), 439–451.

Baskin-Sommers, A. and Sommers, I. (2006). The co-occurrence of substance use and high-risk behaviors. *Journal of Adolescent health* 38(5), 609–611.

Berg, K. C., Crosby, R. D., Cao, L., Peterson, C. B., Engel, S. G., Mitchell, J. E. and Wonderlich, S. A. (2013). Facets of negative affect prior to and following binge-only, purge-only, and binge/purge events in women with bulimia nervosa. *Journal of Abnormal Psychology* 122(1), 111.

Bradley-Adams, K. (2012). Mental health. In B. Kozier, G. Erb, A. Snyder, S. Harvey and H. Morgan-Samuel (eds), *Fundamentals of Nursing: Concepts, Process and Practice* (2nd edn). Harlow: Pearson Education Limited.

Cannon, W. (1929). *Bodily Changes in Pain, Hunger, Fear and Rage* (2nd edn). New York: Appleton.

Cella, D., Riley, W., Stone, A., Rothrock, N., Reeve, B., Yount, S., ... and Cook, K. (2010). The Patient-Reported Outcomes Measurement Information System (PROMIS) developed and tested its first wave of adult self-reported health outcome item banks: 2005–2008. *Journal of Clinical Epidemiology* 63(11), 1179–1194.

Chesney, E., Goodwin, G. M. and Fazel, S. (2014). Risks of all-cause and suicide mortality in mental disorders: a meta-review. *World Psychiatry* 13(2), 153–160.

Clement, S., Schauman, O., Graham, T., Maggioni, F., Evans-Lacko, S., Bezborodovs, N., ... and Thornicroft, G. (2015). What is the impact of mental health-related stigma on help-seeking? A systematic review of quantitative and qualitative studies. *Psychological Medicine* 45(1), 11–27.

Coppel, D. (2014). Post-concussion syndrome. In *Mind, Body and Sport: Understanding and Supporting Student-Athlete Mental Wellness* (pp. 65–68). Indianapolis, IN: National Collegiate Athletic Association.

Corrigan, P. W., Druss, B. G. and Perlick, D. A. (2014). The impact of mental illness stigma on seeking and participating in mental health care. *Psychological Science in the Public Interest* 15(2), 37–70.

Corrigan, P. W. and Wassel, A. (2008). Understanding and influencing the stigma of mental illness. *Journal of Psychosocial Nursing and Mental Health Services* 46(1), 42–48.

Demirci, K., Akgönül, M. and Akpinar, A. (2015). Relationship of smartphone use severity with sleep quality, depression, and anxiety in university students. *Journal of Behavioral Addictions* 4(2), 85–92.

Eisenberg, D., Downs, M. F., Golberstein, E. and Zivin, K. (2009). Stigma and help seeking for mental health among college students. *Medical Care Research and Review* 66(5), 522–541.

Ellerby, M. (2015). Schizophrenia: stigma and the impact of literature. *Schizophrenia Bulletin* 44(3), 466–467.

Engel, G. L. (1977). The need for a new medical model: a challenge for biomedicine. *Science* 196(4286), 129–136.

Eysenck, M. W. and Keane, M. T. (2013). *Cognitive Psychology: A Student's Handbook*. Philadelphia: Psychology Press.

Geddes, M. R., Tie, Y., Gabrieli, J. D., McGinnis, S. M., Golby, A. J. and Whitfield-Gabrieli, S. (2016). Altered functional connectivity in lesional peduncular hallucinosis with REM sleep behavior disorder. *Cortex* 74, 96–106.

Goldstein, K. (1939). *The Organism: A Holistic Approach to Biology Derived from Pathological Data in Man*. New York: American Book Company.

Grossman, M. and Markowitz, S. (2002). *I Did What Last Night?!!! Adolescent Risky Sexual Behaviors and Substance Use* (No. w9244). Cambridge, MA: National Bureau of Economic Research.

Guerdjikova, A. I., Mori, N., Casuto, L. S. and McElroy, S. L. (2017). Binge eating disorder. *Psychiatric Clinics* 40(2), 255–266.

Judd, F., Komiti, A. and Jackson, H. (2008). How does being female assist help-seeking for mental health problems? *Australian and New Zealand Journal of Psychiatry* 42(1), 24–29.

Kao, Y. C., Lien, Y. J., Chang, H. A., Tzeng, N. S., Yeh, C. B. and Loh, C. H. (2017). Stigma resistance in stable schizophrenia: the relative contributions of stereotype endorsement, self-reflection, self-esteem, and coping styles. *The Canadian Journal of Psychiatry* 62(10), 735–744.

Kaye, W. (2008). Neurobiology of anorexia and bulimia nervosa. *Physiology & Behavior* 94(1), 121–135.

Keel, P. K. and Brown, T. A. (2010). Update on course and outcome in eating disorders. *International Journal of Eating Disorders* 43(3), 195–204.

Kozier, B., Erb, G., Berman, A., Snyder, A., Harvey, S. and Morgan-Samuel, H. (2012) *Fundamentals of Nursing: Concepts, Process and Practice* (2nd edn). Harlow: Pearson Education Limited.

Lachenmeier, D. W. and Rehm, J. (2015). Comparative risk assessment of alcohol, tobacco, cannabis and other illicit drugs using the margin of exposure approach. *Scientific Reports* 5, 8126.

Livingston, J. D. and Boyd, J. E. (2010). Correlates and consequences of internalized stigma for people living with mental illness: a systematic review and meta-analysis. *Social Science & Medicine* 71(12), 2150–2161.

Mansel, B. and Bradley-Adams, K. (2017). 'I AM A STAR': a mnemonic for undertaking a mental state examination. *Mental Health Practice* 21(1), 21.

Maslow, A. H. (1943). A theory of human motivation. *Psychological Review* 50(4), 370–396.

McManus S., Bebbington P., Jenkins R. and Brugha, T. (eds) (2016) *Mental Health and Wellbeing in England: Adult Psychiatric Morbidity Survey 2014*. Leeds: NHS Digital.

Miller-Keane, O. T. M. and O'Toole, M. T. (2003). *Miller-Keane Encyclopedia and Dictionary of Medicine, Nursing, and Allied Health: A Book* (7th edn). Philadelphia: Saunders.

MIND (2013). Mania & hypomania. Available at: www.mind.org.uk/information-support/types-of-mental-health-problems/hypomania-and-mania/#.W1g-rMIna70 25/07/18

Mountjoy, R. L., Farhall, J. F. and Rossell, S. L. (2014). A phenomenological investigation of overvalued ideas and delusions in clinical and subclinical anorexia nervosa. *Psychiatry Research* 220(1–2), 507–512.

O'Connell, K. (2017). Eccentricity: the case for undermining legal categories of disability and normalcy. *Continuum*, 31(3), 352–364.

Preti, A., Rocchi, M. B., Sisti, D. et al. (2011). A comprehensive meta-analysis of the risk of suicide in eating disorders. *Acta Psychiatrica Scandinavica* 124(1), 6–17.

Radford, B. (2010). Belief in witchcraft widespread in Africa. *Live Science*. Available at: www.livescience.com/8515-belief-witchcraft-widespread-africa.html

Reber, A. S. (1995). *The Penguin Dictionary of Psychology*. Harmondsworth, Middlesex: Penguin Press.

Rethink Mental Illness (2017) Schizophrenia Advice Sheet. Available at: www.rethink.org/advice

Rogers, A. and Pilgrim, D. (2014). *A Sociology of Mental Health and Illness*. Maidenhead: McGraw-Hill Education (UK).

Rogers, C. (1951). *Client-Centered Therapy: Its Current Practice, Implications and Theory*. London: Constable.

Roper, N. (2000). *The Roper–Logan–Tierney Model of Nursing: Based on Activities of Living*. Edinburgh: Churchill Livingstone.

Royal College of Psychiatrists (2015) Depression and men. Available at: www.rcpsych.ac.uk/healthadvice/problemsanddisorders/depressionmen.aspx

Schnall, S. (2011). Affect, mood and emotions. *Social and emotional aspects of learning,* 59.

Seidler, Z. E., Dawes, A. J., Rice, S. M., Oliffe, J. L. and Dhillon, H. M. (2016). The role of masculinity in men's help-seeking for depression: a systematic review. *Clinical Psychology Review* 49, 106–118.

Selye, H. (1974). *Stress without Distress*. Philadelphia: P.A. J.B. Lippincott, Co.

Shinew, K. J. and Parry, D. C. (2005). Examining college students' participation in the leisure pursuits of drinking and illegal drug use. *Journal of Leisure Research* 37(3), 364–386.

Singleton, N. and Lewis, G. (2003). *Better or Worse: A Longitudinal Study of the Mental Health of Adults Living in Private Households in Great Britain*. London: Office for National Statistics.

Smith, D. T., Mouzon, D. M. and Elliott, M. (2018). Reviewing the assumptions about men's mental health: an exploration of the gender binary. *American Journal of Men's Health* 12(1), 78–89.

Starr, C. and Taggart, R. (1992) *Biology: the Unity and Diversity of Life* (6th edn). Belmont, CA: Wadsworth.

Steel, Z., Marnane, C., Iranpour, C., Chey, T., Jackson, J. W., Patel, V. and Silove, D. (2014). The global prevalence of common mental disorders: a systematic review and meta-analysis 1980–2013. *International Journal of Epidemiology* 43(2), 476–493.

Tew, J. (2005). *Social Perspectives in Mental Health; Developing Social Models to Understand and Work with Mental Distress*. London: Jessica Kingsley.

Treasure, J. and Alexander, J. (2013). What is anorexia nervosa? In *Anorexia Nervosa* (pp. 17–22). London. Routledge.

Tucker, S. D. (2015). *Great British Eccentrics*. Gloucester: Amberley Publishing Limited.

Vos, T. et al. (2013) Global, regional, and national incidence, prevalence, and years lived with disability for 301 acute and chronic diseases and injuries in 188 countries, 1990–2013: a systematic analysis for the Global Burden of Disease Study. *The Lancet* 386 (9995), 743–800.

Walsh, L. (2009) *Depression Care across the Lifespan*. Chichester: Wiley-Blackwell.

Walters, K., Rait, G., Griffin, M., Buszewicz, M. and Nazareth, I. (2012). Recent trends in the incidence of anxiety diagnoses and symptoms in primary care. *PloS one* 7(8), e41670.

Waxman, S. E. (2009). A systematic review of impulsivity in eating disorders. *European Eating Disorders Review: The Professional Journal of the Eating Disorders Association* 17(6), 408–425.

Westerhof, G. J. and Keyes, C. L. (2010). Mental illness and mental health: the two continua model across the lifespan. *Journal of Adult Development* 17(2), 110–119.

Westmoreland, P., Krantz, M. J. and Mehler, P. S. (2016). Medical complications of anorexia nervosa and bulimia. *The American Journal of Medicine* 129(1), 30–37.

Whiteford, H. A., Degenhardt, L., Rehm, J., Baxter, A. J., Ferrari, A. J., Erskine, H. E., ... and Burstein, R. (2013). Global burden of disease attributable to mental and substance use disorders: findings from the Global Burden of Disease Study 2010. *The Lancet* 382(9904), 1575–1586.

World Health Organization (2010) *ATLAS on substance use (2010) Resources for the prevention and treatment of substance use disorders*. Available at: www.who.int/substance_abuse/activities/msbatlasfrontncont.pdf?ua=1

World Health Organization (2014). www.who.int/features/factfiles/mental_health/en/

World Health Organization (2018). *International Classification of Diseases* (11th revision). Geneva: WHO.

Zipfel, S., Giel, K. E., Bulik, C. M., Hay, P. and Schmidt, U. (2015). Anorexia nervosa: aetiology, assessment, and treatment. *The Lancet Psychiatry* 2(12), 1099–1111.

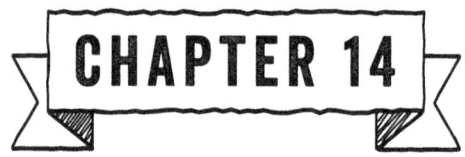

CHAPTER 14

DETERMINANTS OF POOR MENTAL HEALTH AND THE ROAD TO RECOVERY

Keith Bradley-Adams

OVERVIEW

This chapter will build on the previous chapter and further develop understanding of the complexities of mental health care. It begins by focusing upon the factors that may predetermine the likelihood of an individual developing a mental disorder including extrinsic factors such environmental and social influences as well as the intrinsic factors which may be unique to the individual.

The chapter then discusses the concept of case formulation which enables the practitioner to examine the historical experiences and ongoing events which may be influencing the client's current problems. This holistic assessment develops a collaborative approach to care which leads into a partnership approach to recovery.

The chapter concludes with the examination of a model for recovery which focuses on the activities the client and therapist can undertake in partnership to promote recovery and well-being.

LEARNING OUTCOMES

By the end of this chapter you will be able to:

- Identify potential influences on the mental health and well-being of individuals
- List the key determinants to mental health
- Identify the factors which underpin case formulation
- Discuss how to promote recovery

INTRODUCTION

The World Health Organization (2010a) describe a set of individual, societal and environmental factors that may determine the occurrence of disease or infirmity in individuals and communities: the social and economic environment, the physical environment and the person's individual characteristics and behaviours. These circumstances combine together to increase susceptibility to poor health. Whilst we often think of these conditions as determinants of poor physical health they are the determinants of poor mental health too. Factors such as income, housing, education, physical environment, genetics, gender and availability of services are major influences on health.

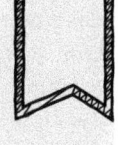

PAUSE FOR THOUGHT 14.1

The World Health Organization (2008) describe the determinants of health as 'the conditions in which people are born, grow, work, live, and age, and the wider set of forces and systems shaping the conditions of daily life. These forces and systems include economic policies and systems, development agendas, social norms, social policies and political systems.'

When you read this statement how do you think the mental health of you, your family and your friends may be influenced by where you live, your socio-economic status and the lifestyle choices you make? What about government interventions such as introducing legislation or increasing or reducing spending in some areas – would these have an impact?

Check the end of the chapter for an answer to this activity.

Evidence from a number of studies around the world suggests that your physical health and mental health will be compromised if you have a low income, poor housing, lower educational attainment, and so on (Bambra et al., 2010; Phelan et al., 2010). Persons who experience these hardships are more likely to have poor health and will die younger than their more affluent neighbours (Mackenbach et al., 2011).

Mental disorders are an 'equal opportunities' set of illnesses which affect everyone irrespective of age, gender, ability or ethnicity (Steen and Thomas, 2016). However, there are some socio-demographic determinants to poor mental health which suggest that social causation is at least in part involved in the development of disorder. The World Health Organization (2014) state that mental disorder is influenced by the social, economic and physical environment with inequalities in socio-demographic factors correlating strongly with the inequalities in mental health. Much of the data focuses on morbidity (the rates of a disease or disorder) and mortality (the rates of death). The following groups appear to experience disparity in both these paradigms and may therefore be considered vulnerable.

GENDER

It has long been believed that the incidence of mental disorder in both genders is closer than the reported rates suggest. There are many explanations for this but one is alexithymia, the lack of an ability to express emotions. Men are more likely to experience alexithymia than women (Zaidi et al., 2015) and as such are less able to describe symptoms of psychological distress. Conversely, women are likely to be better able to recognise emotional distress, seek help and report symptoms thus creating an imbalance in reported incidence of distress (Leising et al., 2009). Men are more likely to exhibit 'limited self-disclosure', a set of behaviours which limit one's ability to discuss thoughts and feelings with others. In the UK evidence on suicide suggests that men are three times more likely to commit suicide than women (Office for National Statistics, 2018).

Whiteford et al. (2015) found that whilst serious mental illness occurs more frequently in males common mental health problems are more prevalent in females which would support the alexithymia hypotheses. Another contributory factor to disparity in mental health between males and females is the gender pay gap, which results in women having an increased risk as they are also more likely to be in lower income groups (Fortin et al., 2017).

SEXUALITY AND ORIENTATION

Contemporary mental health services should treat all persons with equality irrespective of their sexuality, a far cry from the appalling treatment meted out in the past when men like Alan Turing were 'treated' with enforced cures for homosexuality, considered a mental disorder in the UK until the 1960s and in the USA until 1987. Although American psychologists and psychiatrists were encouraged by the APA to view homosexuality as a normal lifestyle choice the American National Association of Social Workers was a little slower to adopt this stance, although by 1993 they too accepted that homosexuality is not a mental disorder. Wider society too has a more enlightened view yet still today we see higher rates of mental disorder in gay men and women. Storholm et al. (2013) found that sexually active young gay men are at greater risk of anxiety, depression, post-traumatic stress disorder (PTSD) and suicidality than their straight peers, although interestingly as they grow older the figures are similar. This is supported by Bolton and Sareen (2011) who suggest that gay and bisexual individuals are three times more likely to attempt suicide than straight individuals and show increases in diagnosis of most other mental disorder.

Kidd et al. (2011) found that lesbian, gay, bisexual and transsexual (LGBT) persons experiencing mental disorder also experienced increased stigma from being members of two minority groups – the LGBT group and the mental disorder group – which increases their vulnerability and also the length of treatment. Storholm et al. (2013) also found rates of mental disorder in black and Hispanic gay men to be higher than in white gay men.

RACE

Jackson et al. (2010) report that there is a disproportionate level of black males in the mental health system in the UK. They attribute this to several factors including other social factors such as poor housing, low levels of educational attainment, unemployment, and so on, but also suggest that at some level there may be unconscious race bias. It is also evident that black men are less likely to engage with services than their already poorly engaging white peers and are more likely to come to the attention of services via the criminal justice system (Jackson et al., 2010). Afro-Caribbeans are four times more likely to be sectioned under the mental health act than white Anglo-Saxon persons exhibiting the same symptoms (Smyth, 2018). Once involved with services Afro-Caribbeans are more likely to receive medication than psycho-social interventions, such as counselling; are more likely to be cared for in secure environments; and more likely to experience control and restraint (Jackson et al., 2010). Older black women, who fall into three vulnerable groups (age, gender and race), have very high rates of depression in comparison to their white peers and are significantly over-represented compared to younger white women or white men of any age (Seaton et al., 2010).

This disparity in representation in national statistics is not limited to persons of Afro-Caribbean origin, however. Bradby and Nazroo (2010) found that UK citizens who classed their ethnicity as 'white Irish' have higher levels of morbidity and mortality for most illnesses, both physical and psychological. This is supported by Weich et al. (2004) who found significantly higher levels of common mental disorders (see previous chapter) in persons who identified themselves as white Irish. Persons identifying as white Irish, like those identifying as Afro-Caribbean, have been subject to discrimination in many other areas in the past and, possibly, in the present too so higher levels of mental disorder are no surprise.

EDUCATION AND INCOME

Reiss (2013) found that there was an increase in reported rates of mental disorder in children with lower educational attainment. This finding is not surprising as an association between mental disorder and educational attainment in adults is well documented (WHO, 2014). It is unclear why this should be the case but as, generally, persons with mental disorder are subject to the influence of a range of socio-economic influences, housing and income, and so on, it may be these that contribute to educational attainment rather than the mental disorder. It is also possible to argue that the correlation in lower educational attainment and mental disorder is effect rather than cause and that the disorder is influencing education rather than vice versa. Breslau et al. (2008) found that there is a link between mental disorder in childhood and low educational attainment, particularly for those experiencing serious mental illness.

These factors reduce opportunities in later life, with persons with mental disorder likely to be employed in low-skilled and low-paid jobs (Dunn et al., 2008). Quite simply, poor people suffer mental disorder disproportionally (Elliot, 2016). This is a vicious circle as poverty not only causes mental disorder but in turn is also a result of mental disorder (Elliot, 2016) with persons with poor mental health struggling to secure well-paid employment, if able to work at all. Delgadillo et al. (2016) found that persons living in poverty had increased incidence of mental disorder and also lower recovery rates. Allen et al. (2014) describe a gradient of disadvantage where a correlation between income and mental health can be made with those in the lowest socio-economic groups suffering the highest levels of mental disorder and those in the higher brackets suffering the least. Hudson (2005) reports a symbiosis between mental disorder and poverty stating that mental disorder may be linked to poverty as both a symptom and cause with poverty both causing and being caused by disorder.

Marmot et al. (2010) report that persons in the 20 per cent lowest income bracket are three times more likely to develop a mental disorder than those in the top 20 per cent. Loibl (2017) found that persons from lower socio-economic groups not only had poorer mental health than their more affluent neighbours but also were more likely to engage in risky activities such as binge eating or drug and alcohol use which are also believed to contribute to poor mental health. Hart (1971), in his seminal work on the inverse care law, first pointed out that the needier the population the fewer services are provided, thus trapping individuals in a cycle of poverty and mental disorder. Historically rates of mental disorder increase during times of austerity, particularly when cuts to health and social services and the benefits system occur (Reeves et al., 2016).

DISABILITY

McManus et al. (2016) report that there is an increase in physical health conditions in persons experiencing common mental health problems, 38 per cent compared to 25 per cent of those not experiencing common mental health problems. Conversely Matheson et al. (2014) suggest that rates of mental disorder increase in persons with chronic physical conditions such as chronic obstructive pulmonary disease (COPD) and diabetes. Scott et al. (2009) assert that both chronic physical illness and chronic mental disorder are disabling, arguing that they should be considered equally disabling. They go on to point out that a significant number of people will experience comorbid occurrence of physical disability and mental disability and that these individuals have their life chances severely impaired.

Thornicroft (2011) asserts that those living with mental disorder live an average of 20 years less than individuals not experiencing mental disorder and that comorbid poor physical health is a significant factor in this. De Hert et al. (2011) agree with this view, but point out that much of the mortality and morbidity may be attributed to 'poor lifestyle choice' factors such as smoking, substance abuse, and so on. Thornicroft (2011) suggests that a key factor is the iatric effect; that is the side effects and complications of medication used to treat mental disorder such as the risk of obesity and type 2 diabetes in persons prescribed second-generation antipsychotics.

Thompson et al. (2011) found that engaging in physical activity has a beneficial effect on psychological well-being, a view supported by Carek et al. (2011) who found that exercise improves symptoms of depression and anxiety; and by Acil et al. (2008) who report similar findings for persons experiencing psychosis. These measures would also help manage the physical symptoms associated with mental disorder and should be encouraged in all persons diagnosed with a mental disorder, particularly those prescribed medication.

HOMELESSNESS

Kyle and Dunn (2008) report that persons with mental disorder require the security and comfort of good-quality housing to manage their symptoms and reduce relapse rates. However, evidence suggests that individuals with mental disorder are more likely to be housed in poor or sub-standard accommodation (Kyle and Dunn, 2008). Persons who are homeless have higher than average levels of mental disorder (Fazel et al., 2014) although it is unclear in many cases if persons become homeless as a result of their disorder or vice versa. Hwang and Burns (2014) report that homeless adults have higher rates of mental disorder and substance misuse than housed individuals and also require specialised services to maintain engagement and concordance. Social deprivation is seen as a major influence in developing disorder and in inhibiting recovery (Walters et al., 2012).

ACTIVITY 14.1

Imagine you are caring for the following person. As well as any biological or physiological concerns what are the socio-economic factors (age, gender, income, housing, employment education, sexuality, relationship status, etc.) and social dynamics (the pluralistic relationship between the individual and the wider society, i.e. how an individual influences the world around them and how they are influenced by the environment) you would need to consider?

Steve is a 23-year-old former soldier who is experiencing symptoms of post-traumatic stress disorder (PTSD). Steve was brought up in care following the suicide of his lone-parent mum. Since leaving the army Steve has been 'sofa surfing' or sleeping rough. He does not actively engage with services but 'self-medicates' on alcohol and cannabis to cope with pervasive thoughts and feelings of anxiety. Steve has lost 4 kilograms in recent weeks and seldom eats three meals a day. He wishes to turn his life around and has asked for support in finding some form of education or training to help him become a painter and decorator.

Check the end of the chapter for an answer to this activity.

When assessing the mental health of individuals and preparing a care and treatment plan to manage mental illness health professionals have to adopt a biopsychosocial approach, taking cognisance of both positive and malign factors which could be causing or perpetuating ill health and factors which may support recovery.

CASE FORMULATION

Macneil et al. (2012) suggest that in a person-centred and holistic approach to care of persons experiencing mental disorder a formal diagnosis only tells half the story and that in order to fully understand underlying causes to a disorder the clinician has to understand their client and their idiosyncratic life. This nosological approach (i.e. to adopt a whole-person approach which looks at not only the biological or pathological causes of illness but also the psychological, sociological and spiritual elements) to the care of persons with mental disorder has gained wide support in contemporary psychiatry, providing further proof of the acceptance that the medical model is limited. This is an important consideration as it reminds clinicians of the need to develop individual care and treatment plans which recognise the unique nature of each person they care for. To do otherwise would be to develop a 'standardised' package of care and expect everyone in society, irrespective of factors such as education, employment, housing, income, relationship status, and so on, to follow the same pathway to recovery. Case formulation proposes that there are five paradigms which should be investigated in order to develop a strategy for planning and delivering care which meets the unique needs of each and every person. By identifying these factors and working in collaboration with the client the clinician is better able to develop a person-centred and holistic approach to care based on the development of a therapeutic relationship.

Presenting problem: *the main issues which are impacting negatively on the client at the given time.* This would include signs and symptoms of any illness along with any other phenomena (substance use, etc.) which may be the key concerns of the client. These difficulties may not always be apparent to the client and sometimes the role of the clinician is to raise awareness of concerns and to influence the client's perceptions or beliefs (e.g. if the person has little insight into their condition). Resolution of these difficulties would form the basis of a care and treatment plan which would provide structure to the interventions to be employed. They do not necessarily involve specifically targeting the diagnosed condition; for example, the client may be diagnosed with schizophrenia but may identify their main concern as unemployment, poor housing or even side effects of medication such as weight gain. Interventions could involve working with the client to meet these needs rather than simply prescribing and administering medication for the more obvious symptoms.

Predisposing factors: *a historic holistic examination of the person's lived experiences from birth to the present day.* This includes biological, psychological and sociological factors such as maternal difficulties during gestation; the absence of 'normal' birth; organic brain injury; genetic factors including mental health issues in a close family member; witnessing or experiencing abuse in childhood: and environmental and socio-economic factors which may predispose a person to an increased risk of developing mental health problems. These events may be traumatic or stressful to have lived and to retell and sensitivity is important when revisiting this history. Often predisposing factors are divided into sub-categories of childhood experiences, historic adult experiences and recent experiences. An individual event in itself may not be considered as a precipitating factor; however, when taken as a whole, a catalogue of events could predispose an individual to mental disorder.

Precipitating factors: *the recent events that may be the triggers to the current problem.* Including substance use or withdrawal; non-concordance with prescribed medication; poor physical health; changes in socio-economic status (such as divorce, unemployment, homelessness, etc.); changes to sleep or diet; involvement with criminal justice system as a victim or perpetrator; etc. These changes are the catalyst for the current presentation and again may be the result of a body of events rather than attributable to a single cause.

Perpetuating factors: *the factors that 'feed' the problem and keep it going.* These may include symptoms of disorders such as anankastic or compulsive behaviours; ongoing substance use; ongoing non-concordance; disengagement from support networks such as family or mental health services; risk taking; ongoing changes to sleep or diet. Perpetuating factors would also include poor response to treatment and unresolved predisposing and/or precipitating factors.

Protective factors: *these are the factors which may lessen or reduce distress or behaviours.* They are the areas of strength in the individual's life such as family; social relationships; hobbies and interests; spirituality; employment; financial security etc. Resilience and coping skills are protective factors that can be improved through the development of a therapeutic alliance between the person experiencing the disorder and the clinician. Joint working to identify protective factors also creates increased hope in both the clinician and patient, and this in itself can become a factor that strengthens the therapeutic relationship.

PAUSE FOR THOUGHT 14.2

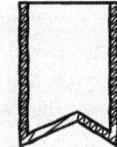

When we look back at the former soldier (Steve) we discussed earlier in this chapter what do you think may be some of the predisposing, precipitating and perpetuating factors which contribute to his current mental disorder? What protective factors may influence Steve's recovery?

Check the end of the chapter for an answer to this activity.

VULNERABILITY AND RISK

The World Health Organization (2010b) assert that persons with mental disorder are vulnerable. They are vulnerable to exploitation and harm (including sexual, physical and financial abuse) from others in society and often receive less favourable treatment from those in authority (e.g. restrictions to their rights to freedom and choice; direct and indirect discrimination; exclusion; reduced access to services, including education, housing, health, etc.; and less favourable treatment when involved with the criminal justice system). Persons with mental disorder are very vulnerable and as well as the risks they pose to themselves are at risk of physical abuse, sexual abuse, financial abuse, and so on (Fazel et al., 2014; Jones et al., 2012; Kyle and Dunn, 2008).

The greatest risks in mental disorder are to the sufferers themselves and not to the wider society. Time to Change (2018) report that as few as 1 per cent of assaults are carried out by persons diagnosed with a recognised disorder whilst conversely 70 per cent of suicides are persons diagnosed with a mental disorder. The Mental Health Act 1983/2007 also considers this and states that persons should be detained under the act if they are a danger to themselves or others, themselves listed first as this is the most common presentation. Haw et al. (2001) report that a survey of persons who presented at accident and emergency departments across the UK following an episode of self-harm found that 92 per cent of patients had a diagnosed mental disorder, with 47 per cent having two or more disorders. However, Singhal et al. (2014) suggest that suicide is not unique to mental disorder as persons with a range of chronic somatic conditions including asthma and eczema are at increased risk. Indeed the highest suicide rate with any disorder is associated with trigeminal neuralgia which is often referred to as the 'suicide disease' in the US (Jin et al., 2015; O'Connor and Dworkin, 2009).

PAUSE FOR THOUGHT 14.3

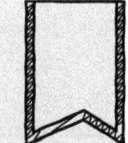

Think of a time when you have cared for a person experiencing mental disorder. Did you think about the risks posed to them by others or by the symptoms of their illness? What can you do to protect service users who are vulnerable?

Check the end of the chapter for an answer to this activity.

RESILIENCE, HOPE AND RECOVERY

Resilience is the ability to 'bounce back' following adversity. It may refer to people having the mental fortitude to avoid periods of mental ill-health or to recover from an episode of mental ill-health. Resilience requires skills of adaptability to changed circumstances, such as loss or reduced status. Resilience is evident when comparing persons who have broadly similar experiences and backgrounds where one develops a mental disorder whilst the other remains well. The factors which are pre-determinants of poor mental health are also inversely associated with resilience; that is, persons with good social links, good physical health, good income, and so on, are likely to be more resilient than persons who have not had those advantages. There is some limited evidence to suggest that neurological factors such as the presence of higher levels of some chemicals or organic differences in regions of the brain may also influence resilience (Chan et al., 2016; Levone et al., 2015). Much of the evidence on resilience also points towards some individuals having greater capacity to recover from, or delay the progression of, serious physical health conditions including cancer and HIV too.

One factor known to improve recovery is hope. Where persons experiencing mental disorder are able to recognise that recovery is a possibility and are given more autonomy in working toward recovery then outcomes are greatly improved. Marino (2015) takes this concept further by suggesting that hope should not only be hope of recovery but hope of once more being able to contribute actively to society through work, education, social relationships, and so on. Where mental health services are able to offer hope the prospect of recovery is greatly increased.

It was long assumed that there is no hope of recovery in mental disorder, particularly for those experiencing the serious mental illnesses. In the 1950s the first effective medications were introduced but these only served to hide symptoms and could not cure the underlying disorder. The term 'palliative care' was used to describe this approach, taken from the Latin *pallium* or cloak. Anthony (1993) dispelled this myth arguing that the closure of large institutions that began in the 1980s and the attempts to rehabilitate persons with mental disorder could bring in a new period of mental health care which he referred to as the recovery-focused mental health movement. In contemporary mental health care Anthony's vision is still being built upon, and recovery and hope are the guiding principles of care. The guiding principle today is that complete medical recovery, the absence of all symptoms, may not be achievable for many but that the chance to live a full and meaningful life despite these symptoms, or social recovery, is achievable (Perkins and Slade, 2012; Repper and Perkins, 2003).

Kidd et al. (2015) report that despite moves worldwide in the last 30 years to promote the ethos of recovery many governments are still not providing an atmosphere where recovery can flourish. Their research highlights the exclusion of the patients' voice in setting the agenda for recovery and note that where the views of the patient are respected and where service delivery involves open dialogue between service users and service providers recovery is more likely to occur.

Although it is generally accepted that medical recovery (i.e. the complete absence of all symptoms) may be unrealistic for many individuals experiencing serious mental illness, there is no reason why individuals cannot hope to achieve 'personal recovery' or 'social recovery'. Personal recovery is defined by the person experiencing the mental disorder and is their perception of their relative wellness which may include living with some symptoms but doing so in a way which does not stop the individual from feeling satisfied, hopeful and of value (Slade and Wallace, 2017). Social recovery is not simply being able to live independently and not to be 'a burden' on society but to enjoy the meaningful life enjoyed by those whose lives are not affected by mental disorder (Ramon, 2018). In contemporary terms it is common to discuss recovery 'in illness' as opposed to the earlier perception of recovery 'from illness' (Perkins and Slade, 2012).

Recovery involves enabling the person to regain their personal identity as a separate entity from an illness. It requires others to perceive you not as an illness but as a person who has had, and may still exhibit some symptoms of, an illness. Recovery differs from rehabilitation which confers more of a medical approach to recovery and fails to recognise the individual nature of the journey. Recovery is more holistic in meaning than rehabilitation as it recognises the whole person and their journey toward re-establishing a life with meaning and purpose which need not necessarily be symptom free but where they are able to reconnect with society, restore lost skills and remediate deficits in functioning. Social inclusion and acceptance are core components within this so the role for wider society is to accept persons with mental disorder for who they are in an non-judgemental, anti-discriminatory environment which focuses on the strengths and achievements of the individual rather than simply labelling them as 'mad'.

There are many models of recovery which focus on either the actions which those caring for a person recovering from mental disorder should adhere to or to the autonomous behaviours an individual with a mental disorder should themselves engage in. These models often focus on the mechanisms and stages of recovery but do not always acknowledge the environment necessary for recovery to occur. Existing models focus on individuals rather than on partnership approaches and fail to describe the attitudes and beliefs required for a clinician and a person in recovery working collaboratively to promote optimum recovery. The model in Table 14.1, the Swansea University Recovery Framework (SURF) proposes such a model.

PAUSE FOR THOUGHT 14.4

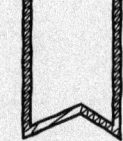

Focusing on Steve (discussed previously) or a client you are currently working with, how may the model in Table 14.1 support your approach to promoting recovery? If you reflect on other clients, are there elements of this framework that may have improved your relationship and/or outcomes?

Check the end of the chapter for an answer to this activity.

Table 14.1 SURF – Swansea University Recovery Framework.

SURF – Swansea University Recovery Framework		
R	RESPECT	Both the clinician and the service user should have mutual respect for one another. The service user should respect the professionalism and experience of the clinician (who must earn such respect) and their wish to do what they believe to be in the service users' best interests.
E	EMPOWERMENT	The clinician should respect the individuality of the service user, their rights to make informed decisions, to be involved in decisions about their care, to be the expert in 'themselves', etc.
C	CONGRUENCE	Service users must be able to be accepting of themselves, i.e. that their beliefs about who they are, are compatible with the reality of who they are.
O	OPENNESS	The clinician must have an 'open' personality in that they must possess creativity and imagination, be able to undertake self-analysis and disclosure and possess intellectual curiosity.
V	VERACITY	Clinicians must provide service users with full and frank information in a timely manner in order to enable service users to make informed choices. If there are valid reasons why the truth is to be withheld in a service user's best interest then these must be documented and form a part of the care and treatment plan.
E	EMPATHY	The clinician should be able to recognise when the service user is suffering and be attuned to their feelings. They should have an emotional resonance with the service user and use their experience and knowledge to understand what it must feel like to be them.
R	RESILIENCE	The clinician must be able to put aside personal beliefs and to deliver unconditional positive regard to the service user no matter how challenging that may be on occasions. They require a capacity to be able to cope with disappointments and to carry on delivering care in the person's best interests.
Y	YARDSTICK	Recovery is measurable. Clinicians require an objective, collaborative and ongoing assessment of the service user to be able to identify and celebrate recovery. The good clinician may also be the yardstick by which their colleagues measure their care.

CONCLUSION

Having completed this chapter you should have greater understanding of the complexities of contemporary mental health care. Your understanding of factors which may influence development of, or resistance to, mental ill-health and which may also influence recovery should be broadened. This should in turn influence your appreciation of individual, needs-led approaches to care and to the importance of working in partnership with clients.

GO FURTHER ACTIVITY

Having read this chapter how important is hope in the care of persons experiencing mental disorder and their families? If you reflect on a previous care experience where a positive outcome occurred was it person-centred, holistic and collaborative? Conversely if you reflect on an episode of care which went less well was the opposite true? As you move forward how important will instilling hope in your clients be to you?

Check the end of the chapter for an answer to this activity.

ANSWERS TO THE CHAPTER 14 ACTIVITIES

———— Pause for Thought 14.1: Answers

From reading the WHO description of determinant of health, you may decide that it is likely that where you live, socio-economic status and lifestyle choices may play a large part in determining your (and others') mental health. Government spending to increase lifestyle, community services, and socio-economic status may have a beneficial impact on improving the mental health of a community.

———— Activity 14.1: Answers

As a male, Steve may have greater difficulties in labeling his emotions (a condition called alexithymia, which is more frequent in males) which may prevent him from expressing himself well. He may also feel that his mental health will be stigmatised by his peers, thus resist the support he is offered. As he does not have parental support, he may have to further depend on friends. He may feel he has very little ability to change his circumstances and that there is little support on offer to get himself back on his feet.

——— Pause for Thought 14.2: Answers

Predisposing factors which relate factors which relate to Steve's mental health, maybe the enormous stress and traumatic events of serving in the army and perhaps issues growing up as his parents separated. Precipitating factors may include Steve's ongoing recent substance abuse and living situation (e.g., not having his own home). Perpetuating factors may involve his ongoing substance abuse. Protective factors may include Steve's friends who are helping him and Steve's motivation to find support and education.

——— Pause for Thought 14.3: Answers

A person experiencing mental health disorders are much more likely to cause themselves harm as opposed to others in society. You may have thought about this. Perhaps more support, personalised care, and monitoring of service users could reduce self-harm or suicide.

——— Pause for Thought 14.4: Answers

Having respect for the client, helping to empower them, having empathy, and being unbiased (as well as all the other aspects of the framework) may be useful in the case of a mental health practitioner developing a relationship with Steve and helping him achieve certain mental health outcomes. It is vital to adopt a holistic approach to Steve, taking cognisance of biological, psychological and social factors.

——— Go Further Activity: Answers

This activity requires you to reflect on your own thoughts and experiences.

REFERENCES

Acil, A. A., Dogan, S. and Dogan, O. (2008). The effects of physical exercises to mental state and quality of life in patients with schizophrenia. *Journal of Psychiatric and Mental Health Nursing* 15(10), 808–815.

Allen, J., Balfour, R., Bell, R. and Marmot, M. (2014). Social determinants of mental health. *International Review of Psychiatry* 26(4), 392–407.

Anthony, W. A. (1993). Recovery from mental illness: the guiding vision of the mental health service system in the 1990s. *Psychosocial Rehabilitation Journal* 16(4), 11–23.

Bambra, C., Gibson, M., Sowden, A., Wright, K., Whitehead, M. and Petticrew, M. (2010). Tackling the wider social determinants of health and health inequalities: evidence from systematic reviews. *Journal of Epidemiology & Community Health* 64(4), 284–291.

Bolton, S. L. and Sareen, J. (2011). Sexual orientation and its relation to mental disorders and suicide attempts: Findings from a nationally representative sample. *The Canadian Journal of Psychiatry* 56(1), 35–43.

Bradby, H. and Nazroo, J. Y. (2010). Health, ethnicity, and race. *The New Blackwell Companion to Medical Sociology*, 113–130.

Breslau, J., Lane, M., Sampson, N. and Kessler, R. C. (2008). Mental disorders and subsequent educational attainment in a US national sample. *Journal of Psychiatric Research* 42(9), 708–716.

Carek, P. J., Laibstain, S. E. and Carek, S. M. (2011). Exercise for the treatment of depression and anxiety. *The International Journal of Psychiatry in Medicine* 41(1), 15–28.

Chan, S. W., Harmer, C. J., Norbury, R., O'Sullivan, U., Goodwin, G. M. and Portella, M. J. (2016). Hippocampal volume in vulnerability and resilience to depression. *Journal of Affective Disorders* 189, 199–202.

De Hert, M., Cohen, D. A. N., Bobes, J., Cetkovich-Bakmas, M., Leucht, S., Ndetei, D. M., … and Gautam, S. (2011). Physical illness in patients with severe mental disorders. II. Barriers to care, monitoring and treatment guidelines, plus recommendations at the system and individual level. *World Psychiatry* 10(2), 138–151.

Delgadillo, J., Asaria, M., Ali, S. and Gilbody, S. (2016). On poverty, politics and psychology: the socio-economic gradient of mental healthcare utilisation and outcomes. *The British Journal of Psychiatry* 209(5), 429–430.

Dunn, E. C., Wewiorski, N. J. and Rogers, E. S. (2008). The meaning and importance of employment to people in recovery from serious mental illness: results of a qualitative study. *Psychiatric Rehabilitation Journal* 32(1), 59–62.

Elliott, I. (2016). *Poverty and Mental Health: A Review to Inform the Joseph Rowntree Foundation's Anti-Poverty Strategy*. London: Mental Health Foundation.

Fazel, S., Geddes, J. R. and Kushel, M. (2014). The health of homeless people in high-income countries: descriptive epidemiology, health consequences, and clinical and policy recommendations. *The Lancet* 384(9953), 1529–1540.

Fortin, N. M., Bell, B. and Bohm, M. (2017) Top earnings, inequality and the gender pay gap; Canada, Sweden and the United Kingdom. *Labour Economics* 47, 107–123.

Hart, J. T. (1971). The inverse care law. *The Lancet* 297(7696), 405–412.

Haw, C., Hawton, K., Houston, K. and Townsend, E. (2001). Psychiatric and personality disorders in deliberate self-harm patients. *The British Journal of Psychiatry* 178(1), 48–54.

Hudson, C. G. (2005) Socioeconomic status and mental illness; tests for the social causation and selection hypotheses. *American Journal of Orthopsychiatry* 75(1) 3–18.

Hwang, S. W. and Burns, T. (2014). Health interventions for people who are homeless. *The Lancet*, 384(9953), 1541–1547.

Jackson, J. S., Knight, K. M. and Rafferty, J. A. (2010). Race and unhealthy behaviors: chronic stress, the HPA axis, and physical and mental health disparities over the life course. *American Journal of Public Health* 100(5), 933–939.

Jin, H. S., Shin, J. Y., Kim, Y. C., Lee, S. C., Choi, E. J., Lee, P. B. and Moon, J. Y. (2015). Predictive factors associated with success and failure for radiofrequency thermocoagulation in patients with trigeminal neuralgia. *Pain Physician* 18(6), 537–545.

Jones, L., Bellis, M. A., Wood, S., Hughes, K., McCoy, E., Eckley, L., … and Officer, A. (2012). Prevalence and risk of violence against children with disabilities: a systematic review and meta-analysis of observational studies. *The Lancet* 380(9845), 899–907.

Kidd, S., Kenny, A. and McKinstry, C. (2015). The meaning of recovery in a regional mental health service: an action research study. *Journal of Advanced Nursing* 71(1), 181–192.

Kidd, S. A., Veltman, A., Gately, C., Chan, K. J. and Cohen, J. N. (2011). Lesbian, gay, and transgender persons with severe mental illness: negotiating wellness in the context of multiple sources of stigma. *American Journal of Psychiatric Rehabilitation* 14(1), 13–39.

Kyle, T. and Dunn, J. R. (2008). Effects of housing circumstances on health, quality of life and healthcare use for people with severe mental illness: a review. *Health & Social Care in the Community* 16(1), 1–15.

Leising, D., Grande, T. and Faber, R. (2009). The Toronto Alexithymia Scale (TAS-20): a measure of general psychological distress. *Journal of Research in Personality* 43(4), 707–710.

Levone, B. R., Cryan, J. F. and O'Leary, O. F. (2015). Role of adult hippocampal neurogenesis in stress resilience. *Neurobiology of Stress* 1, 147–155.

Loibl, C. (2017). Living in poverty: understanding the financial behaviour of vulnerable groups. *Economic Psychology* 421–434.

Mackenbach, J. P., Meerding, W. J. and Kunst, A. E. (2011). Economic costs of health inequalities in the European Union. *Journal of Epidemiology & Community Health* 65(5), 412–419.

Macneil, C. A., Hasty, M. K., Conus, P. and Berk, M. (2012). Is diagnosis enough to guide interventions in mental health? Using case formulation in clinical practice. *BMC Medicine* 10(1), 111.

Marino, C. K. (2015). To belong, contribute, and hope: first stage development of a measure of social recovery. *Journal of Mental Health* 24(2), 68–72.

Marmot, M., Allen, J., Goldblatt, P., Boyce, T., McNeish, D., Grady, M. and Geddes, I. (2010). Fair society, healthy lives: strategic review of health inequalities in England post 2010. Available at: institute of healthequity.org/projects/ fair-society-healthy-lives-the-marmot-review (accessed 7 November 2016).

Matheson, F. I., Smith, K. L. W., Fazli, G. S. et al. (2014). Physical health and gender as risk factors for usage of services for mental illness. *Journal of Epidemiological Community Health* 68, 971–978.

McManus, S., Bebbington, P., Jenkins, R. and Brugha, T. (eds) 2016). *Mental Health and Wellbeing in England: Adult Psychiatric Morbidity Survey 2014*. Leeds: NHS Digital.

O'Connor, A. B. and Dworkin, R. H. (2009). Treatment of neuropathic pain: an overview of recent guide-lines. *The American Journal of Medicine* 122(10), S22–S32.

Office for National Statistics (2018). *Suicides in the UK: 2017 Registrations*. London: ONS.

Perkins, R. and Slade, M. (2012). Recovery in England: transforming statutory services? *International Review of Psychiatry* 24(1), 29–39.

Phelan, J. C., Link, B. G. and Tehranifar, P. (2010). Social conditions as fundamental causes of health inequalities: theory, evidence, and policy implications. *Journal of Health and Social Behavior*, 51(1_ suppl.), S28–S40.

Ramon, S. (2018). The place of social recovery in mental health and related services. *International Journal of Environmental Research and Public Health* 15(6), 1052.

Reeves, A., Clair, A., McKee, M. and Stuckler, D. (2016). Reductions in the United Kingdom's govern-ment housing benefit and symptoms of depression in low-income households. *American Journal of Epidemiology* 184(6), 421–429.

Reiss, F. (2013). Socioeconomic inequalities and mental health problems in children and adolescents: a systematic review. *Social Science & Medicine* 90, 24–31.

Repper, J. and Perkins, R. (2003). *Social Inclusion and Recovery: A Model for Mental Health Practice*. London: Elsevier Health Sciences.

Scott, K. M., Von Korff, M., Alonso, J., Angermeyer, M. C., Bromet, E., Fayyad, J., ... and Haro, J. M. (2009). Mental–physical co-morbidity and its relationship with disability: results from the World Mental Health Surveys. *Psychological Medicine* 39(1), 33–43.

Seaton, E. K., Caldwell, C. H., Sellers, R. M. and Jackson, J. S. (2010). An intersectional approach for understanding perceived discrimination and psychological well-being among African American and Caribbean Black youth. *Developmental Psychology* 46(5), 1372–79.

Singhal, A., Ross, J., Seminog, O., Hawton, K. and Goldacre, M. J. (2014). Risk of self-harm and suicide in people with specific psychiatric and physical disorders: comparisons between disorders using English national record linkage. *Journal of the Royal Society of Medicine* 107(5), 194–204.

Slade, M. and Wallace, G. (2017). Recovery and mental health. In M. Slade, L. Oades and A. Jarden (eds), *Wellbeing, Recovery and Mental Health*, 24–34. Cambridge: Cambridge University Press.

Smyth, C. (2018). Black people are four times more likely to be sectioned. *The Times*, 1 May.

Steen, M. and Thomas, M. (2016). *Mental Health across the Lifespan: A Handbook*. London. Routledge.

Storholm, E. D., Siconolfi, D. E., Halkitis, P. N., Moeller, R. W., Eddy, J. A. and Bare, M. G. (2013). Sociodemographic factors contribute to mental health disparities and access to services among young men who have sex with men in New York City. *Journal of Gay & Lesbian Mental Health* 17(3), 294–313. DOI: 10.1080/19359705.2012.763080

Thompson Coon, J., Boddy, K., Stein, K., Whear, R., Barton, J. and Depledge, M. H. (2011). Does participating in physical activity in outdoor natural environments have a greater effect on physical and mental wellbeing than physical activity indoors? A systematic review. *Environmental Science & Technology* 45(5), 1761–1772.

Thornicroft, G. (2011). Physical health disparities and mental illness: the scandal of premature mortality. *The British Journal of Psychiatry* 199(6), 441–442.

Time to Change (2018) Violence & mental health. Available at: www.time-to-change.org.uk/media-centre/responsible-reporting/violence-mental-health-problems (accessed 25 July 2018)

Walters, K., Rait, G., Griffin, M., Buszewicz, M. and Nazareth, I. (2012). Recent trends in the incidence of anxiety diagnoses and symptoms in primary care. *PloS one* 7(8), e41670.

Weich, S., Nazroo, J., Sproston, K., McManus, S., Blanchard, M., Erens, B. et al. (2004). Common mental disorders and ethnicity in England: the EMPIRIC Study. *Psychological Medicine* 34(8), 1543–1551.

Whiteford, H. A., Ferrari, A. J., Degenhardt, L., Feigin, V. and Vos, T. (2015). The global burden of mental, neurological and substance use disorders: an analysis from the Global Burden of Disease Study 2010. *PloS one* 10(2), e0116820.

World Health Organization (2008). *Closing the Gap in a Generation: Health Equity through Action on the Social Determinants of Health. Final Report of the Commission on Social Determinants of Health* Geneva: WHO.

World Health Organization (2010a). Mental health: strengthening our response. Fact sheet, 220.

World Health Organization (2010b). *Mental Health and Development: Targeting People with Mental Health Conditions as a Vulnerable Group*. Geneva: WHO.

World Health Organization (2014). Mental health: a state of well-being. Available at: www.who.int/features/factfiles/mental_health/en/

Zaidi, S. M. I. H., Arshad, M. and Yaqoob, N. (2015). Gender distinction in alexithymia among graduation students of Pakistan. *European Journal of Research in Social Sciences* 3(4), 99–103.

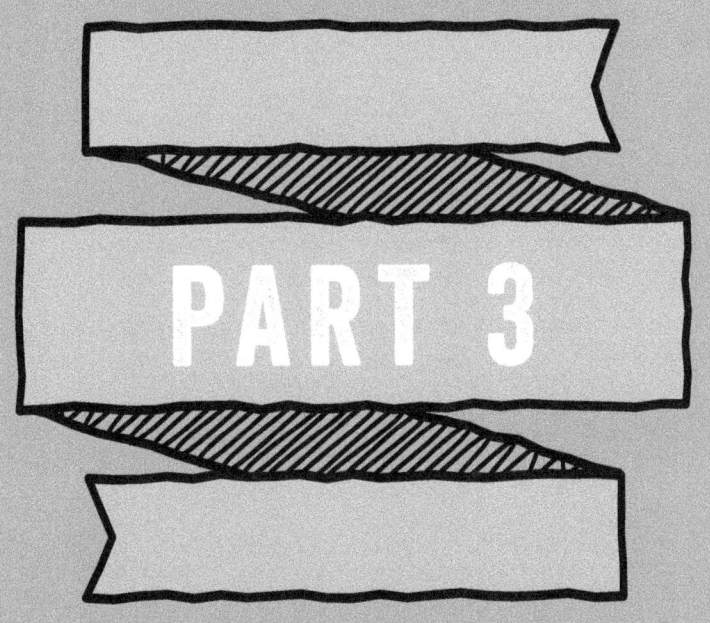

PART 3

CONTEMPORARY
TOPICS

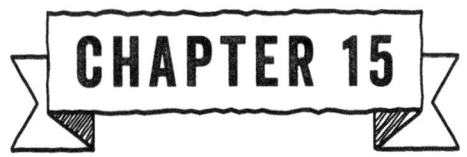

CHAPTER 15

USING AND DEVELOPING EVIDENCE IN HEALTH AND SOCIAL CARE PRACTICE

Hazel M. Chapman

OVERVIEW

This chapter outlines the processes of developing evidence-based practice and carrying out research, and highlights the similarities and differences between the two. This chapter aims to increase your skills and motivation in utilising research evidence to improve your practice, introduce you to the process of research and develop your research skills.

LEARNING OUTCOMES

By the end of this chapter you will be able to:

- Critique research papers
- Share best practice with your colleagues
- Assist with research in practice
- Develop your research skills with a view to becoming a researcher

INTRODUCTION

Professional health and social care practice is complex, and people often have different views about what is important and how they or their loved ones should be cared for. Other factors, such as sharing resources fairly, delivering value for money, treating people as individuals and respecting their choices, as well as the practitioner's knowledge and skill in providing care, mean that it is difficult to prescribe exactly how each practitioner should manage a particular situation. Through reflecting on your own experience, you can sometimes identify what works well for some scenarios. However, where a situation is rare, or where your analysis is never challenged, your practice will not advance. Without an evidence base, you might not achieve the best experience or outcome for service users, or you might squander resources or damage the person's trust in your care.

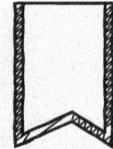

PAUSE FOR THOUGHT 15.1

Reflect on an everyday aspect of your professional practice. Try to identify what elements of that practice are based on habit and common practice and what elements are based on evidence and theoretical understanding. Can you give a clear rationale for every element? What are the gaps in your knowledge about this aspect of your practice?

WHAT IS EVIDENCE-BASED PRACTICE?

Sometimes, you are interested in an aspect of practice and need to know more – that often means you need to find and understand existing knowledge to inform your practice. Finding, evaluating and applying relevant knowledge to your practice is called evidence-based practice. You use different types of evidence to support your practice, gained from areas of knowledge such as ethics, biosciences, psychology and sociology. You may need to start by reading relevant sections or chapters in textbooks, just to gain a background knowledge of the topic. You often learn and update your practice through policies and protocols that are based on research evidence. However, this may not give you sufficient depth of knowledge and understanding to question and develop practice. Sometimes, you may act without questioning the evidence to support your practice. Practice can become habitual, based on observation of others and ill-considered assumptions. As an accountable professional, you should understand the knowledge on which your practice is based. This includes being able to question the evidence and appraise its quality and value to our practice. You must be able to determine where, how and to what extent you should use evidence in your practice. Since you depend on so many different knowledge bases, it is unlikely that you would be expert in all of them. However, by following the process outlined in this chapter, you will be able to evaluate and apply evidence that is relevant to your practice.

It is important to remember that any changes to practice should always consider existing processes, and must not compromise ethics and the safety of the service user. Any significant changes should be discussed with senior colleagues before implementation.

ACTIVITY 15.1

List aspects of your practice that you would like to know more about or to show improvement in. Identify some topics so that you can start finding and reading the relevant evidence.

EVIDENCE-BASED PRACTICE AND RESEARCH

Using evidence-based practice is different to carrying out research, which is a process that aims to advance the knowledge base for all health and social care professionals. Occasionally, you may find a poorly understood area of practice where research is needed to add to health and social care knowledge. Researchers carry out rigorous studies into different aspects of health and social care so that practitioners can use their findings (the evidence) to support their practice development. As a practitioner in health and social care, you may be asked to assist with data collection in a research study, so it is important that you understand the research process so that you can ask pertinent questions, and carry out your part in the research ethically and to a high standard. To advance in your career, you will need to develop a more questioning approach to assumptions about knowledge and practice in your field, undertaking further degrees that involve developing research skills and knowledge. Whatever profession or academic discipline you work within, the process of finding out new knowledge requires similar sets of research skills. Professionals in health and social care work across academic disciplines and theoretical perspectives, so they need to be able to understand and use research from different perspectives.

As practitioners and consumers of research, we have to weigh up the pros and cons of new information and understand what its implications are. When planning to introduce clinical supervision into our workplace, for example, we check to see how we can manage it within our resources, which approach meets the essential criteria for our purposes and whether it will meet the standard needed for care quality improvement. We would check which approaches are credible and successfully used – perhaps look for reviews or meet with organisations who have already implemented clinical supervision. We would assess some of the key measures to ensure they meet the necessary standards – relevant training and education; adequate workload time; suitable settings; written policy that considers ethico-legal concerns, for example. If we had access to high-quality research, policy and evaluation literature, we would read it. Finally, we would probably discuss different types of clinical supervision and how to manage it with colleagues and potential participants. In other words, all research findings are different in quality, purpose, resource demands and use, and we always need to ensure they meet our professional, organisational and ethical requirements.

It is important to develop the skills and attitudes of enquiry and use of evidence to support your practice. At its most basic level, you should use current policies and guidelines to support your practice. Additionally, you should also use critical reflection and clinical supervision to identify those areas of practice where your knowledge of the evidence base is lacking, so that you can search policies, protocols, government reports, and standards produced by professional bodies and research evidence to improve your own practice and, where applicable, share your knowledge with other members of the team. So, evidence-based practice is all about finding evidence that is relevant to an area of your practice, evaluating its quality and relevance, and developing an understanding of the evidence in order to apply those findings in practice. Research evidence is reviewed by government, health and social care organisations, professional bodies and employer organisations to ensure that policies are evidence-based. Research is needed to create knowledge and evidence for you to use in your everyday practice.

THE PROCESS OF EVIDENCE-BASED PRACTICE

PROBLEM IDENTIFICATION

A problem might be something you have done or observed in practice where you think the process or outcome could be improved for some reason. It might also be part of your practice that you have never questioned but where you are unsure of the reasons or evidence to support it. It is often easier to identify problems when you take part in clinical supervision, a form of supported reflection that focuses on your professional development needs, including:

- Learning needs
- Self-awareness, emotional resilience and coping strategies, awareness of others
- Knowledge of professional and managerial structures and processes and how to use them to enhance care

With practice, by reflecting in a structured way, you will learn to identify problems and ask questions. The problem may be one that needs little more enquiry than simply checking the current policy, but if you are aware of some ambiguity or concern about current practice or understanding within your professional setting, then you may need to review the evidence in more depth.

ACTIVITY 15.2

Choose just one of the topics you considered in Activity 15.1 where you think that your practice, or that of your team, could be improved. Improvement may relate to a specific activity or intervention, but it can also include being able to explain your actions or a procedure to a service user or student or colleague. Explain what you think the problem or query is.

SCOPING CURRENT POLICY AND PRACTICE

The complexity of health and social care practice means that decision-making and interventions are often the result of evaluating, prioritising and synthesising a number of different factors. Organisations develop policies to ensure that care meets a number of legal requirements and ethical standards and uses current evidence to optimise care. Finding local policy should be fairly straightforward – most organisations store and update their policies online, usually on a network that is accessible to all staff. Some local policies will refer to professional codes of ethics or standards produced by other organisations, such as *The Royal Marsden Manual of Clinical Nursing Procedures* (Royal Marsden Hospital, 2015). Once you know what the policy is, unless you think the policy may need updating or improving, you should be able to use it for practice. This does not imply unquestioning obedience, simply that your own professional knowledge and competence should enable you to understand and use policy appropriately.

However, you may identify an area of practice that is not covered by policy, or where the policy is unclear. You may think that the guidance does not specifically apply to the situation you need it for, or that two different policies may apply in one situation and you are not sure which takes precedence. You may observe practice that appears to differ from policy, find it difficult to follow a policy in your own practice, or even find that local policy differs from policy in another organisation. You may have read an article in your professional journals that suggests new evidence requires a change in policy. A service user might ask you a question about their care that you cannot answer. You may see that policy is out of date or even be the person who is asked to update it. In these situations, you need to know how to find the relevant evidence and how to evaluate its relevance, quality and application to your practice.

Before undertaking a search of the research literature published in peer-review journals, it is usual to identify other sources of information that may help you to understand the background to your topic. Colleagues and mentors who are experts in the field may point you to useful sources of information to get you started, for instance classic papers, gold standard guidance (such as the guidance by the British Thoracic Society on administering emergency oxygen; see O'Driscoll et al., 2017), relevant policies, standards, reports by relevant institutions, such as UNICEF (the United Nations' Children's Fund), Public Health England, the Social Care Institute for Excellence (SCIE) and NICE (National Institute for Health and Care Excellence), as well as by the government and by your professional organisations. These and other forms of data and evidence that are not published in journals are collectively known as 'grey literature' and include unpublished dissertations (master's and doctoral research), online reports and publications from reputable sources and conference presentations (Auger, 1998). Since studies that do not provide conclusive findings or simply add to existing findings are less frequently published, the use of such data may reduce publication bias (Hopewell et al., 2007). Additionally, it is often useful to search for this type of literature to provide background and context to your identified topic before you carry out a search of the research literature published in journals. Remember that, although research evidence is important, all research builds on a body of established knowledge that you will find in books about your topic – do identify key texts and chapters within them and read them before you look for the research evidence. Having a feel for your subject will make it much easier for you to find and understand relevant research.

ACTIVITY 15.3

Search for the grey literature relevant to your topic and use it to identify some background to your topic and the current guidelines or policies that apply. List any controversies/ differences between policy and practice or aspects of practice that are not supported by guidelines.

Once you have organised this information and narrowed down your topic or question, you will need to search the peer-reviewed research literature to help you identify best practice or current state of knowledge to support your practice in relation to your focused topic or question.

LITERATURE SEARCHING AND RECORDING

You need to find all the literature that is relevant to your question or topic. When you look for literature of any kind, it is important to keep a record of when you searched, which electronic databases or catalogues you accessed, what search terms you used and in what combinations, what your inclusion criteria were, what limiters or exclusions you used in your initial search (such as publication time period, language, age of participants), then any further exclusion criteria you adopted to reduce your initial results down to the final articles for your review. (Many databases have an option to save your search if you are signed in, and even alert you to new publications that meet your search criteria.) At this point, you also need to identify how many duplicates there were, note the number and cite your final articles chosen for review (see Table 15.1). The way that you combine terms with Boolean operators (AND, OR, NOT or AND NOT) is important – using AND means that both terms must be in the papers, reducing the number of hits, while OR means one or the other terms must be in, increasing the number of hits. Whether you use a term as a major heading, subject heading or key word also affects the number of hits, so do keep a record of this as well.

Table 15.1 Literature search

Date searched:

Database used:

- Search terms 'patient-centred care' AND 'nursing'; 'client-centred care' AND 'nursing'; 'patient-focused care' AND 'nursing' (all key words)

  o Scope note: 'Patient care in which health resources and health personnel are organized around the needs and priorities of the patient ...'

- Limiters used:

  o Date published January 2011 onwards
  o English language only
  o All adult
  o Abstract available
  o Scholarly (peer-reviewed) journals only

- 28 results

- Exclusion criteria:

  o No reference to patient-centred care in abstract – 2
  o No reference to patient-centred care in text – 11
  o Child focus – 1

14 results: Ahern et al. (2011); Bradley & Falk-Rafael (2011); Chenoweth et al. (2011); Doss et al. (2011); du Toit & Surr (2011); McCormack et al. (2011); Mullay et al. (2011); Rokstad et al. (2012); Rollin (2011); Thornton (2011); Tse et al. (2012); Utriainen et al. (2011); van Mossel et al. (2011) and Wagner et al. (2011).

This process sounds fairly straightforward, but unless you are familiar with background theory and evidence, finding the relevant search terms can be quite difficult. The databases all have a thesaurus of the terms that they use, which is important because terminology and spellings differ. As well as looking terms up in the database, you can also have a look at any papers you already have and see what key words they identify or use in their title or abstract that might be useful. Although it is important to keep a record of all your searches (and if you sign into the main databases, you can often save your record electronically), it may take several attempts before you end up with the search strategies that find the most relevant papers. Especially with a scoping review, where you are trying to identify all relevant evidence, you usually need to search several databases using a variety of different search terms to access all the literature you need.

ACTIVITY 15.4

Search for research literature relevant to your topic, recording your searches as you go. Complete one or more literature search records and download or print out your final papers for reading.

DATA EXTRACTION AND CRITICAL APPRAISAL

Once you have identified your papers, you then need to extract the data or findings from them and evaluate the quality of the evidence and conclusions. To standardise this process and limit bias in your analysis, it is usual to use a critical appraisal tool. This is a series of questions or a checklist, appropriate to the type of research being reviewed, that you complete when reading the paper in order to assess the trustworthiness of the evidence and therefore the relative weight that you give to the findings in your review. It is important to use the correct tool, as different types of research need different approaches to establish trustworthiness – generally, you will find tools to appraise quantitative, qualitative, mixed methods and systematic review research (Davies and Logan, 2018), but you will find more specific tools on the Critical Appraisal Skills Programme (CASP) website. This review will then form the basis for future practice, so it is important to ensure that the evidence is sound.

When you are organising the evidence, it is helpful to use a data extraction table (see Table 15.2) so that you can identify similarities and differences between the different studies and evaluate the strengths and limitations of the evidence. This is an important stage in amalgamating the findings to identify common and unusual themes and you will often find such a table in published literature reviews (Chapman et al., 2018).

ACTIVITY 15.5

Read each of your final papers then use a critical appraisal tool to evaluate it and complete the data extraction table.

CRITIQUING, REVIEWING AND PRESENTING FINDINGS

You have now organised your papers, extracted the key information from them and identified their strengths and limitations so that you can work out which findings are more or less credible, and where they are most relevant. The next step is to weave this information into a meaningful narrative that makes sense to you and enables you to explain your conclusions logically and identify their implications for practice. You can organise your thoughts around areas of controversy, common findings and themes, aspects that have not been well researched, or where the research is mainly either qualitative or quantitative. Analysing, evaluating and synthesising ideas are skills that can be learned. Analysis is the process of breaking ideas down into their component parts, to understand where they came from and how they fit together, while evaluation adds the process of judging the strengths and limitations of ideas through reasoned, logical thought and by comparison with related concepts. Synthesis is where you combine a number of different perspectives in order to develop a new understanding of the ideas. This is the aim of a good literature review – it will allow you to create a more advanced understanding of this aspect of your practice. Some findings may be more conceptual and less directly practice-focused, while others may be more tangible, but it is important that you identify their implications for practice.

Table 15.2 Data extraction table

Author, date of publication, study location	Aims of the study	Methods/study design	Findings and recommendations	Comments (including strengths and limitations)
Chapman and Clucas (2014) England	To explore student nurses' understanding and behaviours of respect towards patients in order to inform educational strategies to optimise respectful care.	Hermeneutic phenomenology – interpretative phenomenological analysis. Interviewed 3rd year adult field student nurses (n = 8) to identify and interpret student nurses' behaviours and understanding of respect towards service users.	Respect is a complex concept that is difficult to apply in practice. Students are not always aware of incongruence between their feelings of respect towards service users and their behaviours towards them. Role-modelling of respectful care is variable, and essential care is often learned from health care assistants.	Rigour and transparency of method and analysis – tables to show process and quotations to support themes. Causation cannot be inferred. Gaps: future research could look at effects of educational interventions or service user perspective.

ACTIVITY 15.6

Organise the findings from your data-extraction table into themes and identify areas of agreement and disagreement, gaps in the findings and methods. Summarise your findings into a structure that is meaningful for you.

ACTION PLANNING AND PRACTICE DEVELOPMENT

You have now found, read, analysed and summarised the evidence on your topic, but what are you going to do with it? Here are some suggestions:

- Write an action plan (see Table 15.3) to identify how you can use this knowledge to improve your own future practice.
- Share it with colleagues in a presentation to consider changes to practice.
- Discuss its implications for practice with your line manager.
- Present it at a conference.
- Write it up for a practice journal.
- Use it as the basis of a research project (with appropriate academic support or supervision).

Table 15.3 Action plan example

SMART Objectives	Activity	Time Frame and Resources	Success Criteria
Specific, measurable, achievable, realistic and time-bound goal – write one in each row.	What do you need to do to achieve this goal?	How quickly can you start to do this, how long will it take to achieve it and what do you need to make it happen?	How can you measure whether or not you have achieved your goal?

ACTIVITY 15.7

Think about how the findings relate to your practice in your chosen topic and write an action plan. Discuss your action plan with your clinical supervisor or line manager and work out its potential for personal and organisational quality improvement.

RESEARCH SKILLS IN PRACTICE

Now that you have completed a full scoping review of the literature related to a topic of interest, you will have found a lot of information that you were not aware of and feel more confident that, in that area of practice, you have a clearer understanding of the evidence and how to improve the quality of care. You will also feel more confident in your literature searching and reviewing skills. All of this is essential for you to become an evidence-based practitioner. However, there are always more questions and more development in other areas of science and practice that need researching and evaluating, so health and social care practitioners need to both collaborate with researchers and, ultimately, become producers of research. It is essential that we contribute to the research agenda, both in identifying questions of concern in our professions and in contributing to the ways in which those questions are answered and the findings are interpreted. That is the only way in which we can ensure that the service users' voices are heard, and that our professional expertise is developed to meet future demands. Having read and critically appraised some research, you now have some understanding of research and, with some specific training, could act as a co-researcher on ethically approved and supervised research projects. The next step is to gain some research skills and experience under supervision – this would often be as part of a master's qualification. The next section provides guidance on the key stages of a research study, but it is important to remember that in health and social care research, you may need to revisit previous stages as the project develops.

REVISITING THE LITERATURE REVIEW AND DEVELOPING YOUR RESEARCH QUESTION

Before developing your research question, you need to consider whether or not you intend to carry out research or some other form of enquiry. The *UK policy framework for health and social care research* defines research as 'the attempt to derive generalisable or transferable new knowledge to answer or refine relevant questions with scientifically sound methods. This excludes audits of practice and service evaluations' (Health Research Authority, Health and Social Care in Northern Ireland, NHS Research Scotland, and Health and Care Research Wales, 2017, p. 6). It also outlines the benefits of improved standards of care, service-user education and enhanced staff development that occur within research-active organisations. While they do provide a tool for deciding if your study is research, service evaluation or audit, if it involves service users or their data it is often helpful to seek advice from the HRA.

Writing a literature review prior to carrying out research is very similar to the process already discussed. You may be undertaking this research as part of your role and have less choice about the topic and the goal of this literature review is to identify a research question. The process of identifying a research question may involve some discussion with more experienced researchers because you have to consider several factors:

- What research needs doing (in other words, if it has already been done, it is probably not necessary, unless it needs updating, improving or upscaling)
- What is achievable, especially within the time you have available and the number of participants you can access and recruit
- What is important and relevant to practice
- What is ethical (experimentation on humans is very limited in health and social care for this reason)

The research question should identify what your study will learn and how it will do so. For example, your topic of interest may be attitudes towards older people amongst social carers, but your research question would need to be more specific in order to make it both achievable and clear to participants and users of the research what you are trying to find out and how. So, your research question might be: *Attitudes of paid social carers in elder care towards older people: an exploratory hermeneutic phenomenological study.* This identifies your sample group more clearly, it identifies that the study is interested in the meaning of expressed perceptions, experiences and attitudes towards older people, as interpreted by the researcher, and that this is a small study aiming to identify some themes that could be explored across other, similar settings, to develop a deep understanding of this experience. If the question posed was: *Measurement of attitudes of paid social carers in elder care towards older people using Kogan's attitudes to old people scale (1961)*, then the study and the findings would be very different.

The two questions are very different because they view the world and what can be known about it from different perspectives – in other words, the questions and therefore the methods used to answer them are determined by the paradigm or underlying philosophy of the researcher (see Cronin et al., 2015 for an accessible discussion of research paradigms, methodology and design). The first question comes from a view of the world where multiple realities are possible (a relativist ontology), where each individual's experience and meaning derived from it can only be indirectly and imperfectly understood (an interpretivist epistemology), and where the person is valued as an individual in their own right (a person-centred axiology). The second question comes from an expectation that one reality can be uncovered (an objectivist ontology), where relationships between statements, concepts, attitudes and behaviours can be suggested, measured, tested and generalised (a positivist/post-positivist view of the world) and where the individual is reduced to a set of statistics (a state where values are limited to collecting, analysing and presenting the data without impinging on people's legal and general ethical rights). Health and social care must adhere to strict ethical principles that generally require a person-centred axiology whatever the research philosophy (Health Research Authority et al., 2017; McCormack et al., 2017).

Neither of the perspectives outlined above is necessarily right or wrong, but they may be more or less useful and appropriate in different circumstances. Understanding the effectiveness of a particular type of pain management in people with a certain type of cancer may require a more positivist approach to look at different drug regimes and dosages, but unless other studies look at people's preferences and barriers to adherence with regards to different types of pain management, then they will only find out some of the important information. Increasingly, in health and social care, the importance of using diverse research methods to answer complex questions is being recognised (Waring et al., 2016). Once you decide whether you are using a quantitative, qualitative or mixed methods approach, you will need to narrow it down to a specific methodology. You should use more specialist chapters and texts on your chosen methodology that explain how it affects your study design, including the research question, ethical issues, data collection, data analysis and the possible outcomes of your research.

WHY IS MY QUESTION IMPORTANT AND WHAT IMPACT WILL MY RESEARCH HAVE?

Whatever question you ask, it must have the aim of gaining knowledge in order, ultimately, to improve people's health and well-being or people's health and social care. So, when you write your research question, you need to consider what impact it will have. It is important to identify how the answer to your research question will have an impact on people's lives (National Institute for Health Research, n.d.)

ACTIVITY 15.8

Write out your research question, including the methodological approach you are taking. Keep editing it until the question and the methodology are in alignment. Consider the potential impact of your research when writing your question.

ETHICAL CONCERNS AND PROCESSES IN
HEALTH AND SOCIAL CARE

Ethics, ensuring that your research 'respects the rights, safety and dignity of participants' (Health Research Authority et al., 2017), is a fundamental consideration in the planning, recruitment and process of health and social care research. Historically, there have been situations where research has been unethical (Carmack et al., 2008) and, in addition to harming the participants, their families and communities, this has also led to widespread mistrust of research and a reluctance to take part in it.

There are some clear ethico-legal issues to consider in your research, such as anonymity and confidentiality of participants, including protection of all the data gathered ('Data Protection Act', 2018), protecting participants from harm, benefiting society and ensuring that people have equal access to being able to take part in and benefit from research. Refusal to take part and ability to withdraw from research without ill-effects to the person or their life chances is a fundamental right. Consideration of the Human Tissue Act (United Kingdom Government, 2004) is relevant if you are using any body parts (including teeth) or fluids, while knowledge of the Mental Capacity Act (2005) is essential for research involving people with learning disabilities, mental health disorders or illness that may affect their capacity to give informed consent. Research with children involves complex ethical issues and initial access to HRA advice (2018) is advised. It is important to consider how the whole research process takes into account the perspective of the service user and the effects that taking part in the research may have upon them (McCormack et al., 2017). Health and social care can only meet the needs of people who use these services if it is based on their own experiences, wishes and beliefs. Some groups may be under- or over-researched; the former suggests their needs and views may not be considered when formulating policy; the latter can reduce participation and over-burden communities. It is also important to consider the rigour, credibility and value of the research itself – collecting data and reaching conclusions can only be a worthwhile and ethical endeavour if the research is carried out according to the standards required by the chosen methodology and produces credible findings that are then shared with practitioners and academics in order to move knowledge and practice forward. If the findings are based on flawed research, they could be misleading.

Students and employees of universities commonly need to apply for ethical approval from their university. You would also need to liaise with any organisations where you might access or recruit participants, or whose data or resources you might use, to gain any necessary permissions or ethical approval in order to carry out research within their organisation. It is good practice to involve people who represent potential participants in your study at the planning stage. As a general principle, ethical approval is only given by one organisation. If your research requires ethical approval from an external organisation, you would usually require scientific merit approval from the University. National Health Service (NHS) Trusts have a Research and Development Lead and if you are considering research related to any NHS service, it is advisable to contact them early in the development of your study design for advice on any potential difficulties. Similarly, while the HRA provide a decision-making tool (Health Research Authority, 2017) to help you decide whether or not you need ethics permission from them, if there is any possible doubt it is advisable to contact them.

There is an integrated Research Application system (IRAS) (HRA, 2019) through which you would apply for the relevant approvals/permissions from the following review bodies:

- Administration of Radioactive Substances Advisory Committee (ARSAC)
- Confidentiality Advisory Group (CAG)
- Gene Therapy Advisory Committee (GTAC)
- Health Research Authority (HRA) for projects seeking HRA Approval
- Medicines and Healthcare products Regulatory Agency (MHRA)
- NHS/Health and Social Care in Northern Ireland (HSC) R&D offices
- NHS / HSC Research Ethics Committees
- National Offender Management Service (NOMS)
- Social Care Research Ethics Committee

Principal researchers normally have, or are undertaking, a doctorate, but you may undertake research under supervision as a master's student or as part of a larger research team. While ethical considerations mean that research should not be undertaken lightly, it is important to promote research in order to ensure that the evidence base for practice is continuously developed and updated to improve practice for the benefit of all service users.

ACTIVITY 15.9

Find out which ethical approvals and permissions you will need to carry out your research, download the relevant forms and read through them.

HOW CAN I ANSWER MY QUESTION? APPROACH, SAMPLING AND AVOIDANCE OF ERROR

While some beliefs about the world and what can be known about it are implicit within your chosen methodology , it is generally helpful to choose the approach that will answer your question – that will in turn resolve an initial problem for practice. In health and social care, the service-user experience is often central to questions about interventions and outcomes (such as pain or reduced quality of life associated with some interventions). This requires a qualitative approach, focusing on individual experience. Nonetheless, measurable outcomes (such as five-year survival rates following different interventions) are also important, and for these a quantitative approach would be used. Both types of data would be taken into account when developing guidance and policy, which are evidence based. Sometimes, particularly when researchers work together to collect sufficient data in a more complex study design to try to answer a question in one study, they will use a mixed methods approach – this is often used where a question is complex and, if used correctly, can make findings more robust (Creswell, 2015). Whichever approach you use, it is important to make it clear in your research question. For instance, you might carry out a quasi-experimental matched pairs study comparing quality of life outcome measures and times to healing between two different ways of managing venous leg ulcers, which would be a quantitative study. You might carry out a phenomenological study of the lived experience of a specific type of leg ulcer management for service users in a specialist leg ulcer outpatient service, which would be a qualitative study. You might carry out a convergent parallel design study exploring the experience of venous leg ulcers in two different treatment groups, and measuring contributing factors, severity of ulcer and outcomes – this would be a mixed methods study to understand how factors relating to severity, service-user experience and outcome are related.

Whichever approach you use, it is important to recruit an appropriate sample from your target population, using inclusion criteria (such as adults who have experienced being children in care) and exclusion criteria (such as children, people who cannot give informed consent) to answer your question and ensure that your findings are credible.

QUANTITATIVE STUDY DESIGNS EXPERIMENTS AND QUASI-EXPERIMENTS

In an experimental study, you need to posit a theory (a hypothesis) that if you change one thing (the independent variable) it will alter another thing (the dependent variable) – this aims to demonstrate that one event causes another (causality) and is common in the natural sciences, such as physics. To achieve this, samples are randomly generated and allocated to treatment groups to reduce bias and ensure that the sample is representative of the general population. This enables the findings to be generalised and is called probability sampling. The experimental group will experience the changed variable (for example an experimental drug) and the other group will belong to a control group (receiving a placebo or dummy drug). In a true experiment, neither the person who administers the drug nor the participant would know which group they were in. This is called a double-blind, randomised control trial (RCT). In health and social care, this type of experiment is not often carried out in humans for ethical reasons. It is difficult to justify carrying out experiments on humans where the outcomes are unknown or potentially harmful. Also, while it is useful in comparing outcomes between clearly defined and easily replicable interventions, it is rarely possible to control for all the confounding variables (other factors that might affect the outcome), making the findings meaningless. Consequently, quasi-experiments are more common.

Quasi-experiments also attempt to measure the outcome of a specific intervention or variable, but the sampling is often non-probability, since the research is often carried out with existing groups (for example, comparing the outcomes of asthma management from a nurse-led outpatient service and a consultant-led outpatient service). Since people have not been randomly assigned to these groups, other lifestyle, general health and severity of illness factors may also affect outcome measures, meaning that cause and effect cannot be established.

NON-EXPERIMENTAL QUANTITATIVE STUDIES

Sometimes, we can only try to understand what causes something through measuring outcomes and then comparing two groups on the basis of a factor that already exists. In other words, while we have an outcome measure (dependent variable) and a potential causal factor (independent variable), we cannot randomly assign someone to a group (manipulate the variables). Instead, we look at people already belong to one or other group and compare outcomes between the two groups. This is called a causal-comparative design. For example, various studies have looked at the time to union (healing) following a tibial shaft fracture in people who smoke and those who do not by measuring outcomes in some way and then comparing the outcomes between the two groups to see if there is a statistically significant difference (Patel et al., 2013). Again, cause and effect cannot be established in this way, meaning that it is one piece of evidence amongst many that lead to a more robust model of the role of cigarette smoking in fracture healing.

Other studies investigate potential relationships between two or more variables by measuring both sets of variables and analysing how they change in relation to each other. For example, if we measure the average consumption of red meat in a large number of people and also the frequency of cardiovascular disease in the same population, we might see that the two variables increase or decrease together (this is a positive correlation). A relationship where one factor increases as the other factor falls is called a negative correlation. However, a correlation does not mean there is a causal relationship between the two because other factors that could confound the findings have not been ruled out.

Descriptive studies aim to enhance understanding of a specific phenomenon, such as the incidence of HIV infection in a given population – this might be important for planning services and providing a rationale for carrying out research, as well as being able to evaluate the effectiveness of public health interventions.

Surveys and questionnaires are a form of data collection that often involves quantitative data analysis. They may be purely descriptive, having face validity – that is they appear to measure what they say they are measuring – so a questionnaire that asks people what times of day and days of the week they prefer their outpatient appointments for a warfarin clinic might be useful in planning services. A scale has been designed to measure something that may include questions that experts in the field think are important in defining and measuring that concept – it is said to have content validity. Kogan's scale measuring attitudes to older people (Kogan, 1961) uses a series of questions that try to identify different aspects of attitudes towards older people, including thoughts, feelings and behaviours towards and experiences of older people. The findings of these scales are then compared with other uses of that construct (the defined phenomenon that we are trying to measure) in order to validate the scale. In other words, checking that it does measure what it is supposed to measure. Reliability is assessed by identifying whether the same results will be gained when measured at other times and that different ways of asking similar questions produce the same results. This scale has construct validity, which means that it has both content validity and is in agreement with other measures of similar or related constructs.

RESEARCH SKILLS TO COLLECT AND ANALYSE DATA: QUANTITATIVE APPROACHES

Much of the work in quantitative research is involved in designing the study to answer the question – once you have chosen the correct study design, sample, data-collection tools and methods of analysis, the findings and discussion should be reasonably straightforward. This is because you will generally have narrowed down your question and the possible answers before you collect your data so that the options are fairly narrow. You will need to think about how to recruit people in order to gain the most responses in an ethical fashion. For instance, mailshot surveys generally have very low response rates, while asking people face-to-face has a much higher response rate. If you are aiming for a specific population, for example psychiatric emergency social workers, you might recruit via a dedicated website or through presentations to groups at conferences or through introductory letters, or even via colleagues or representatives in the workplace. In these instances, particularly, it is important to ensure that people do not feel pressured to take part.

The advantage of surveys and questionnaires is that they are easily anonymised and data can be collected and analysed quite quickly (see Andres, 2012 for an accessible introduction to designing surveys). Online surveys are easy to distribute and, even if the response rate (the number of people responding divided by the sample) is low, it is generally higher than a postal survey and may produce more data than a telephone or face-to-face survey because of the ability to access large numbers at a low resource and financial cost (Evans and Mathur, 2005). For most research, it is preferable to use a scale or questionnaire that has been previously validated, since this will add credibility to your study. If you develop your own tool, you will need to start by designing, testing and piloting the tool, then evaluating its validity and reliability as part of your study. However, although face-to-face and telephone interviews take longer, the response rate is often higher and you may be able to recruit people to follow-up interviews. Surveys are useful for providing a simple answer to a positivist question, but they lack the depth and understanding that can be gained from interviewing people either individually or in groups.

Collecting other kinds of quantitative data can be more complex than it would seem from papers in academic journals. For instance, when collecting data from electronic records, the coding may be incomplete or inaccurate, while papers can go missing from written records or be misplaced. If a longitudinal study involving collecting data related to health is carried out, during that time people may miss an appointment or drop out of the study, making the sample smaller and less representative. Studies that analyse audio-recordings or video-recordings for different types of communication or interaction may yield different amounts if two scorers are involved, so training and testing for inter-observer reliability is essential. For every type of data collection, there will be points to consider – use of reliable measurement tools, safe management, testing and storage of data sources and data (everything from human tissue to video-recordings to case note records to observation notebooks) and the choice of data analysis.

Analysis involves reducing and organising data to answer the question (or at least part of it). Quantitative data are generally analysed using statistics to describe a phenomenon or to test a hypothesis or to evaluate a new measurement tool. In order to carry out a statistical analysis, we have to decide what type of data we are using, as that determines which tests we can apply. The four types of data are:

- **Nominal** – a simple category, such as male = 1 and female = 2. Each category is identified by a number but they cannot be treated mathematically. This is categorical data.
- **Ordinal** – this might be a ranking system, such as: 1 = appears calm; 2 = displaying mild agitation/withdrawal; 3 = expressing feelings of anxiety/depression; 4 = expressing self-harming thoughts; 5 = expressing suicidal thoughts. They suggest that each level is higher than the previous one, but there is no insight into the distance between each level, so their use is generally limited to descriptive statistical analysis. Again, this is categorical data.
- **Interval** – this is numerical data that represents ranking and distance between two measures, which means you can add or subtract them. For instance a temperature of 20 degrees centigrade is the same distance from 40°C as 40°C is from 60°C. However, in centigrade, there is no absolute zero and you cannot sensibly divide and multiply the measures; i.e. 60°C is not twice the temperature of 30°C. (However, if you use the Kelvin (K) scale, which starts at absolute zero, that can be used as ratio data.) You can use interval data for some types of inferential statistics as it is a continuous variable.

- **Ratio** – as with the Kelvin scale, or with weight, you have an absolute zero and it makes sense to say that 200°K is twice 100°K, or 200 kilogrammes is twice 100 kilogrammes. Again, this is a continuous variable, amenable to multiplication and division as well as subtraction and addition, and is suitable for use in inferential statistics.

We have briefly discussed statistical testing of a measurement tool and will now focus on descriptive and inferential statistics.

Descriptive statistics are generally used to enable us to see the 'big picture' – in other words, they clarify something by reducing it down to numbers, without actually testing a theory or hypothesis. Nominal data can be displayed in a frequency table (for example to show how many males or females hold senior management positions within an organisation) or a bar chart (perhaps to illustrate the different types of admission by medical specialism to an acute admissions ward). Nominal data can also be shown as a pie chart. For example, if you want to know how and where a service user spends their time during the day so that you can work out how to enrich their lifestyle, you might collect nominal data every hour on where they are and what they are doing. You could then produce frequency tables and pie charts to show where they spend most of their time and how they fill it. The central tendency of this type of data is the mode, or the most common category, which might be sleeping and in the bedroom, or standing and in the day room. Although very basic data, this would be a useful start for understanding a person's lived experience.

Inferential statistics not only reduce and organise data, but they are used to make predictions about the world and how different conditions can lead to different outcomes. Ordinal data can sometimes be used to compare difference between two groups, but no assumptions can be made about the mean average of the data because it is not interval data. Consequently, only statistical tests that are based upon the median of the data can be used. The median is literally the mid-point of a dataset. If you have a range of 61 numbers from 0 to 35, you would order them from 0 to 35 and find the number that is at 31st place in the list. Median-based tests are called non-parametric tests. Non-parametric tests can still be used to describe a phenomenon quantitatively and to compare two groups if the data are ordinal. You can also use ordinal data to explore the relationship between two variables and see if they correlate negatively or positively.

Interval and ratio data that have a normal distribution (that is, when plotted in a histogram, the data form a bell curve shape) can be used to predict much stronger and more complex relationships between groups and variables, ranging from multiple group comparisons, parametric correlations (where a normal distribution around the mean can be assumed), regression analysis (where a number of variables are analysed in relation to an outcome variable, to see which has a significant correlation, then ranked from highest to lowest order so that, while cause and effect cannot be assumed, relative predictive strength can be). Finally, if continuous variables are used in experimental conditions as outcome measures, they can be used to attribute cause and effect and can either support or disprove a hypothesis. While you need to understand some basic principles in statistics, the important points are:

- Choose or design a data capture tool that is appropriate to your research question.
- Include your statistical analysis when you design your study, so that you understand what type of data you need to collect and how many participants/samples you will need.
- Rule out confounding variables where possible, and where the data type is suitable, either by using an experimental study design or by including them in a multiple regression analysis.
- Seek statistical and ethical advice before planning your study.

For more detailed discussion of quantitative statistical analysis, please see 'An introduction to data analysis: quantitative, qualitative and mixed methods' by Tiffany Bergin (2018).

RESEARCH SKILLS TO COLLECT AND ANALYSE DATA: QUALITATIVE APPROACHES

With qualitative research, the initial question tends to be more open, prone to change according to the research process and accepting of complexity. It builds inductively from data that are observed and interpreted to construct some interpretation or understanding of an experience. This type of research often involves significant ethical and philosophical thought and, once the data have been collected, the analysis and findings generally take more effort to develop since the process is iterative (searching backwards and forwards for codes, themes or categories), reflexive (requiring constant consideration of one's own position and perspective in relation to the study and construction of findings), based on a deep understanding of the subject matter and academic discipline, but requiring a focus on participants' perspectives, experiences, cultural mores and social drivers and constraints. Qualitative research generally runs along a continuum from the most idiographic (specific to the individual) to the most generalisable (from postmodernist deconstruction to phenomenology to ethnography to grounded theory). Other than grounded theory, most qualitative research does not, on its own, claim to develop theoretical models, but to enhance understanding of experience, perception, cultural meanings or social phenomena. Although this type of research is based on understanding individuals or cultural or social groups, conceptual and thematic analysis of findings from a number of qualitative papers exploring similar concepts or phenomena can lead to the development of theory that is amenable to testing by statistical analysis or experimentation if ethics permit. While there are a multiplicity of methodological approaches, there are similarities in data collection and analysis so that skills in this type of research often overlap. (Accessible information on qualitative research methods can be found in Green and Thorogood, 2018; for examples of more innovative approaches to carrying out research in social work, see Hardwick et al., 2016).

A qualitative researcher needs to learn the skill of self-awareness and of understanding their own views, position and relationships to the study, the data and their role in constructing knowledge. This requires continuous reflection and examination of their own perspectives and how they influence every stage of the study, from development of the research question, study design, data analysis and findings to discussion of the implications of the research. Reflective diaries and memos that are used to explore and analyse insights into the data are required in most methodologies. Since qualitative research generally assumes that social phenomena cannot be observed and understood objectively, and that the researcher interprets all data through their own worldview, this means that they must make that worldview transparent to enable others to gauge its potential effects on the findings.

A qualitative researcher needs to know and understand their methodological perspective so that they can align their study design and methods appropriately, without mixing them up. For example, a phenomenological study would not involve comparisons between participants because the philosophical approach is to understand their existential truths. However, a grounded theory study aims to construct generalisable models of how processes or institutions affect people, often through the effects of the experience on their self-concept, self-esteem and self-efficacy. While a positive perspective, such as the type frequently used in natural science experiments requires little explanation in papers, all qualitative research requires an outline of the world view, type of knowledge, values, methodology and resulting study design, as well as the positionality of the researcher within the study.

Positionality is often along a continuum, with an emic researcher fully belonging and engaging in the culture or situation that they are studying, while an etic researcher sits outside the research and observes others. Many qualitative researchers adopt some kind of insider perspective, but few will fully immerse themselves in the experience being explored unless they already belong to the participant group.

Qualitative researchers need to be able to write and ask appropriate questions that will both capture the type of data that they need to answer their question and ensure that the participants are not inhibited from providing unexpected but relevant insights. Questions should not lead the participants to a particular answer or close down their response, so they should be open, exploratory and allow for different individual response according to the participant's experiences and perspectives. Where possible, questions should be based on a sound theoretical understanding of relevant literature. Even in grounded theory, where reliance on previous research around a specific topic is regarded as potentially undermining the grounded nature of the research, a total lack of relevant theoretical knowledge would not be desirable as some important insights might be missed (although data and findings are compared with the literature towards the end of analysis in order to identify new findings, corroborate or question existing theory and construct new theory to move the discipline forward).

While the approach, terminology, level of detail and focus of analysis is different across different methodological approaches, there are some commonalities in collecting and analysing qualitative data:

- **Data capture** – do write notes of your observations at the time or soon after the time you make them, and record when you made them. We start processing and therefore changing information in the process of collecting, storing and remembering it, so the closer to the source, the more literal our account will be. This is one reason why many observations, situations and interviews are video- or audio-recorded. However, there are some potential hazards – check your equipment is working and, if possible, take spare recorders and certainly spare batteries as appropriate. Always check the recording is happening where possible at the time, and check the data has been recorded immediately afterwards. Check the recorder light occasionally as sometimes power cables can be accidentally pulled from connections. If any recordings fail, do write notes immediately on what you remember so that you do not lose all the data. Where data collection is all manual, try to make your observations as detailed as possible and do not make any assumptions about what you would expect – try to write almost as if you were an alien writing about a new world.

- **Data immersion** – whatever the detailed method or terminology used is, you need to start somewhere, and that is usually by immersing yourself in the data. If you have videoed or audio-recorded interactions, you can watch or listen to them again. Transcribing your own data, while it is time consuming, is very useful in the process of data immersion and is an important stage in the process of learning to carry out research. Write memos, notes or reflections on your impressions and ideas throughout the process so that you do not forget them when you start to reflect on your process and analyse the data.

- **Coding** – Once you have transcribed the data or written up your field notes, you need to go through them looking for key words or phrases; think about how people think, feel and behave and look for explanations of how and why processes, systems and organisations function. At this stage, try not to take anything for granted, but break the data down into small and even apparently simple and straightforward descriptive codes. Depending on your chosen methodology, you will then construct a system of integrating and structuring your initial codes to produce an analysis of the phenomenon under scrutiny – tables, mind-maps and even physical cut-and-pasting to rearrange ideas may all be used as part of this process.

It is very important to follow the specific process for your methodology, and to keep track of the decision-making process, since this will demonstrate rigour in your research.

- **Analysis and discussion of findings and implications** – in qualitative research, it is very important to relate your findings to what is already known. This helps to situate your findings within a body of knowledge so that it can be understood and related back to theoretical principles. It also demonstrates where your findings support, conflict with or add to the sum of knowledge. Since, with the exception of grounded theory, most qualitative research is not regarded as generalisable, any conflicting or new findings should lead to further research aimed at addressing this. Any implication for future practice, policy and education within your discipline and related disciplines should be discussed with a view to supporting continuous quality improvement in health and social care.

Most importantly, qualitative researchers need self-awareness, sensitivity and empathy towards others in order to build trust, achieve understanding and honestly represent the perspectives of participants in order to improve lives. While qualitative surveys are possible, their complexity is in the questionnaire design and analysis (which is similar to other types of qualitative data analysis). The next section will focus on the skills and implications of using particular types of data collection methods.

OBSERVATION

Observational studies will have different levels of immersion and naturalistic approaches, but whether audio-recording a health consultation or observing situations as an outsider or as taking part in them, the qualitative researcher aims to have as little impact upon the situation as possible. Being 'part of the furniture' is the ultimate goal. While an audio-recorder, even if the researcher is not in the room, is quite intrusive and may make interactions a little stilted for a while, a video-recorder is even more likely to affect interactions. Documentary television programmes have secretly filmed situations in order to present a more naturalistic 'fly-on-the-wall' insight into situations, including the 2011 Winterbourne View *Panorama* documentary by the British Broadcasting Corporation filming the abuse of people with learning disabilities. However, although this led to 11 people being sentenced for criminal acts, it would be unlikely to have gained ethical permissions as a research study. This is partly because filming without consent can only be allowed if it is in a public place, does not involve minors or vulnerable people or if it is carried out by reporters and is considered to be in the public interest. Additionally, research is held to high standards of transparency and respect for the rights of participants. Consequently, often the best way to understand situations is to become immersed in a situation so that people know why you are there and learn to trust your humanity and integrity.

While you may keep a notebook on you to record certain observations while you are in the field, it is also important to record impressions and observations in more detail as soon as you leave the situation. Analysis may involve working out relationships between people, groups, processes and notable events and exploring how they relate to relevant theoretical concepts. Again, this often starts with line-by-line analysis of recorded conversations or events, building up codes, themes and the relationships between them to gain an understanding of the situation. Understanding of different types of communication and of how power and control are transacted between individuals and within groups is often involved in collecting and analysing this type of data, so a background in social psychological and sociological theory is useful. Within an ethnographic study, you may experience one or more different roles to better understand them, or because you are already an insider in the situation. It is essential to reflect on your own perspectives as part of this process – where possible, you should use your supervisors or co-researchers to discuss your responses and perceptions of situations you have observed so that you can write about your process of analysis.

ACTIVITY 15.10

Watch a short extract from a television documentary and write notes on what you observe, including the physical, psychological and social environment. Make notes on the possible meanings of the situation for the different participants, how they negotiated the situation and how the outcomes were achieved. Reflect on your insights – where they came from and what informed them. What differences would it have made if you had been in the situation at the time rather than observing a videoed situation?

INTERVIEWING

Most health and social care professionals are fairly confident in their interpersonal and communication skills, but interviewing for research requires a slightly different approach to clinical encounters (although the discipline of thinking about how power in relationships, use of language and body language all affect the way people respond in encounters can be useful in clinical practice). Appropriate seating arrangements and body space to enable the participant to feel comfortable are important, and, before even discussion of consent and timing, it is very important to make the person physically comfortable, explain about toilet facilities and emergency procedures if appropriate, and provide them with water to drink.

Although the questions posed are initially formulated by the interviewer, they need to be written and asked in such a way that the participant feels they have the opening, time and space to consider what the question means to them and how they might answer it as fully and individually as possible. While it is helpful to nod and acknowledge the participant's contributions, since that will encourage them to reflect more deeply and continue contributing, it is important not to show a preferred response or set of values as this will affect the data collected and could alter the outcomes of the research. So do avoid comments that might suggest support or otherwise of any particular comment or observation made by the participant. It is often useful, when someone has answered a question, to ask them for an example from their own experience to illustrate their response – this makes it easier to ensure that you have understood their point and provides supporting data for your analysis. Active listening, checking that you have understood a person's point and allowing plenty of time to allow considered answers all ensure that your findings are more robust because they are based on rich, full data. Remember to allow time to debrief at the end of every interview – ensure that participants have the opportunity to ask questions, to discuss any questions or concerns that they may have and for you to direct them to any support or information they may need. Anticipate any potential distress or knowledge gaps that may be caused to participants when you are planning your study so that you can incorporate appropriate support mechanisms into the process. Remember that you have a duty of care towards your participants, so if they show signs of distress, do halt the process and provide support as appropriate.

FOCUS GROUPS

Focus groups are often a useful way of generating debate and a more complex picture of a specific phenomenon from a group of people, particularly when a pre-existing group can provide deeper insights and a variety or experiences while still supporting each other. Additionally, there may be some interest in observing interactions within a naturally occurring group, such as a multidisciplinary team, to gain insight into their attitudes and approaches to each other. However, some people may find it difficult to express their opinions in a group and there may be a dominant contributor or point of view agreed by the majority that can result in some opinions not being heard. By using focus groups, you increase your number of participants and, to a certain extent, can reduce a potential power difference between you, the researcher and the participants. However, managing a focus group and paying attention to the participants (including bringing in participants who are not contributing) takes a lot of attention and sometimes it is helpful to have assistance from a co-researcher who can keep track of topics discussed on a flipchart or board. This helps to maintain the focus of the group and can help the facilitator to ensure that points are addressed fully. It is useful to take pictures of the board to illustrate the process. People can become frustrated if other people dominate the conversation, so do observe for signs of frustration and try to see that people are given the opportunity to speak. Many of the guidelines for interviews apply in focus groups (especially in recording the interaction), and for a novice researcher it is particularly important to have support to ensure that the group is managed fairly and positively. Service-user groups, self-advocacy groups and pressure groups are often very helpful in understanding a phenomenon or process from a critical perspective and can usually link the researcher to other resources or potential participants.

IMPACT, DISSEMINATION AND PUBLICATION

Having collected, analysed and reached conclusions from your data, it is now time to share it with others. Research is not a personal process; rather, it is generally designed and led by one person for the purpose of adding to the sum of knowledge and improving practice, education and/or policy. This is why it has to be so structured. You should always design and carry out research with a purpose – think about the impact of your research on practice, education and policy.

If you have some status in your field and research credentials, it is much easier to identify the best journal to which you submit your paper, but if you have never carried out research before or never been published, then you should seek advice from your supervisor or mentor or an experienced researcher in your field as to which are the best journals or conferences for sharing your findings. Where possible, publish before presenting at conference so that you can refer people to your work. Your research may not be quite suitable for research in one of the more notable, peer-reviewed academic journals, but is probably still useful for updating professionals and students in your field, so remember that practice journals are worth writing for – they will raise the profile of your work and make it easier for you to make links with other researchers and practitioners in your field. Networking at conference or through professional websites can lead to professional and research collaborations that produce stronger research grant bids and projects. You should also share your research with your work colleagues in small lectures or seminars or use it to develop teaching packs or policy guidance. If you do not write up and share your research in some way, you are not doing justice to your participants and mentors, so always build this stage into your research planning.

This chapter is a very basic introductory guide to evidence-based practice and research, but every time you carry out research you will read more and understand more from the experience. The process can appear quite onerous, but the rewards, in terms of personal satisfaction and practice development, are worth it. Follow the process as carefully as possible and document any decisions or difficulties along the way. Take it step by step, accept that sometimes you will have to retrace your steps to go forward in a slightly different direction and think carefully about the ethical aspects of your research. Refer to the key texts in your chosen methodology for specific advice and access support from your supervisor or research support network. Even if you decide not to carry out research, understanding the process and how evidence is created and disseminated gives you the tools to advance your own practice and improve quality within your own setting. That, after all, is the goal of research in health and social care.

GO FURTHER ACTIVITY

Answer the following questions:

- What do you hope to find out in your research?
- Why and how will that help to advance your field of interest?

    o   *Knowledge*
    o   *Practice*
    o   *Education*
    o   *Policy*

- Who is your audience (who will use your research) and how will they access your work?

ANSWERS TO CHAPTER 15 ACTIVITIES

The questions posed in this chapter are meant to be for reflection – answers will be dependent on the reader's own experiences and research around needs and purposes. Information to support reflection can be found in the sections they relate to.

REFERENCES

Andres, L. (2012) *Designing and Doing Survey Research*. London: Sage.

Auger, C. P. (1998). *Information Sources in Grey Literature*. London: Bowker-Saur.

Bergin, T. (2018). *An Introduction to Data Analysis: Quantitative, Qualitative and Mixed Methods*. London: Sage.

Carmack, H. J., Bates, B. R. and Harter, L. M. (2008). Narrative constructions of health care issues and policies: the case of President Clinton's apology-by-proxy for the Tuskegee syphilis experiment. *Journal of Medical Humanities* 29(2), 89–109. doi:10.1007/s10912-008-9053-5

Chapman, H. M. and Clucas, C. (2014). Student nurses' views on respect towards service users — an interpretative phenomenological study. *Nurse Education Today* 34(3), 474–479.

Chapman, H. M., Lovell, A. and Bramwell, R. (2018). Do health consultations for people with learning disabilities meet expectations? A narrative literature review. *British Journal of Learning Disabilities*, 0–18. doi:https://doi.org/10.1111/bld.12222

Creswell, J. W. (2015). *A Concise Introduction to Mixed Methods Research*. Thousand Oaks, CA: Sage.

Critical Appraisal Skills Programme (CASP) (2018).

CASP Checklists. Available at: https://casp-uk.net/casp-tools-checklists/

Cronin, P., Coughlan, M. and Smith, V. (2015). *Understanding Nursing and Healthcare Research*. London: Sage.

Data Protection Act, legislation.gov.uk (The Stationery Office 2018).

Davies, B. and Logan, J. (2018). *Reading Research: A User-Friendly Guide for Health Professionals* (6th edn). Milton, ON: Elsevier.

Evans, J. R. and Mathur, A. (2005). The value of online surveys. *Internet Research* 15(2), 195–219. doi:http://dx.doi.org/10.1108/10662240510590360

Green, J. and Thorogood, N. (2018). *Qualitative Methods for Health Research* (4th edn). London: Sage.

Hardwick, L., Smith, R. and Worsley, A. (2016). *Innovations in Social Work Research: Using Methods Creatively*. London: Jessica Kingsley.

Health Research Authority (October 2017). Is my study research? Retrieved from www.hra-decision-tools.org.uk/research/

Health Research Authority (19 March 2018). Research involving children. Retrieved from www.hra.nhs.uk/planning-and-improving-research/policies-standards-legislation/research-involving-children/

Health Research Authority (2019). Integrated Research Application System. Retrieved from www.myresearchproject.org.uk/

Health Research Authority, Health and Social Care in Northern Ireland, NHS Research Scotland & Health and Care Research Wales (2017). *UK Policy Framework for Health and Social Care Research*. London: (HRA).

Hopewell, S., McDonald, S., Clarke, M. J. and Egger, M. (2007). Grey literature in meta-analyses of randomized trials of health care interventions. *Cochrane Database of Systematic Reviews* (2). doi:10.1002/14651858.MR000010.pub3

Kogan, N. (1961). Attitudes toward old people: The development of a scale and an examination of correlates. *Journal of Abnormal and Social Psychology* 62, 44–54.

McCormack, B., van Dulmen, S., Eide, H., Skovdahl, K. and Eide, T. (ed.) (2017). *Person-Centred Healthcare Research*. Chichester: Wiley-Blackwell.

Mental Capacity Act, www.legislation.gov.uk/ukpga/2005/9/contents (The Stationery Office 2005).

National Institute for Health Research (NIHR). Our policies. Retrieved from www.nihr.ac.uk/about-us/who-we-are/our-policies/

O'Driscoll, B. R., Howard, L. S., Earis, J., Mak, V., British Thoracic Society Emergency Oxygen Guideline Group and B. T. S. Emergency Oxygen Guideline Development Group (2017). BTS guideline for oxygen use in adults in healthcare and emergency settings. *Thorax* 72(Suppl 1), ii1–ii90.

Patel, R. A., Wilson, R. F., Patel, P. A. and Palmer, R. M. (2013). The effect of smoking on bone healing: a systematic review. *Bone & Joint Research* 2(6), 102–111. doi:10.1302/2046-3758.26.2000142

Royal Marsden Hospital (2015). *The Royal Marsden Manual of Clinical Nursing Procedures* (9th edn). Available at: www.rmmonline.co.uk/

United Kingdom Government (2004). Human Tissue Act, www.legislation.gov.uk/ukpga/2004/30/contents

Waring, J., Allen, D., Braithwaite, J. and Sandall, J. (2016). Healthcare quality and safety: a review of policy, practice and research. *Sociology of Health & Illness* 38(2), 198–215. doi:10.1111/1467-9566.12391

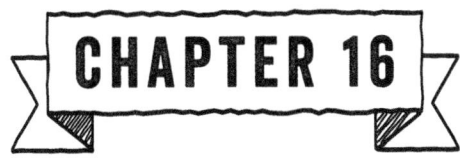

CHAPTER 16

LEADERSHIP AND MANAGEMENT

Stephanie Best

OVERVIEW

Many students interested in health and social care do not immediately recognise that leadership and management relates to them or their subject area. This chapter aims to address this gap and will open by considering what leadership and management is and their relevance in contemporary health and social care. The debate around leadership and management will be explored and, in the age of populist leaders, the need to consider theory will be discussed. The chapter will offer a guide to some of the numerous approaches to examining leadership and finally will introduce some of the skills required for leadership and management in health and social care today.

LEARNING OUTCOMES

By the end of this chapter you will be able to:

- Identify the relevance of leadership and management in health and social care
- Identify key areas of leadership and management
- Identify multiple approaches to viewing leadership
- Identify some of the skills a leader and manager needs in health and social care today

INTRODUCTION

Just about everyone uses, or has family members that use, health or social care services. In the UK these services are funded via the national governments led by varying political ideals. Regardless of political party, funding available for health and social care is finite. Understandably, service users, tax payers and governments, demand that health and social care is delivered as efficiently and effectively as possible. However, our and our loved ones' health and well-being is personal and important to us, which leads to a delicate balance between services provided (both availability and quality) and resources available.

Leadership and management plays a vital role in this balancing act, facilitating the delivery of complex health and social care within a limited budget. The fast moving political, social and economic context of health and social care requires people with an understanding of management, leadership and health and social care delivery to deliver this balance. The need to manage people, establish an appropriate culture and deliver change count amongst the many abilities required from leaders and managers in health and social care. Balancing stakeholder expectations where there are powerful voices, many with opposing interests, often under intense scrutiny (for example, from politicians and the media), can be a challenging role.

When health and social care fails the role of leaders and managers is often found to be lacking. Unfortunately, there are too many examples where this has happened. From Bristol at the turn of the century to Mid Staffs, and Winterbourne, the failings are never simplistic but always include a failure in leadership and management.

ACTIVITY 16.1

What additional pressures will be placed on health and social care in the future?

Check the end of the chapter for an answer to this activity.

CASE STUDY 16.1 MORECOMBE BAY INVESTIGATION

The investigation into Morecombe Bay Maternity Unit was as a result of a series of babies dying alongside a series of other significant failings. It took some years for the alarm to be raised. The report by Bill Kirkum in 2015 found that the maternity unit had a culture of not acknowledging failings, poor record keeping, missed opportunities for investigation and care being clinically substandard. In addition, the regulator (Nursing and Midwifery Council) was identified as failing families. The report highlights the lack of leadership both clinical and organisational: 'it was difficult to identify evidence of strong and decisive leadership' (p. 59).

Lessons learnt include: A review of clinical skills, knowledge and competencies for maternity staff, a new risk assessment process, and a programme to raise awareness of incident reporting and ensuring managers are clear on their responsibilities for quality. Wider recommendations include establishing clear standards for incident reporting and investigation in maternity service and the introduction of a duty of candour for all NHS professionals.

Look up a failure in either a health or social care setting. What were the reasons behind the breakdown in care? What can be learnt from this event?

Check the end of the chapter for an answer to this activity.

The chapter will be split into three main areas:

What is leadership and management? In this section we will look at some of the different views on leadership and management, exploring the ongoing debate and considering how theory fits in an era of the guru leader.

How can we look at leadership and management? There are many ways to explore leadership and management and, in this section we will explore some of these including theoretical perspectives.

What practical skills do leaders and managers in health and social care need to have? Leading and managing in health and social care requires many 'hands on' skills. In this section we will introduce some of these including teamworking, communication and relationship building.

WHAT IS LEADERSHIP AND WHAT IS MANAGEMENT?

There are myriad views on what comprises leadership and what management entails today. Thoughts on leadership and management have evolved over the years, though not necessarily arrived at a consensus. The term management predates leadership and was created around the time of industrialisation to bring order to the mass changes occurring at the time. Henri Fayol (1841–1925) was a French engineer who first started developing a theory of management. He laid out six primary functions of management: forecasting, planning, organising, commanding, co-ordinating and controlling. At this time there was no focus on health or social care.

Much of the leadership and management literature/debate has been developed from business and industry. With this in mind, views commonly associated with leadership and management can be seen in Table 16.1. Management is often linked with process and routine, not thinking beyond the remit of the prescribed role/job. By contrast leadership is often considered to be dynamic and exciting, driving through change and seizing opportunities. This stereotypical view

Table 16.1 Traditional views of leaders and managers (after Northouse 2016, Storey 2004, Zimmerman, 2001)

Leaders	Managers
Visionaries	A safe pair of hands
Transformational	Transactional
Empower	Control
Negotiate	Monitor results
Take a long-term view	Focus on the short term
Seek to challenge and develop new	Seek to maintain the status quo
Expert status and knowledge	Specialist knowledge not required

Table 16.2 Contemporary leadership and management characteristics for health and social care

Leaders	Managers
Clarity of vision/strategy	Reliable and consistent
Showing the way forward	Efficient and effective use of resources
Galvanising action	Skilled in ensuring fair process is followed equitably
Taking a long-term view	Focus on immediate priorities with a view to the long-term implications of actions

risks losing the essential skills inherent in effective management essential for the smooth running of health and social care services. Table 16.2 offers an evolved view with characteristics for contemporary leaders and managers.

While much of the management role will fall to those sitting in a 'management' post, the expectation for leadership today is far broader. Mindful of the failings outlined in the case study earlier, the need for leadership in health and social care is no longer the preserve of traditional senior positions such as chief executive officers. To deliver care in the contemporary health and social care setting, and balance demands and resources requires leadership at all levels of the health and social care system.

Leadership:	Is an activity and not dependent on role or seniority
Management:	Is an activity dependent on role and includes seniority

The reality in health and social care today is that the same people often perform the two roles. Increasingly there is a need for leadership in management roles, for example, with change management.

> If an organisation is overmanaged and underled, it eventually loses any spirit or purpose. A poorly managed organisation with a strong charismatic leader may soar briefly – only to crash shortly thereafter … The challenges of today's organisations require the objective perspective of managers as well as the brilliant flash of creativity that wise leadership provides. (Bolman and Deal, 2013, p. viii)

Management and leadership can be considered as distinct but complementary activities and roles with a large degree of overlap. It is the degree of overlap that is at the heart of debate.

The rise of leadership in health and social care emerged with the seminal texts *To Err Is Human: Building a Safer Health System* (IoM, 1999) and *Crossing the Quality Chasm* (IoM, 2001). Published in the USA, the learnings spread to the UK and beyond. Here they identify ten steps for safe and effective service care delivery, focusing on the collaboration of those commissioning services, health and social care organisations that provide care, health and social care professionals and service users. The need for leadership is highlighted at all levels.

Over the years the call for leadership has grown so much that there is a shift in NHS policy away from management to the more exciting leadership (Ford and Harding, 2007). While this may be appropriate there is a need to ensure we don't throw the baby (i.e. management) out with the bathwater. There will only be so much that leadership can achieve and the need for sound underlying practices remain.

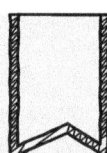

PAUSE FOR THOUGHT 16.1

Think about who can be a leader in health and social care?

Check the end of the chapter for an answer to this activity.

THE ROLE OF THEORY

So far we have discussed the very practical nature of leadership and management which can bring to mind the question of 'why bother with theory?' As the place of leadership rises within and beyond health and social care we come across the 'guru' leader. These exciting people have often transformed a failing sector and have interesting experiences to share. The challenge is that without a theoretical basis it makes it difficult to transfer learnings from one context to another. Leadership and management, especially in health and social care, is particularly context specific. A theory is a model or framework that allows us to make sense of what we see and how we see things. It allows us to understand 'truth' or 'reality' and can offer guidance on how to behave.

Theories;

i) Help us answer questions and understand what is going on; e.g. theory of gravity
ii) Provide guidance on how to behave; e.g. theory of conformity

Without a theory behind an experience, applying learning to a new setting is challenging. In the next section we will consider some of the leadership theories available to guide or explain our actions in the health and social care context.

MULTIPLE LENSES TO VIEW LEADERSHIP

Confusion can often arise when trying to explore leadership in the health or social care setting. There are multiple potential viewpoints, and in this section we will consider different perspectives, from the organisation to the individual, classical leadership theories and alternative views.

PERSPECTIVES

ORGANISATIONAL

Leadership is provided (or not) by organisations. We talk about how well an organisation is led and the implications of this (see Case Study 16.1). Leadership from an organisational level will set the culture employees experience and so set the expectations around ways of working. Organisational culture is often expressed as 'the way things work around here' and is developed through shared experiences. Culture arises from three factors: i) the beliefs, values and assumptions within an organisation; ii) the experiences of people within the organisation; and iii) beliefs, values and assumptions brought in by new members (Schein and Schein, 2017). It is the leaders who set the tone by establishing their beliefs, values and assumptions, and a positive correlation has been shown between organisational culture, the behaviour of leaders and job satisfaction (Tsai, 2011). This correlation indicates the significance of organisational leadership for the individual's experience.

TEAM

While the culture of an organisation is set from the top we are all influenced by the team we work in. Teams are interdependent groups of people and exist throughout organisations; for example a senior management team, a community resource team or drug rehabilitation team. Effective leadership of the team will lead to successful outcomes and ineffective leadership will result in failure. Key leadership influences on team processes include; clarifying objectives (providing the vision), encouraging participation, enhancing commitment to quality and supporting innovation (West et al., 2003).

INDIVIDUAL

Our own perspectives will also impact on leadership. *What do you think is the right thing to do?* This area is sometimes referred to as personal or self-leadership. Everyone develops their own leadership and management style over time. It helps us (and others) know how we deal with change, manage a crisis, motivate ourselves and others. Vision is commonly associated with leadership and applies at the individual level (as well as at the team and organisational level). Table 16.3 provides some areas associated with personal leadership.

Table 16.3   Areas associated with personal leadership

Area	Ask yourself
Values	What is important to you?
Curiosity	What interests you?
Motivation	What drives you?
Integrity	What do you want your track record to be?
Kindness	Is how you treat others important to you?
Personal resilience	What is your support network like?

PAUSE FOR THOUGHT 16.2

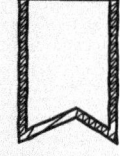

Reflecting on the areas in Table 16.3, what do you want to achieve over one year, five years and ten years?

CLASSICAL LEADERSHIP THEORY

The leadership literature refers to a range of classical leadership theories, so it is helpful to have an understanding of some of the main theories.

PAUSE FOR THOUGHT 16.3

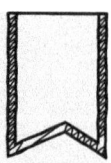

As you read through each theory try to think of one positive and one negative of using each of these leadership approaches in health and social care today.

TRAIT THEORY

Early leadership theory originated around the concept of the 'Great Man'. Thomas Carlyle (1795–1881) proposed that some people were born to be leaders and held innate characteristics such as charisma, intelligence, masculinity and confidence. These ideas largely reflected the characteristics of white, male leaders of the time. In fact, in his paper 'The Hero as King', Carlyle suggested people respect 'able and noble' leaders as they will know what will be in their best interests (in Stippler et al., 2011).

BEHAVIOURAL THEORIES

Attention shifted from the personal characteristics of leaders around the 1950s to consider leaders' behaviour. Several theories sit within this umbrella, including Blake and Mouton's managerial grid. This leadership approach concentrated on leaders 'concern for people' and 'concern for production'.

CONTINGENCY OR SITUATIONAL THEORIES

As leadership theory progressed around the 1960s we started to see some acknowledgement of followers. Up till now all the attention had been on the leader rather than the context they found themselves in. Hersey and Blanchard (1969) developed a Situational Leadership Curve that identifies that leadership style is dependent on the readiness of the followers (in particular their willingness and their ability). See Figure 16.1 for a visual representation of Hersey and Blanchard's Situational Leadership Curve.

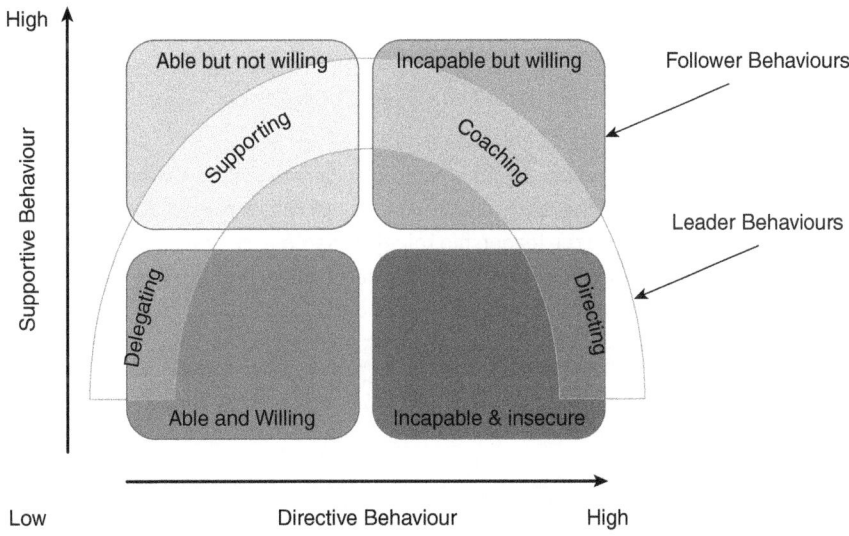

Figure 16.1 Situational leadership curve (after Hersey and Blanchard, 1969)

TRANSFORMATIONAL AND TRANSACTIONAL THEORY

Moving into the 1970s and beyond, transactional and transformational leadership emerged (Bass, 1985 built on Burns, 1978). Transactional leadership views leadership as an exchange between leader and worker with a reward for the work done. It is associated with an emphasis on following rules and regulations so staying with the status quo. In contrast transformational leadership looks to engage the worker and is associated with a more entrepreneurial approach with charismatic leaders who stimulate workers and work for the benefit of the organisation rather than themselves.

This brief timeline of leadership theory demonstrates how approaches to leadership have evolved over time. Each of the theories has pros and cons to their use (some harder to identify than others).

ALTERNATIVE LEADERSHIP THEORIES

Many of the classical leadership theories place the leader at the centre of activity with little consideration of the team working with them. More recently, leadership theories have been emerging that offer a 'post-heroic' view of leadership (King's Fund, 2011), in particular working with the health and social care sector (Hartley and Bennington, 2010). Many of the recent failings in health and social care have been attributed to the nature and role of leadership (Francis, 2010, 2013; Learmonth, 2015). With this there has been a call for a new style of leadership that engages directly with frontline practitioners. Here we consider two relatively new styles.

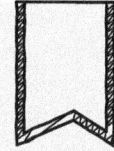

PAUSE FOR THOUGHT 16.4

What do you think post-heroic leadership would look like?

Check the end of the chapter for an answer to this activity.

DISTRIBUTED LEADERSHIP

The theory of distributed leadership argues that no one person can be the best leader in all circumstances. The focal point of the leadership role does not follow the traditional organisational hierarchy, so anyone can take up the leadership role (for example, chairing meetings, leading case conferences). Here, there is a difference made between leaders and leadership (Bolden, 2007). Other terms found in the literature for distributed leadership include collective, shared and collaborative. West et al. (2014) provide a useful discussion on collective leadership and the Health Foundation (2011) offer some applied examples of shared leadership to influence care for people from black and minority ethnic groups.

AUTHENTIC LEADERSHIP

The ethos of authentic leadership is to encourage transparency and integrity to develop values and beliefs that align with the organisation. Avolio et al. (2004) in early work on authentic leadership offer a definition as 'a process that draws from both positive psychological capacities and a highly developed organizational context, which results in both greater self-awareness and self-regulated positive behaviours on the part of leaders and associates, fostering positive self-development'. Some of the key attributes are given as clarity, integrity, courage, service, trust, humility, compassion and vulnerability (Irvine and Reger, 2006). These can be challenging characteristics to demonstrate when immersed in the busy day-to-day work of leading and managing in health and social care teams, departments and organisations.

ALTERNATIVE PERSPECTIVES

There are other ways of viewing leadership. For example, Northouse (2016, p. 6) defines leadership as 'a process whereby an individual influences a group of individuals to achieve a common goal' with these four components: Leadership is a process; leadership involves influence; leadership occurs in groups, and; leadership involves common goal (see Table 16.4).

Table 16.4   Leadership components from Northouse (2016)

Leadership...	
...is a process	Therefore leadership cannot be dependent on a trait or individual behaviour. Rather it is an interaction between leaders and followers
...involves influence	Leadership requires influence – if there is no influence there will be no followers
...occurs in groups	Influencing followers happens with groups of people from just a few people to entire organisations (leading yourself is not considered within this approach).
...involves common goals	Having common goals highlights the need for leaders and followers to be working together and starts to introduce the idea of leadership that is ethical.

So, when we are thinking or discussing leadership we need to be clear what we mean and how we are talking about it. Whose viewpoint are we talking about and how is it impacting on our work?

PRACTICAL CONSIDERATIONS

CHANGE

'Change is the only constant in life' (Heraclitus, Greek philosopher, 535–c. 475 BC)

Health and social care is always changing. Some of the reasons for this will have been identified in Pause for Thought 16.1. Managing change is an essential role of any manager or leader in health and social care. As fiscal constraints grow the demand for more innovation in practice is called for. This requires: i) an element of creativity to identify new ideas (see Horizon NHS and the Centre for Creative leadership white papers); and also ii) a means to make decisions. Two well-known and well-used tools are the SWOT analysis and Lewin's driving forces model.

SWOT

A SWOT (strengths, weaknesses, opportunities and threats) analysis can be used at the individual, team or organisational level. They can be completed by one person or by a group. The idea is to identify the various internal and external positives and challenges to embarking on a course of action.

You can undertake a SWOT analysis about yourself but this example considers whether to try a new treatment approach. Strengths may include: the cost, enhance the reputation of the team, preferred model by staff. Weaknesses may include: lack of in-house availability of appropriately skilled practitioners, requires specific facilities. Opportunities may include lack of any competition or use of new technology. Finally, threats may involve non-alignment with local/government policy or demographic changes in the population. Each of these strengths and weaknesses are put into the SWOT chart for easy analysis (and communication) of the key assets or areas of concern (Figure 16.2).

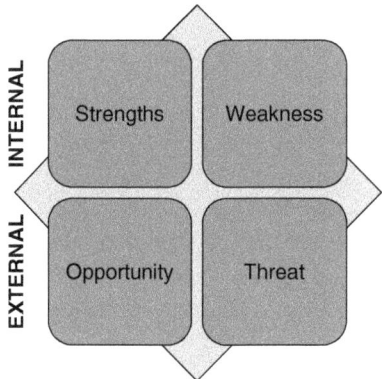

Figure 16.2   SWOT analysis chart

LEWIN'S FIELD ANALYSIS

Lewin's approach provides a framework for assessing different factors that may sway a decision (Figure 16.3). First all the different reasons for and against undertaking a change are identified. Then there is the opportunity to score them (out of 10) – you decide how important each factor is. This helps recognise that some factors may be more emotionally laden than other areas. The example in Figure 16.3 considers changes to the provision of childcare services.

Score	Forces for change	Aim	Forces against change	Score
9	Cost		Families won't like it	7
5	Easier to manage	REDUCE THE NUMBER OF STAFF PER CHILD	Staff won't like it	5
7	Government policy change		Fewer people at the Christmas party	2
21	Total		Total	14

Figure 16.3   Lewin's field analysis applied example

The way this analysis has been completed suggests the forces for change are stronger than the forces against change and so may help with decision-making. However, it is important to recognise that both tools will only be as useful as the information that is put into them. You will need to consider the views of your stakeholders.

STAKEHOLDER ENGAGEMENT

When considering decisions about change there is value in identifying who the stakeholders may be. Stakeholders are anyone who have an interest in the activity. Not every stakeholder can be or will want to be involved with every decision.

Power and interest: Different stakeholders will have different impacts on the proposed change. Some people will hold great power while others may have influence. Either can be for or against your idea. You can plot people's power and interest in your proposed change on a grid (Figure 16.4).

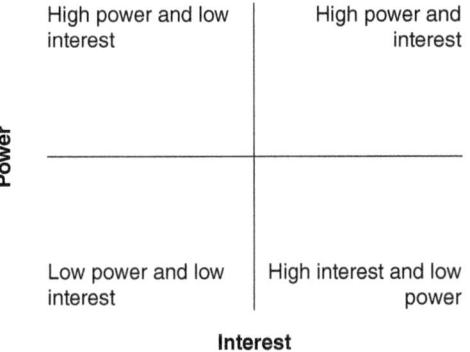

Figure 16.4 Stakeholders' power and interest grid

ACTIVITY 16.2

- Think of a change you are aware of that would be a good idea (it can be from your day-to-day life or set in health and social care). Think of the stakeholders who may be involved and place them on the power/interest chart.
- Who would you make sure you engaged first and why?
- Who would be more challenging but just as important to engage?

Check the end of the chapter for an answer to this activity.

One vital point to note is that change is not a linear process. We have to recognise that we live in an era where 'intervention A does not predictably lead to outcome B. ... Things get in the way. Something we could not have predicted pops up—and gives an initiative a boost' (Braithwaite et al., 2017). This means working in health and social care will demand an element of resilience – personal and organisational.

TEAMWORK

Successful leadership and management in health and social care requires effective teamwork. Many barriers can be put in the way of ensuring a team achieves its goal. These include different professional groups having different agendas, team members having different terms and conditions of employment, difficulties with communication, lack of awareness of other team members' roles and responsibilities, or lack of support and help to develop teamworking (West et al., 2012). Carter et al. (2009) identified eight essential components for teamworking:

1. Clear team leadership and identity – inspiring vision
2. Clear objectives – shared vision
3. Involvement in decision-making and constructive debate – commitment to delivering excellent care
4. Effective communication and team members working interdependently
5. Accurate and timely feedback on performance
6. Managing conflict
7. Positive attitudes to diversity and positive, supportive relationships
8. Inter-team co-operation and effectiveness and organisational loyalty

These eight success factors highlight a range of skills including leadership requiring relationship building, communication and feedback. We will now focus on these three skills.

RELATIONSHIP BUILDING

Building relationships is a key component of leadership in health and social care. Good relationships depend on several factors including communication and mutual trust and respect. Open and honest dialogue helps develop trust and demonstrate respect. Emotional intelligence plays a role in relationship building. Emotional intelligence is 'the ability to monitor one's own and others' feelings and emotions, to discriminate among them and to use this information to guide one's thinking and actions' (Salovey and Mayer, 1990, p. 189). Having emotional intelligence enables effective communication, empathising with others and so helps overcome day-to-day work-based challenges. There are four principal components of emotional intelligence: self awareness, self-management, social awareness and relationship management. Figure 16.5 shows the four areas of emotional intelligence and what lies behind them.

Each of these components are interdependent and will develop confidence in leadership skills (Goleman, 2013).

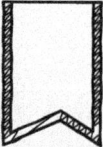

PAUSE FOR THOUGHT 16.5

How could you develop your self-awareness?

Check the end of the chapter for an answer to this activity.

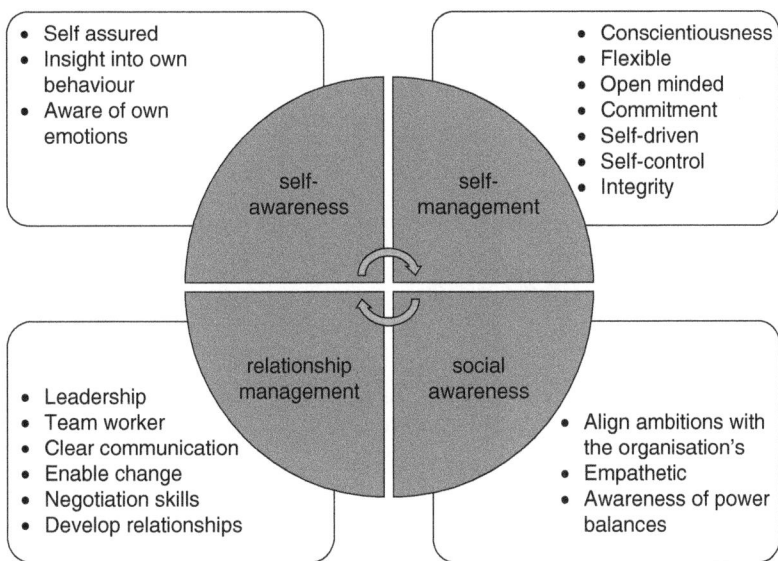

Figure 16.5 Four components of emotional intelligence

COMMUNICATION

An important component of teamworking in health and social care is building shared under-standing of the work, and appropriate processes for delivering high-quality service provision. This takes time. A good example of actively working on communication to improve service-user outcomes is the World Health Organization pre-operative checklist. Amongst important questions such as patient's name and procedure is: 'Have all the team members introduced themselves by name and role?' (NHS Institute for Innovation and Improvement, 2009). This is important to ensure staff can feel confident in speaking up during an operation potentially avoiding accidents.

Communication can be verbal (e.g. face to face with peers or service users), written (e.g. emails), visual (e.g. presentations) or non-verbal (e.g. body language). These skills can be interde-pendent and here we focus principally on verbal skills.

- **Interpersonal skills**: Interpersonal skills are required when we communicate face to face, either one to one or with groups. These skills can be impacted on by how confident we feel (or how confident we can portray ourselves to be). The purpose of the communication may set the climate (for example negotiating an agreement) and can influence the emotional setting and expectation of participants.
- **Talking**: What you say matters. The content of your message will need to vary dependent on the context you find yourself in from the speech at the leaving do of a long-standing employee to a disciplinary meeting. In any situation the clarity of what you want to convey needs to be unambiguous. In some scenarios it is appropriate to ask the other person what they understand from what you have said. Finally, the tone of your voice has an impact on how your message is taken. There can be great benefit in getting feed-back from others about tone as we don't always hear how we sound to others (see 'Feedback' below).

- **Listening**: Taking the time to actively listen to what is being said is a skill. You need to pay attention to what is said, ask questions and clarify what you think is meant. Asking open-ended questions (How do you …?, What if …? Why does …?) that encourage the other person to share and lets them know you understand what they are saying.

PAUSE FOR THOUGHT 16.6

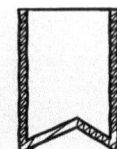

Think of two occasions: one where you communicated effectively and one where it didn't go so well. Reflecting on the communication section, can you identify why things went well or not?

FEEDBACK

- **Feedback:** is a subset of communication and a vital part of developing knowledge. Good leaders need to be able to give good critical feedback and receive feedback. Done well, feedback can help motivate and progress skills, knowledge and behaviour so maximising people's potential.
- **Self-feedback**: Drucker (2005) suggested that whenever you make a key decision make a note of what you expect the outcome to be. A year or so later compare the results with your expectations. If you do this consistently over several years it will help you determine where some of your key strengths are.
- **Giving feedback**: Providing critical feedback can be hard to do but without it we don't know how we have performed. We need to balance what has been done well while identifying areas for improvement. Table 16.5 provides some areas to consider when providing critical feedback.

Table 16.5 Giving critical feedback

Checklist	Areas to consider
Be clear about why you are providing feedback	Exactly what is the point(s) you want to share? Prioritise two or three points
Ensure you are ready to provide feedback	Do you have all the details (and evidence if appropriate), and do you have the time to feedback properly?
Ensure the setting is appropriate for the person	Relaxed environment, away from others may be appropriate
Ensure the person has time to give their viewpoint	Do they need time to prepare their thoughts?
Identify potential outcomes	What are you expecting as a result of giving this feedback?

- **Receiving feedback**: Equally, we are not always good at taking feedback (good or bad). This is something that can be developed over time. It is worth practising some phrases and behaviours to use whenever you are given feedback. See Box 16.1.

BOX 16.1   GIVING CRITICAL FEEDBACK

Positive – try these statements:

- 'It's great to hear – thanks'
- 'It's an area I have been trying to focus on improving – thanks'
- 'I picked this up at my last review'

Negative – think about these actions:

- Let the person commenting finish before you respond.
- Try to listen with an open mind and reflect on whether you think it is a valid comment (you may only be able to do this later on). Try to be as honest as you can.
- If you are not sure what the other person means then ask for specific feedback. They should be able to give you examples to reflect on.

PAUSE FOR THOUGHT 16.7

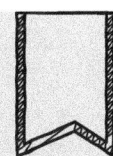

Are there times you have been given feedback and not handled it as well as you might have liked? Can you think of how you might respond when you are given feedback in the future?

CONCLUSION

In this chapter we have introduced some of the key features in theory and practice of leadership and management in health and social care. As well as exploring some leadership theory we have introduced some theoretical concepts from organisation and management such as organisational culture and emotional intelligence. Having a sound understanding of some of the basics of leadership and management will help you further explore areas that are of interest to you. You may not wish to be a manager but working in health and social care you will be managed. Gaining an understanding of leadership and management will enable you to get the most from this relationship.

GO FURTHER ACTIVITY

Having read this chapter what areas do you want to find out more about?

How will you go about doing this?

Is there anyone who can help you?

What is your timeframe?

ANSWERS TO CHAPTER 16 ACTIVITIES

—— Case Study 16.1: Answers

Examples of failures in health and social care you may wish to look at include;

- Mid Staffordshire NHS Trust
- Winterbourne

Sadly, there are numerous other examples and if you search for examples of failures in health and social care you will find many others.

—— Pause for Thought 16.1: Answers

Examples include those in formal roles but also others who may not typically be thought of as leaders:

- Chief executives
- Managers
- Clinicians
- Technicians
- Union representatives
- Patients/clients
- Advocacy groups

—— Pause for Thought 16.4: Answers

No one person in charge, no single expert, emphasis on all team members contributing, encouraging flexible approaches to challenges in the workplace.

——— **Activity 16.1: Answers**

You may think about:

- Changing demographics
- User expectation
- Technological advances
- Rising costs
- Media
- Politics

——— **Activity 16.2: Answers**

1   Think of the stakeholders who may be involved and place them on the power/interest chart.
2   High power and interest
3   High power and low interest

——— **Pause for Thought 16.5: Answers**

How could you develop your self-awareness?

Activities may include:

- Creating time to think – slow down
- Keep a journal
- Seek out feedback
- Reflection

FURTHER READING

Northouse, P. (2016). *Leadership: Theory and Practice* (7th edn). Los Angeles: SAGE Publications.
Swanwick, T. and McKimm, J. (2011). *ABC of Clinical Leadership* (ABC Series.) Chichester: Wiley Blackwell.
Walshe, K. and Smith, J. (2011). *Healthcare Management*. Maidenhead: Open University Press.

USEFUL WEBSITES

Kings Fund: www.kingsfund.org.uk

Institute of Health Care Managers: www.ihm.org.uk

Health Foundation: www.health.org.uk

Nuffield Trust: www.nuffieldtrust.org.uk

Bevan Foundation: www.bevanfoundation.org

Bevan Commission: www.bevancommission.org/en

Social Care Institute for Excellence: www.scie.org.uk

REFERENCES

Avolio, B. J., Gardner, W. L., Walumbwa, F. O., Luthans, F. and May, D. R. (2004). Unlocking the mask: a look at the process by which authentic leaders impact follower attitudes and behaviors. *The Leadership Quarterly* 15(6), 801–823.

Bass, B. M. (1985). Leadership: good, better, best. *Organizational Dynamics* 13(3), 26–40.

Bolden, R. (2007). Distributed leadership. Exeter: University of Exeter Centre for Leadership Studies. Available at: http://business-school.exeter.ac.uk/documents/discussion_papers/management/2007/0702.pdf

Bolman, L. and Deal, T. E. (2013). *Reframing Organizations: Artistry, Choice, and Leadership* (5th edn). Chichester: Wiley.

Braithwaite, J., Churruca, K., Ellis, L. A., Long, J., Clay-Williams, R., Damen, N., . . . Ludlow, K. (2017). *Complexity Science in Healthcare: Aspirations, Approaches, Applications and Accomplishments*. A White Paper. Available at http://aihi.mq.edu.au/resource/complexity-science-healthcare-white-paper

Burns, J. M. (1978). *Leadership*. New York: Harper & Row.

Carter, M., West, M., Dawson, J., Richardson, J. and Dunckley, M. (2009) Developing team based working in NHS Trusts, Summary Report. Aston University: Birmingham. Available at: https://research.aston.ac.uk/portal/files/4859699/Summary_report.pdf

Drucker, P. F. (2005). Managing oneself. *Harvard Business Review* (January): 100–109.

Ford, J. and Harding, N. (2007). Move over management – we are all leaders now. *Management Learning* 38, 475–493. doi: 10.1177/1350507607083203

Francis, R. (2010) *Independent Inquiry into Care Provided by Mid Staffordshire NHS Foundation Trust January 2005 – March 2009*. London: Stationery Office.

Francis, R. (2013) *Report of the Mid Staffordshire NHS Foundation Trust Public Inquiry*. London: Stationery Office.

Goleman, D. (2013) The focused leader. *Harvard Business Review*. Available at: https://hbr.org/2013/12/the-focused-leader

Hartley, J. and Bennington, J. (2010). Recent trends in leadership thinking and action in the public and voluntary service sectors. Available at: www.kingsfund.org.uk/sites/default/files/Recent-trends-in-leadership-Thinking-action-in-the-public-voluntary-service-sectors-Jean-Hartley-John-Benington-Kings-Fund-May-2011.pdf

Health Foundation (2011) Shared Leadership for Change. Available at: www.health.org.uk/sites/health/files/SharedLeadershipForChange.pdf

Hersey, P. and Blanchard, K. H. (1969). Life cycle theory of leadership. *Training & Development Journal* 23(5), 26–34.

IoM (Institute of Medicine) (1999). *To Err is Human: Building a Safer Health System*. National Academy Press: Washington.

IoM (Institute of Medicine) (2001), Committee on Quality of Health Care in America and Institute of Medicine Staff, 2001. *Crossing the Quality Chasm: A New Health System for the 21st Century*. National Academies Press.

Irvine, D. and Reger, J. (2006). *The Authentic Leader: It's about PRESENCE, Not Position*. Washington, DC: DC Press.

King's Fund (2011). The future of leadership and management in the NHS. No more heroes. Report from The King's Fund Commission on Leadership and Management in the NHS. Available at: www.

kingsfund.org.uk/sites/default/files/future-of-leadership-and-management-nhs-may-2011-kings-fund.pdf

Learmonth, M. (2015). Who doesn't want to be a leader? Leaders are such wonderful people; Comment on 'Leadership and Leadership Development in Healthcare Settings – A Simplistic Solution to Complex Problems?' *International Journal of Health Policy Management* 8(4), 45–47.

Morecombe Bay Investigation (2015). www.gov.uk/government/publications ISBN 9780108561306 ID 26021502 03/15 47487 19585

NHS Institute for Innovation and Improvement. (2009). Saving lives in surgery. Available at: http://testing.chfg.org/resources/09_qrt02/NHSIII_Checklist_for_Chief_Execs.pdf

Northouse, P. G. (2016). *Leadership. Theory and Practice* (7th edn). London: Sage.

Salovey, P. and Mayer, J. D. (1990). Emotional intelligence. *Imagination, Cognition, and Personality* 9, 185–211.

Schein, E. and Schein, P. (2017). *Organizational Culture and Leadership* (5th edn). Hoboken, NJ: Wiley.

Stippler, M., Moore, S., Rosenthal, S. and Doerffer, T. (2011). *Leadership. Approaches – Development – Trends.* Gütersloh, Germany: Verlag Bertelsmann Stiftung.

Storey, J. (2004). Changing theories of leadership and leadership development. In J. Storey (ed.), *Leadership in Organizations: Current Issues and Key Trends* (pp. 11–37). London: Routledge.

Tsai, Y. (2011). Relationship between organizational culture, leadership behavior and job satisfaction. *BMC Health Services Research* 11, 98. doi: 10.1186/1472-6963-11-98

West, M., Borrill, C. S., Dawson, J. F., Brodbeck, F., Shapiro, D. and Haward, B. (2003). Leadership clarity and team innovation in health care. *The Leadership Quarterly* 14(4–5), 393–410.

West, M., Alimo-Metcalfe, B., Dawson, J., El Ansari, W., Glasby, J., Hardy, G. et al. (2012). Effectiveness of Multi-Professional Team Working (MPTW) in Mental Health Care. Final report. NIHR Service Delivery and Organisation programme. www.netscc.ac.uk/hsdr/files/project/SDO_FR_08-1819-215_V01.pdf

West, M. Eckert, R. Steward, K. and Pasmore, B. (2014) Developing collective leadership for health care. Available at: www.kingsfund.org.uk/sites/files/kf/field/field_publication_file/developing-collective-leadership-kingsfund-may14.pdf

Zimmerman, E. L. (2001). What is under the hood? The mechanics of leadership versus management. *Healthcare Executive* 16(6), 26.

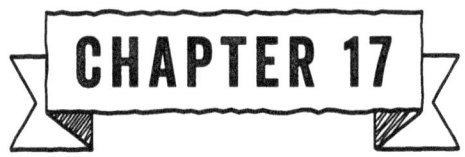

CHAPTER 17

LEGAL AND ETHICAL CONSIDERATIONS IN HEALTH AND SOCIAL CARE

Hugh Upton and Angela Smith

OVERVIEW

This chapter will focus on providing discussion of some key legal and ethical issues that occur in the area of health and social care in modern society. The chapter will focus on issues that are contentious and particularly open to debate, which are often those where recent cases have been brought to court. It will aim to show how ideas in law and ethics have to be combined in order to produce regulation. However, not only does work on legal and ethical principles frequently overlap in this area, but the outcome often remains controversial. Clearly, the viewpoints of both the judiciary and society on the best way to help those in various kinds of need are not static but continue to develop and to resist any final resolution. Topics for discussion include beginning of life issues such as abortion, in vitro fertilisation (IVF), surrogacy and end of life issues such as dementia care, truth telling, mental capacity, euthanasia and assisted suicide.

LEARNING OUTCOMES

By the end of this chapter, you will be able to:

- Discuss some of the theoretical approaches to ethical issues in health and social care
- Identify some of the key legal and ethical issues at the beginning of life
- Identify some of the key legal and ethical issues relating to the end of life
- Identify some of the key legal and ethical problems in providing care for those lacking full capacity

INTRODUCTION

In the past hundred years, the health and social care system in England and Wales has seen massive medical advances. Often this has led to ethical debate over whether the fact that a practice or procedure can be done means that it should be done. Absenting legislation in many areas of health care law, decisions in controversial cases have been left to the judiciary, who effectively have been making life and death decisions in respect of patients. This has led to legal precedents being set which then have to be followed in later cases until that particular principle is overturned by a higher court or can be distinguished on a point of law (in that the legal principle is not the same and therefore the precedent need not be followed) or until Parliament creates legislation on the matter.

It has become evident that the judiciary, whether interpreting legislation or having to apply legal principles to cases where there is no legislation to rely upon, have faced difficulties in making equitable decisions that are satisfactory to society. One can only commend the judgments for the detailed discussion they provide and illustrating the struggle involved in reaching the decision.

In the controversial field of health and social care, there is a need not just for legal regulation but for a systematic and defensible way of involving our moral values as well. These values may play a part in many contexts, including justifying changes in medical law, drawing up and interpreting professional codes of ethics, or defending a personal conviction (perhaps to the point of conscientious objection) that is contrary to current practice. Thus, the various ethical principles and theories need consideration when looking at any aspect of care and /or treatment for individuals, as well as at wider issues of policy and regulation.

ETHICAL THEORIES AND PRINCIPLES

We mention just some of the best-known approaches to ethical decision-making below.

UTILITARIANISM

Simply put, this is an ethical theory that focuses on the consequences of our actions with respect to achieving what we regard as the ultimate good (see Driver, 2006). The best-known suggestion for this good is happiness, as proposed by John Stuart Mill (1806–1873). With this proposal adopted, utilitarianism states that the morally right course of action is that which will maximise the overall total of happiness. Thus, it might turn out that if there is £50,000 available, it should be spent on improving the health of 50 patients in some way, as opposed to maintaining the life of one terminally ill patient, on the grounds that the first policy produces a greater overall total of benefit than the second.

DEONTOLOGY

While utilitarianism relates to the effects of our actions, deontology draws upon a different aspect of our ordinary moral beliefs: the idea that doing the right or wrong action is not always a matter of achieving a beneficial outcome (see Davis, 1993). In particular it supports avoiding actions that are disrespectful or unfair to people even if we think the overall effects would be good. The prominent duties are typically negative (do not lie, do not kill) though others may be positive (help those in need) and any of them may be regarded as very strong, perhaps even absolute requirements. In deontological ethics the writings of Immanuel Kant (1724–1804) have been very influential.

VIRTUE ETHICS

Whilst the above two theories focus on consequences and actions respectively, virtue ethics looks rather at the characters of those who are acting, at their dispositions to behave in certain ways and how these dispositions might fit into our conception of a good way of life for a human being (see Driver, 2006). It looks, for example, at what would count as being charitable, or courageous, or just, in the relevant circumstances.

THE FOUR PRINCIPLES

The Four Principles approach to medical ethics was originally devised by Tom Beauchamp and James Childress in their 1977 textbook *Principles of Biomedical Ethics*, now in its seventh edition (2013). The principles can be given in summary as follows:

Respect for autonomy: the requirement that the decision to consent to or to refuse treatment should be that of the patient alone, albeit subject to certain exceptions when dealing with children (aged under 18), those without capacity and those detained under the Mental Health Act 1983. Patients with capacity should be given the facts regarding treatment without any pressure or duress being exerted and then make an autonomous decision whether to consent or refuse. This must be respected, even if refusal would ultimately lead to the patient's death. This principle is also enshrined in law (*Montgomery v. Lanarkshire Health Board* [2015] UKSC 11).

Beneficence: the health care professional should undertake actions that are for the benefit of the patient. Although seemingly obvious, what actually constitutes a benefit to a particular patient at a particular time may be hard to judge; perhaps even for the patients themselves.

Non-maleficence: the requirement to do no harm. Again, whilst this principle may appear obvious in that (a few deplorable cases aside) all health care professionals seek to avoid causing harm, the fact is that some treatments may have harmful consequences or side effects. Thus, whether an intervention leaves the patient better or worse off overall (benefited or harmed) may be uncertain.

Justice: all patients should be given what is due to them, treated fairly and without discrimination. Whilst this may apply straightforwardly in an ideal world, in the real world there are limited resources available to the NHS and difficult decisions to be made.

LEGAL AND ETHICAL ISSUES AT THE BEGINNING OF LIFE

ABORTION

Whilst the legal principles in respect of termination of pregnancy have remained in place more or less untouched since 1967 (Abortion Act 1967 (AA 1967) as amended by the Human Fertilisation and Embryology Act 1990 (HFEA 1991)), such challenging issues as women's rights and the status of the embryo mean that the ethical debate continues, and hence so does the issue of possible changes to the law.

England, Wales and Scotland have one of the most liberal abortion laws in the world. The AA 1967 allows termination of pregnancy up to 24 weeks provided it is performed by a registered medical practitioner, having been agreed by two medical practitioners, in good faith, that to continue the pregnancy 'would involve risk, greater than if the pregnancy were terminated, of injury to the physical or mental health of the pregnant woman or any existing children of her family' (s1(1) AA 1967). In England, Scotland and Wales there were some 202,469 terminations carried out in 2016. Of this number, 192,635 (95 per cent) were carried out under this section of the Act (Department of Health, 2017; National Services Scotland, 2017). It is perhaps this area that is ethically most contentious, since this ground for terminations comprises what are considered 'socio-economic' reasons, such as being unable to afford to bring up a child or becoming pregnant at an inconvenient time.

In Northern Ireland the law is much more restrictive. The Abortion Act 1967 does not apply to Northern Ireland which means that they are still governed by the Offences Against the Person Act 1861 (OAPA 1861) although since 1945, the Infant Life (Preservation) Act 1929 (ILPA 1929) has been extended to Northern Ireland which means that terminations may be carried out if to preserve the life of the mother or to prevent permanent and serious damage to her physical or mental health (s1(1) ILPA 1929). Thus, reasons of foetal abnormities (terminations may be carried out at any stage of the pregnancy on this ground under the AA 1967), rape or incest would not be sanctioned. In 2017 only 13 terminations were carried out in Northern Ireland (Department of Health, 2018). As a consequence of this, women regularly travel to mainland UK for terminations, such that 721 terminations were carried out in England and Wales in 2016 to women from Northern Ireland (Department of Health, 2017).

ACTIVITY 17.1

Debate the issue of abortion for socio-economic reasons – should termination of pregnancy be allowed? Try to weigh up both sides of the argument, considering both the mother and the foetus. Should an unborn child be given the right to life or should the mother's rights and wishes be the priority?

Check the end of the chapter for an answer to this activity.

ACTIVITY 17.2

Look at the cases of Gillick v. West Norfolk and Wisbeck Area Health Authority [1986] AC 112 and Axon R (on the application of) v. Secretary of State for Health and Anor [2006] EWHC 37 and consider whether you think that children should be able to make a decision on the issue of abortion without parental knowledge and agreement. Try to look at the arguments from both sides.

Check the end of the chapter for an answer to this activity.

IN VITRO FERTILISATION (IVF)

In 1978, the world's first 'test-tube' baby, Louise Brown, was born. At this time, there was no legislation in place governing this practice. In 1982, the Warnock Committee was set up with a remit to look at assisted reproduction (please note that the actual Terms of Reference of the Committee were to consider recent and potential developments in medicine and science related to human fertilisation and embryology; to consider what policies and safeguards should be applied, including consideration of the social, ethical and legal implications of these developments; and to make recommendations). The Committee reported its findings in 1984. Consequently, the Human Fertilisation and Embryology Act 1990 was created and the Human Fertilisation and Embryology Authority (HFEA Authority) was set up to regulate treatment and research in respect of human embryos. Despite initial misgivings, IVF is now widely accepted worldwide, and in 2018 the Human Fertilisation and Embryology Authority reported that over 300,000 children have been born in the UK through IVF since licensed fertility treatment became available in 1991 in the UK (HFEA, 2018). However, whilst the principle of IVF in general has ethical considerations, the issue chosen for debate in the remainder of this section is whether embryos should be created with a view to them becoming human beings for a specific purpose, i.e. that of saving a sibling.

In the case of *Quintavalle (on behalf of Comment on Reproductive Ethics) v. Human Fertilisation and Embryology Authority* [2005] UKHL 28 the House of Lords (as it then was) was asked to consider the case of Zain Hashmi, a six-year-old child who suffered from Beta thalassaemia major (a serious genetic disorder). Zain, with a stem cell transplant from a compatible donor, could be restored to a normal life, but his three elder siblings were found to be not compatible and although his mother had become pregnant naturally with a view to giving birth to a child who could then donate the umbilical cord, she aborted the first child as it was found that the foetus had the same condition as Zain, and a later pregnancy resulted in her giving birth to a child who was not compatible and therefore was unable to donate the required cells. The question being asked before the court was whether the relevant legislation (HFEA, 1990) would allow Mr and Mrs Hashmi to initially create an embryo through IVF, to then test the newly created embryo for genetic disorders through a process known as pre-implantation genetic diagnosis (PGD). If that process could identify whether the embryo was disease free then a further process would examine the Human Leukocyte Antigens (known as HLA Typing) to test whether the tissue of the foetus would be compatible with that of Zain, and therefore, could, at birth, donate cells from the umbilical cord to save the life of his/her brother. The court decided that this procedure could be used. However, due to Mrs Hashmi's age and the quality of her eggs, the treatment was never successful.

ACTIVITY 17.3

Discuss the process above in relation to IVF, PGD and tissue typing from an ethical perspective. You may wish to consider the unborn child, the existing child, and the parents. Also, is testing for other types of disability morally legitimate?

Consider also if the process outlined above would satisfy the principle of beneficence? Will it cause psychological harms? Is it fair and just to use resources to save the life of someone who would otherwise die? Consider if it was your child who had an illness that could be potentially cured.

Check the end of the chapter for an answer to this activity.

SURROGACY

Whilst IVF may be an option for some infertile people wishing to have children, it has to be acknowledged that not all women are able to carry a foetus. One option that has become available to such women is that of surrogacy whereby a woman carries a foetus and then, upon the birth of that child, gives the child to a commissioning couple who can then obtain a Parental Order resulting in a new birth certificate identifying the commission couple as the parents (the foetus must have been created either through IVF or by artificial insemination, which can include the process being undertaken at home). This has changed the way we have traditionally viewed motherhood, where it is evident who is the mother of the child. Whilst the Surrogacy Arrangements Act 1985 and the Human Fertilisation and Embryology Acts 1990 and 2008 have addressed some of the issues surrounding such an arrangement, there is no doubt that there remain serious ethical concerns in respect of this matter, which in itself would warrant a whole chapter being devoted to it. This discussion will be limited to a consideration of some of the ethical concerns in respect of surrogacy without being a full discussion of the biological process (which can be either partial or full surrogacy). For more detailed information you may wish to consult the UK government website (www.gov.uk/legal-rights-when-using-surrogates-and-donors) and also the Human Fertilisation and Embryology Authority (www.hfea.gov.uk/treatments/explore-all-treatments/surrogacy/).

In 1985, Kim Cotton became the first surrogate mother in the UK. She received payment in a commercial agreement, both from the commissioning couple and also from the media, to whom she sold her story. As a reaction to this, the UK government quickly enacted the Surrogacy Arrangements Act 1985 which outlawed commercial surrogacy. Effectively this means that whilst reasonable expenses are allowed to be paid for such an arrangement (and one might consider what is meant by 'reasonable expenses') any contract made between the surrogate mother and a commissioning couple is legally unenforceable. Therefore, no arrangement is enforceable by or against any of the persons making it. The Warnock committee (discussed above) looked at assisted reproduction and considered that surrogacy had far reaching consequences and should be discouraged. Since that time however, it is indisputable that society has changed and attitudes have become more tolerant and accepting of such intervention. It is still, however, a matter of concern from an ethical perspective and some of the following issues are particularly pertinent when looking at such an arrangement.

BOX 17.1   SURROGACY

- Why would a person initially agree to be a surrogate if a birth mother will carry the foetus for nine months and then give her child away? Could this be considered true altruism or may there be other motives?
- Developing that point, might some women feel emotionally pressurised from childless relatives to perform such a process? One would have to consider too how the birth mother would cope with seeing her child being brought up by relatives, or is this preferable to giving a child away to strangers?
- Although only reasonable expenses can be paid, this might be viewed as an inducement to those less wealthy in society which may be seen as discrimination.

(Continued)

- There is emotional vulnerability to be considered by all parties involved in the process.
- One has to consider the balance of power in this type of situation. Is it the surrogate or a commissioning couple? If the surrogate changes her mind and chooses to not give up the child on birth, then the commissioning couple may face an uphill legal battle, having to go through the courts and apply for parental responsibility based on what would be in the child's best interests. Similarly, there is the possibility that the commissioning couple may wish to monitor the surrogate's behaviour during pregnancy.
- Risks associated with pregnancy remain, involving the physical and emotional state of the mother during pregnancy and birth, as well as after giving birth. There are also risks to the foetus, some of which may be identified prior to or after birth. What if the commissioning couple wish the surrogate to have a termination if the foetus is identified as being disabled in some way in utero? What if the disability is not identified in utero but the child is born disabled in some way resulting in neither the commissioning couple nor the surrogate wanting to keep the child?

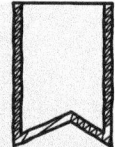

PAUSE FOR THOUGHT 17.1

In the USA the process of surrogacy is more highly regulated than in the UK. You may wish to consider whether tighter regulation in this area is necessary or whether this would potentially be seen as commercialisation of the reproductive process and to be avoided.

Check the end of the chapter for an answer to this activity.

LEGAL AND ETHICAL ISSUES AT THE END OF LIFE

CHARLIE GARD: WHO SHOULD MAKE THE DECISION?

Many legal and ethical issues arise at the end of life; sometimes a very short life. In a highly publicised case that was recently heard through the judicial system, the plight of Charlie Gard became the focus of discussion worldwide, with offers of intervention being made by the President of the United States of America and the Pope. Charlie was born in August 2016 and was considered to be a normal healthy child. However, as time progressed he became unwell and he was diagnosed with a rare inherited disease known as infantile onset encephalomyopathy mitochondrial DNA depletion syndrome (MDDS). In summary, Charlie's parents wished him to undergo experimental nucleoside therapy, against the advice of his medical team at Great Ormond Street Hospital. Funding was raised through a crowdfunding page for Charlie to undertake this treatment in the USA. However, due to delays, prompt treatment was not forthcoming. Eventually, MRI scans were carried out, and the medical profession concluded that Charlie was beyond any help, even from experimental treatment. It should be noted that the experimental treatment proposed had never been tried on mice, let alone on humans. Ultimately, the court declared that it would be in Charlie's best interests to allow him to die, and life support was removed. He died on 28 July 2017 (*Great Ormond Street Hospital v. Yates, Yates and Gard* [2017] EWHC 1909).

The decision raised a number of legal and ethical concerns, many of which were not satisfactorily addressed in the case, and will continue to be debated as further cases come forward. Please see in particular the case of *Alder Hey Children's NHS Foundation Trust v. Evans & Anor* [2018] EWHC 308.

Some concerns raised include the rights of the parents in making decisions on behalf of their children. It is not in dispute that capable adults are entitled to make their own decisions in respect of health care, despite the wishes or guidance given by family, friends and the medical profession. This is based upon the ethical principle of autonomy. By contrast, if an adult is deemed incapable of making his/her own decision then generally the medical team providing the care and treatment will make the decision based upon the 'best interests' of the patient. However, when discussing children the law is not as clearly defined, which in itself leads on to ethical concerns. Children pass through three stages prior to becoming an adult as far as the law on consent is concerned. To briefly summarise (and as stated above, there are anomalies within the system, it is currently far from clear), children fall within three categories prior to them becoming autonomous adults:

Children of tender age (birth until they are considered Gillick competent – see Activity 17.2)

Gillick competent (when a child is considered mature enough to make his/her own decisions in respect of health care). There is no strict age as to when a child is considered Gillick competent, it will depend on the child, the process and the circumstances surrounding the required treatment. However, the legal system is less likely to regard a child as being competent if they refuse treatment – please see *Re E (A Minor)(Wardship: Medical Treatment)* [1993] 1 FLR 386

16–17-year-olds who under the Family Law Reform Act 1969 are generally entitled to provide consent for treatment.

For the purpose of this discussion, the focus will be on children of tender age. Generally speaking, for those children who are of tender age (and Charlie Gard fell into this category) the parents will make treatment decisions on behalf of their children. However, in some instances, there may be dispute between the parents, or a dispute between the parents and the medical profession (as in this case), and it will then fall to the courts to make the decision. Without complicating the matter further from a legal perspective, you may like to consider the following from an ethical viewpoint.

ACTIVITY 17.4 TREATMENT DECISIONS

- Who should make the decision in respect of children who are unable to make treatment decisions themselves? Should these decisions be made by the parents who love and know their children or should it be the medical profession who are more knowledgeable of the probability of harms and benefits? Or should it be the courts, which will look at the matter from an objective viewpoint and weigh up all the evidence provided? If it is the courts, will they tend to rely more on the medical viewpoint than that of the parents?
- What of experimental treatments? Consider that in this case, Charlie had arguably nothing to lose but everything to gain from the experimental treatment. Should it have been denied him?

Whilst in this instance funding of the treatment was not an issue, in the majority of instances it will raise the issue of NHS resources. Should expensive treatments, with little or unknown benefit be attempted on patients, to the detriment of other patients in need of treatment?

Consider too the effect that a prolonged court hearing will have on all parties. The prolonged anguish and uncertainty in this case cannot be disregarded.

Finally, and perhaps the key question in this debate: is the quality or quantity of life more important? Despite the fact that there was no hope for Charlie to survive, his parents continued to fight on his behalf to keep him alive.

EUTHANASIA AND ASSISTED SUICIDE

Euthanasia is a topic that has long generated debate, perhaps especially since the advances in medicine that make it possible to keep people alive when 50–100 years ago they would have died from their illnesses much sooner. Again the question arises: is quality or quantity of life more important? Although the law is clear that suicide is no longer illegal (i.e. I am legally entitled to end my own life if I so choose), bringing about the death of another (euthanasia) or helping others to kill themselves (assisting a suicide) remain illegal. Despite many legal challenges and attempts to amend the relevant legislation in this area, the current law remains confusing and at variance with much of mainland Europe.

The term 'euthanasia' is derived from Greek and literally means 'easy death' or 'dying well'. In general terms, it is the process whereby A's life is intentionally ended by B to avoid A suffering the distressing effects of an illness. However, the problem with this is that legally it constitutes murder, namely 'causing the death of a human being with malice aforethought'. Whilst this definition is now outdated in its language, in simple terms it means that if a person has the intention to cause death or serious harm to another and actually causes the death of that person then he/she is guilty of murder. Motive is irrelevant and therefore, despite the fact that a person might kill for a humane reason (to end someone's suffering), intention would still be found. The serious implications of attempting to amend this definition in law, together with the difficulties in clarifying the distinction between active euthanasia (killing) and so-called passive euthanasia (allowing to die), perhaps partly explain why recent attention has moved instead to the possibility of legalising assisted suicide. Even here, the focus has been narrowed to 'assisted dying', in which assistance with suicide would be legally restricted to helping those already diagnosed as terminally ill.

ASSISTED DYING

Whilst with euthanasia a person is killed by another to end their suffering, assisted dying involves supplying a person with the means to end their own lives, usually providing that person with drugs which they then take themselves. However, as stated above, whilst suicide is no longer illegal, S2 (1)(a) of the Suicide Act 1961 is still specific in that it states that it is an offence if a person, with the intent to do so, encourages or assists another to attempt or to commit suicide. Such an offence is punishable by up to 14 years' imprisonment. In the UK this has been successfully circumvented by taking patients to Switzerland, to the Dignitas clinic, where they can be legally provided with drugs which they then take to end their own lives. Although UK law is intended to protect vulnerable persons from being pressurised into killing themselves by unscrupulous family or friends, one might consider whether, based on respect for autonomy, a capable adult should be entitled to make that decision themselves. Despite high-profile cases in recent years which you may wish to look at (*Pretty v. UK* [2002] 2346/02 ECHR 427; *R (on the application of Purdy) v. Director of Public* Prosecutions [2009] UKHL 45; *Nicklinson & Lamb v. UK* [2015] 2478/15 & 1787/15 ECHR 709; *Conway v. The Secretary of State for Justice* [2018] EWCA Civ 16) and despite many bills being heard in Parliament (the most recent being the Assisted Dying Bill [HL] 2016–17), Parliament has still not amended the law on this issue.

However, the Director of Public Prosecutions has issued guidance to prosecutors (CPS, 2014), which is intended to help them when deciding whether or not to prosecute a person who has assisted another to die in some way. The guidance does not decriminalise assistance and the policy is clear that the guidance cannot be taken as an undertaking that a person will be immune from prosecution if he/she does assist another. What it does, though, is provide 16 factors that would tend to favour prosecution (these include factors such as 'the suspect pressurised the victim to commit suicide'; 'the suspect was paid by the victim or those close to the victim for his or her encouragement or assistance') and six factors that tend against prosecution (for example 'the suspect was wholly motivated by compassion'; 'the suspect had sought to dissuade the victim from taking the course of action which resulted in his or her suicide').

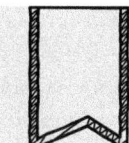

PAUSE FOR THOUGHT 17.2

You may wish to consider some of the ethical arguments both in favour of and against legalising assisted suicide in the UK. Why are we so reluctant to allow this procedure? You may wish to refer back to the ethical theories and principles at the beginning of this chapter to inform your rationale.

Check the end of the chapter for an answer to this activity.

LEGAL AND ETHICAL ISSUES IN THE CARE OF THOSE LACKING FULL CAPACITY

TRUTH-TELLING IN THE CARE OF DEMENTIA PATIENTS

This is an increasingly important area of work and one that highlights the possibility of moral disagreements arising over the best form of care, in this case regarding adult patients whose capacity is compromised. Inevitably there will be differences from the care of those with full capacity.

A sadly typical circumstance is that of an elderly female patient who, unable to retain the information that her husband has died, suffers a frequently recurring conviction that she must leave the care home to prepare a meal for him (see Cutcliffe and Milton, 1996). She may become agitated and distressed at being unable to do so. However, if she is once again reminded of the truth, that there is no need to leave because he has died, she will hear it as if for the first time and suffer the anguish of bereavement. This suffering will be repeated every time she forgets, wants to leave and is reminded of the truth. How should her carers deal with this?

Many will probably think that the normal moral requirement to tell the truth is inappropriate here, perhaps even cruel, leading only to pointless unhappiness. What though of telling a lie?

Suppose that the patient can be calmed by telling her that her husband has rung to say that he will cook for himself this evening. Could that be justified?

Not surprisingly, perhaps, many prefer to avoid both truth-telling and lying and to explore instead techniques of distraction and discussion that enable the issue of her desire to leave to be avoided rather than directly confronted. In any event, there remains a practical, ethical problem regarding the degree to which carers can legitimately leave the delusion in place, perhaps even making use of it, in order to avoid doing more harm than good.

DECEPTION AND MEDICATION

Deception may also be an important issue where patients who lack capacity resist taking their medication. For example (see Mitchell, 2014) suppose that patients resist taking anti-psychotic medication when it is described as such. Is it then morally acceptable to give it to them with the help of the benevolent falsehood that it is needed for their blood pressure? Or, turning to non-verbal deception, may it be given covertly, perhaps hidden in their food?

Clearly there are moral issues both for and against in these cases. Turning to legal guidance, this is provided in the format of the Mental Capacity Act 2005 (please note that a more detailed discussion of the Act is included in Chapter 5). The starting assumption should always be that a person has capacity. If a health care professional has a concern about the patient's decision-making ability (note that age, appearance or behaviour should not lead to an assumption that the patient lacks capacity) then all practicable steps should be taken to assist that person to make a decision. Even if a person makes what may be viewed as an unwise decision (i.e. refusing to take medications for whatever reason), this should not necessarily be taken as illustrating a lack of capacity but should be respected as illustrative of a patient demonstrating autonomy. If, on balance, it is decided that a person does indeed lack capacity to make their own decisions, then any actions taken by a health care professional should be in the patient's best interests. As far as covert medication is concerned, this should only be administered in this manner if the patient lacks capacity, that it is in his/her best interests, that all other methods of administration have been attempted, that the prescriber and the administrator of the medication agree on the format by which it will be administered, and that it is safe and appropriate to administer covertly.

Please note also that for those patients being treated for their mental health, that even if a patient has capacity to consent, refusal to do so may be overridden in some instances in accordance with the Mental Health Act 1983. This is further discussed in Chapter 5.

CASE STUDY 17.1   MARY

Mary, aged 93, has led an active and dignified life. When she was in her mid-eighties she needed a pacemaker fitted. This was done with Mary's consent and it has worked well ever since. Unfortunately, when Mary was in her late eighties she developed dementia and now has lost capacity to make decisions in respect of her care and treatment. The battery on her pacemaker is failing and it needs replacing to keep her alive. She lives in a care home but is completely unaware of her surroundings although physically well. Her GP considers her able to tolerate the general anaesthetic necessary for the battery replacement and believes that she would survive for at least one year if replaced.

Consider the four ethical principles and three ethical theories as to whether Mary should have the battery replaced.

Check the end of the chapter for an answer to this activity.

CONCLUSION

The intention in this chapter has been to introduce the reader to some of the relevant legal and ethical issues that may be encountered when working in the field of health and social care. Inevitably, given the range and complexity of the problems, it can only be an overview of selected issues rather than a comprehensive text. Also, as this area of law is constantly developing in line with changes in practice, it can only be a snapshot of this time in history. It should, however, enable readers to develop their understanding and provide a basis for further discussion. The point should be made here that where judicial decisions have been discussed in this chapter, learners should actively seek to take it upon themselves to further digest the full judgment from cases rather than rely solely on the parts that we have chosen to discuss.

One major underlying problem should be evident even on a brief discussion of the legal and ethical issues in health and social care. Firstly, decision-making in the relevant law, regulations and codes of professional practice needs to be publicly defensible and socially acceptable. Secondly, these decisions clearly have a large moral component. Thirdly, our own moral judgements are often uncertain and lacking in any coherent and systematic basis. Fourthly, what we might call our collective or social judgements inherit this individual uncertainty and have additional sources of disagreement based on our different upbringings and backgrounds. To conclude, then, we seem to need agreed methods and results in ethics yet we have neither, or not to a sufficient degree. We thus need to acknowledge this situation while nevertheless accepting the importance of moral values in the regulation of health care and service provision. We have to do our best to reach consensus where we can and a manageable disagreement where we cannot.

GO FURTHER ACTIVITY

Please look up the case of *ABC v. 1) St George's NHS Trust*; 2) *South West London St George's Mental Health NHS Trust*; 3) *Sussex Partnership NHS Foundation Trust* [2017] EWCA Civ 336 (www.bailii.org/) and consider the case, using different ethical approaches – should the medics have revealed the sensitive medical information to the patient's daughter? Please also consider this case in conjunction with Chapters 5 and 6 and the issue of confidentiality – would it be in the public interest to reveal the information?

Check the end of the chapter for an answer to this activity.

ANSWERS TO CHAPTER 17 ACTIVITIES

—— Activity 17.1: Answers

Arguments in Favour of Termination for Socio-Economic Reasons

Process is not considered to be dangerous; allows woman to carry on her life as she wishes; unwanted child not brought into the world (could have further consequences if has to be taken into care system – financial implications for the state and child knowing he/she was not wanted); principle of autonomy (woman decides what to do with her own body); beneficence and non-maleficence – will benefit the woman who terminates the pregnancy, harm may be caused to her physically and emotionally by having to carry a foetus she does not want; a foetus is not a person until delivered – therefore has no rights, mother should be able to do as she wants.

Arguments against Termination for Socio-Economic Reasons

Religious argument, a foetus becomes a morally significant entity once created; sanctity of human life (subject to legal argument that a foetus is not a human being until born); woman should bear the consequences of her behaviour; can hand over for adoption (many childless couples want to adopt children) so termination deprives other people of a family life.

—— Activity 17.2: Answers

Child: provided they are seen as competent then they should be allowed autonomy; If they are mature enough to engage in sexual activity then they should be considered as mature enough to make a decision about the consequences of this decision; the person carrying the foetus would have the ultimate responsibility for the birth/upbringing of that child so should make the initial decision as to whether to have it.

Parent: have more experience of life than a child; will know their children well and how they will be able to cope/not cope with pregnancy/birth/upbringing; may have to contribute to a baby's upbringing (both in time and money) and so should have a voice in the decision; children are not adults and their decisions may not weigh up all of the material considerations (but equally on this point adults are not necessarily rational beings who consider every decision carefully).

—— Activity 17.3: Answers

Artificial interference with the reproduction process may be seen as interference that is not warranted. Although IVF initially triggered this line of thinking, the procedure is now widely accepted in society, although it has to be acknowledged that it is an unnatural interference with the reproductive process. This in itself lends itself to the question – if something can be done scientifically, does this necessarily mean that it should be done? When considering the process referred to in the Zain Hashmi case, this was one step further on from that of testing for disability, but for the sole purpose of allowing a person to be potentially cured. Look at this from all viewpoints:

Unborn child: Consider how a child would feel knowing that they have been brought into the world for their usefulness to another. On the other hand, might this make them feel special or more valued because of the contribution they have made?

Existing child: Will he/she always feel indebted to their saviour sibling? Would they expect more body parts if needed and compatible?

Parents: How will they treat the siblings – will they love the saviour because of his/her contribution?

Testing for disability is sanctioned, both prior to implantation (through PGD) and by foetal screening (usually around 20 weeks of pregnancy). Are either of these types of testing morally acceptable? Consider:

Morally legitimate: Preferable to bring healthy children into the world; parents may not accept a disabled child; cost to society; stigma of being disabled; a less productive life if disabled (less opportunities, more hurdles to overcome).

Morally wrong to test: the condition is God's will – all children are precious; discrimination – all should be given the opportunity to succeed regardless of disability; all life is valuable; slippery slope – moving towards 'designer babies', what counts as a disability; it has been known to abort foetuses for cleft lip, missing digits.

────── Pause for Thought 17.1: Answers

Arguments for Tighter Regulation

- Anybody involved in the process would know exactly how the process works and their rights and responsibilities; e.g. what if a surrogate changes her mind, what if there is a foetal abnormality?
- It would enable society generally to engage more with the process. Currently it may still be viewed as something which is not strictly validated; if enforced by law then it may be seen as more valid and acceptable within society.
- Law generally is formed as a result of changing views of society and so, if as a society, people are more willing to regard it as acceptable, then perhaps law should be enacted to make it both ethically and legally acceptable?
- If other countries, e.g. USA, have regulated, then should the UK also bring in law so that it is acknowledged and accepted internationally? Currently, people in the UK may feel the need to travel to the USA for such a procedure, so why not regulate in this country?

(Continued)

Arguments to Leave the Status Quo

- It makes children 'objects' to be traded.
- It may make disability more stigmatised, e.g. if legislating to allow surrogate to abort in case of disability.
- What is the value in monetary terms of 'hosting' a foetus child? It may encourage more women to become surrogates for the wrong reasons.
- Just because another country legislates on a matter does not mean that the UK should do so; different countries have different viewpoints on many matters.

———— Pause for Thought 17.2: Answers

In Favour

- It would allow the promotion of a patient's autonomy at the end of life; reduction of suffering and distress; removes an unfair disparity between those able to end their own lives when terminally ill and those unable to do so without assistance; can be seen as a final act of care.

Against

- Some may regard suicide as morally wrong and thus assisting as also wrong; assisting in suicide regarded as contrary to the role of health care professionals; concerns over patients feeling under pressure to request assisted suicide; concerns over misdiagnosis or the possibility of unexpected recovery or cure.

———— Case Study 17.1: Answers

Autonomy: The general principle is that an adult who has capacity should make their own decision in respect of health care (subject to certain provisions within the Mental Health Act 1983). This means that, if she had capacity, Mary could either consent to or refuse treatment (even if refusal would lead to her death). However, she does not have capacity and is therefore unable to make an autonomous decision. She does have a daughter (Jane), but Jane does not have Power of Attorney, so although Jane should be consulted the decision will be made by the health care professionals.

Beneficence and non-maleficence: Health care professionals should act for the benefit of the patient. This principle can be discussed in conjunction with the third principle, non-maleficence or doing no harm. Would the operation, which would involve a general anaesthetic being administered under restraint (with possible resultant pain and distress both before and after the procedure) be of benefit to Mary or would it cause her harm? Note that whilst she may survive for some period with the operation having been conducted (and would die almost immediately the battery failed) we can still ask about her quality of life. Overall, would it be of benefit to her to stay alive, or would she have been harmed? This is the issue that the ethics committee at the hospital where this real life situation occurred had to consider.

Justice: All individuals should be treated fairly, without discrimination, and with limited resources being used equitably. Would Mary's age possibly impact upon the decision being made? Would she be given the operation if she were 45?

Utilitarianism: If one considers the maximising of happiness, then one could say that Mary should not have the operation. Although Mary will probably die earlier in this case, others could benefit from health care resources (time/money/accommodation), and further her family will no longer have to see Mary in an undignified state. Against this, there is the loss of any happiness in Mary's own experience of life, as long as it continues.

Deontology: What are the duties/rules in respect of this issue? There is no suggestion of breaking the rule against killing, so much will depend on the judgements we make regarding harms and benefits.

Virtue: What would a charitable or benevolent person do? Is there in fact just one 'right' thing to do in these circumstances? This is perhaps debatable, and is denied by some writers on virtue ethics.

The committee considered that, as Mary could not make the decision herself, those caring for Mary should make the decision in her best interests. Her daughter was consulted and felt that her mother would not have wanted to have had her life extended in such a way that compromised her dignity and for no valid purpose. The procedure would be unpleasant at least and would involve restraint and sedation before and after the procedure. Her daughter considered that her mother would not have wanted to have had the procedure if she could have made the decision, and that she had led a long and happy life and should not be subject to this intrusion. The committee decided not to operate. The battery lasted for another 18 months before it failed. Soon after, Mary passed away peacefully.

See *Inside the Ethics Committee*, 'Treating Patients with Dementia', series 10, episode 3, Radio 4 (available at www.bbc.co.uk/programmes/b04brpdk#play).

——— Go Further Activity: Answer

When considering the issue of confidentiality, in specific instances information must be divulged (e.g. Notifiable diseases such as Measles and Food poisoning) under specific legislation. However, in this instance there is no mandatory requirement to divulge this information to a third party without patient consent. It would therefore be a matter for the physician to consider as to whether this information should be divulged on the basis that it is in the 'public interest'. One would have to consider the harms that may be caused to all parties if the information is/is not divulged. If the physician were to divulge the information then he/she would need to be able to justify their decision. Not surprisingly, the underlying ethical issues are complex and difficult to resolve. On the one hand is the individual right of the patient to confidentiality, together with the importance of maintaining trust in the profession by upholding such rights in general. On the other is the autonomy of the daughter and her (at least arguable) right to medical information of direct relevance to her life. Is her case crucially strengthened by her decision to become a mother?

FURTHER READING

Inside the Ethics Committee (www.bbc.co.uk/programmes/b007xbtd). A panel of experts discuss a range of ethics issues arising from real life cases.

Rhodes, R., Francis, L. P. and Silvers, A. (eds) (2007). *The Blackwell Guide to Medical Ethics*. Oxford: Blackwell. A particularly useful collection in that it explicitly devotes half its contributions to issues of 'legislative and judicial decisions about social policy'.

Skorupski, J. (ed.) (2010). *The Routledge Companion to Ethics*. Abingdon: Routledge. Introductory articles on almost every aspect of ethics, including famous thinkers, theories and specific moral problems.

Tebbit, M. (2005). *Philosophy of Law* (2nd edn). Abingdon: Routledge. An excellent introduction with material on the relation between ethics and law, including liberty and privacy, responsibility, and insanity and diminished responsibility.

REFERENCES

Beauchamp, T. L. and Childress, J. F. (2013). *Principles of Biomedical Ethics*. Oxford: Oxford University Press.

Crown Prosecution Service (2014). Suicide: Policy for Prosecutors in Respect of Cases of Encouraging or Assisting Suicide. Available at www.cps.gov.uk/legal-guidance/suicide-policy-prosecutors-respect-cases-encouraging-or-assisting-suicide (accessed 26 July 2018)

Cutcliffe, J. and Milton, J. (1996). In defence of telling lies to cognitively impaired elderly patients. *International Journal of Geriatric Psychiatry* 11, 1117–1118.

Department of Health (2017). *Abortion Statistics, England and Wales: 2016*. London: Department of Health. Available at: www.gov.uk/government/uploads/system/uploads/attachment_data/file/679028/Abortions_stats_England_Wales_2016.pdf

Department of Health (2018). *Northern Ireland Termination of Pregnancy Statistics 2016–17*. Stormont: Department of Health. Available at: www.health-ni.gov.uk/news/northern-ireland-termination-pregnancy-statistics-2016-17

Davis, N. (1993). Contemporary deontology. In P. Singer (ed.), *A Companion to Ethics*. Oxford: Blackwell.

Driver, J. (2006). *Ethics: The Fundamentals*. Oxford: Blackwell.

Human Fertilisation and Embryology Act (1990).

Human Fertilisation and Embryology Authority (2018). The UK reaches new milestones for treatments. Available at: www.hfea.gov.uk/about-us/news-and-press-releases/2017-news-and-press-releases/the-uk-reaches-new-milestones-for-fertility-treatments/

Mental Capacity Act 2005.

Mitchell, G. (2014). Therapeutic lying to assist people with dementia in maintaining medication adherence. *Nursing Ethics* 21(7), 844–849.

National Services Scotland (2017). *Termination of Pregnancy Statistics*. Available at: www.isdscotland.org/Health-Topics/Sexual-Health/Publications/2017-05-30/2017-05-30-Terminations-2016-Report.pdf

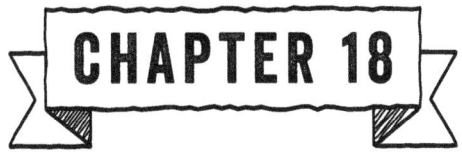

CHAPTER 18

EQUITY, INTERSECTIONALITY AND ANTI-OPPRESSIVE PRACTICE

Sue Bond-Taylor and Ceryl Davies

OVERVIEW

The history of health and social care interventions are littered with examples of professional practice rooted in discrimination and oppression. In recent years, numerous social movements have highlighted the inequalities and divisions that have structured social experience, and the way these intersect with each other to produce discriminatory outcomes. Equality legislation has proliferated, and there is much greater recognition of the need to deliver services in ways that avoid harm, challenge oppression, and seek to promote equity and social justice. Professional ethics within any health and social care field now reflect principles of anti-oppressive practice, and therefore consideration of the theoretical underpinnings and their application to practice is emerging as a crucial dimension of health and social care education. This chapter provides the reader with an introduction to the key issues relating to equity, intersectionality and anti-oppressive practice as a starting point for their professional development.

LEARNING OUTCOMES

By the end of this chapter you will be able to:

- Define key concepts relating to anti-oppressive practice and describe the contributions of important provisions within the legal framework for England and Wales
- Use theory to enhance critical understandings of inequality, discrimination and anti-oppressive practice, including intersectionality and social ecology models
- Identify how legal principles and theoretical frameworks are embedded into the professional responsibilities and everyday practices of health and social care practitioners, in response to a broad range of needs

INTRODUCTION

With an emphasis on the legal framework, key theories and multi-agency working, this chapter begins with an understanding of the key concepts relating to effective anti-oppressive practice. Effective anti-oppressive practice necessitates the requirement for professionals to have knowledge of and apply statutory guidance and key theories/practice models to ensure they work within a professional and legal remit. The key activities, pause for thought and case study discussions create a reflective space for readers from a variety of backgrounds. The aim of this chapter is to provide the reader with the key skills to identify and respond appropriately to issues relating to anti-oppressive practice within a variety of work settings.

THEME 1: EQUALITY, EQUITY AND DIVERSITY

DEFINITIONS

Defining key terms, such as equality, equity, diversity and discrimination, can be a challenge. Here are some helpful definitions for you:

Equality is focused on ensuring that individuals or groups of individuals are not treated differently as a result of specific characteristics (for example, being treated differently based on your gender). The key piece of legislation in the UK is the Equality Act 2010.

Equity is focused on social justice and promoting fairness (for example, equity is making sure that a process has a fair outcome).

Discrimination is focused on treating an individual or group of individuals in an unfair or prejudiced manner based on specific characteristics (e.g. not employing an individual due to his/her disability).

Oppression is focused on treatment that has a negative and harmful impact on individuals or a group of individuals (e.g. a culture where men have more rights than women).

Diversity is focused on promoting a broad spectrum of differences in a positive manner. The aim of a diverse culture is to recognise and celebrate differences within an inclusive culture (e.g. representing cultural diversity within a community or workplace).

Intersectionality is focused on how different needs or social characteristics intersect or overlap to influence each other to determine your position in society and create multiple oppression (e.g. a woman who is oppressed as a result of both her gender and disability).

Social inclusion is focused on ensuring that all citizens have equal opportunity and access to participate as full citizens in our society (e.g. ensuring access to all to health services).

Well-being is focused on several areas of an individual's life, and will be understood and interpreted in a person-centred manner (e.g. emotional or physical well-being).

These terms will be explored further as part of the discussion on the legal framework implemented in the UK to promote equality and diversity.

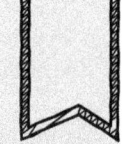

PAUSE FOR THOUGHT 18.1

Making the connection: So, how do these key concepts relate to each other? Pause for thought and reflect on this before reading the summary below.

Check the end of the chapter for an answer to this activity.

LEGAL FRAMEWORK

The role of the Equality and Human Rights Commission (EHRC) is to promote and protect the rights of citizens across the UK, including England, Scotland and Wales. This independent expert body promotes the rights of citizens to ensure that our culture across our society is rights based and promotes dignity, respect and fairness to all. The EHRC has a range of powers to challenge discrimination and unfair practices to enhance the human rights of citizens (www.equalityhumanrights.com/en).

The Equality Act 2010 highlights nine protected characteristics:

- Age
- Gender
- Race
- Disability
- Religion
- Pregnancy and maternity
- Sexual orientation
- Gender reassignment
- Marriage and civil partnership

The Equality Act 2010 states that the discrimination of an individual or a group of individuals as a result of one or more of the characteristics listed above is prohibited, which would be unlawful discrimination. This legislation promotes and protects the rights of all citizens.

The National Health Service and Community Care Act 1990 states that an adult who was eligible to receive required services has the right to have a full assessment of their needs. This Act separates the role of health and local authorities, creating a 'purchaser' and 'provider' split to create a 'market' for services with the aim of achieving best value when providing services. Aligned to the Equality Act, the new UK legislation (e.g. Care Act, 2014 and Social Services and Well-being Act (Wales) 2014) aims to modernise and develop services to deliver health and social care services in a strengths-based manner that promotes independence, social inclusion and community integration. The key principles of the legislative framework in England and Wales are focused on:

- Giving citizens a voice in and control over reaching the outcomes that help them achieve well-being
- Citizens being best placed to understand their own needs and therefore should be fully involved in the decisions made regarding their access to health and social care servcies
- Increasing preventative and early intervention community-based services across the community to promote independence and reduce the need to access acute or critical services

- Supporting people to achieve their own well-being goals
- Including citizens in the design and delivery of services
- Agencies working in a multi-agency manner to protect citizens from abuse and harm

As mentioned, legislation in England and Wales is focused on promoting the voice, choice and control of citizens within our communities, in particular vulnerable citizens. Advocacy is thus an important means of enabling vulnerable adults to have their voice heard in a manner that is independent from statutory services (e.g. health and social care). To ensure a robust and inclusive safeguarding process, the voice of our communities, in particular those vulnerable adults, need accessing and promoting. The focus is on enabling those with limited power to have a voice and role in key decisions influencing their life options and service provision. Empowerment theory (Zimmerman, 2000) promotes the role of those adults receiving care and support services as experts of their own life through a focus on promoting the autonomy and self-determination of all citizens. Self-advocacy is popular within this service area and is focused on individuals bypassing the professional and representing their own interests to achieve changes to circumstances without the dependence on a health or social care practitioner.

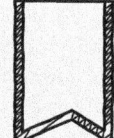

PAUSE FOR THOUGHT 18.2

Look for the key information about the Care Act 2014 and the Social Services and Well-being Act (Wales) 2014. How do these two pieces of legislation compare?

Check the end of the chapter for an answer to this activity.

THEME 2: CRITICAL UNDERSTANDINGS OF INEQUALITY

INTERSECTIONALITY AND MULTIPLE DISADVANTAGE

One of the limitations of the Equality Act is the way that it presents each of these protected characteristics separately as if action to prevent discrimination can be neatly parcelled into these different themes. Whilst s. 14 of the Act refers to the possibility of combined discrimination based on dual characteristics, this element of the legislation has never been brought into force, and legal action remains limited to single characteristics. We now discuss the concept of intersectionality to challenge this assumption and to explore the importance of understanding the interlocking dimensions of inequalities when supporting clients with multiple disadvantages.

INTERSECTIONALITY AND INEQUALITIES

The term intersectionality is attributed to Kimberlé Crenshaw (1989), although its longer history is recognised in the critical writings and activism of multiracial feminists. In her account of the oppression of African-American women, Crenshaw drew an analogy with a crossroads in which traffic poses a threat from multiple directions. A black female positioned at the intersection of race and gender inequalities is therefore vulnerable to discrimination from both directions, on the basis of her biological sex and her race. The impact of this, however, is not simply to emphasise a double discrimination (what has been termed an additive approach) but to produce new and distinctive forms of disadvantage, not experienced by white women or black men. Intersectional theorists therefore reject claims to a universal women's experience, and understand gender to be always shaped through locations of social class, race and other structural and representational identities. Each of these social locations constructs hierarchical systems of power and privilege, rendering them variously advantaged or disadvantaged. Together these hierarchies of power interlock, forming what Patricia Hill Collins has called a 'matrix of domination' (Collins, 2000). This perspective is important because it shifts the focus from the identity itself (*being* female, black, working class, and so on) onto the social relations and inequalities of power in society that attribute identity (patriarchy, colonialism, capitalism, and so on). In the following section, we consider how it might be useful in understanding groups of citizens who present 'multiple disadvantage' and 'complex needs'.

MULTIPLE DISADVANTAGE AND COMPLEX NEEDS

In the field of social welfare practice, Valentine (2016) has described a growing tendency to use the language of 'multiple disadvantage' or 'complex needs' to describe a group of citizens who pose particular challenges because of their social exclusion across a number of areas. Valentine argues that the language of multiplicity is deployed as a way to describe both the means by which people are excluded, and the problems of people themselves. The social problems experienced by those described as 'multiply disadvantaged' are identified as especially intractable, with these individuals often problematically described as 'hard to reach' when in fact they face significant challenges in accessing services due to a failure of health and social care services to meet their individual needs in a bespoke and specialist manner.

Thinking intersectionally can help us to understand this in more critical ways. Multiple disadvantage means experiencing a range of unequal power relations (rather than just identity characteristics), and these intersect to produce distinctive and diverse experiences of disadvantage. Yet services are frequently designed to address singular forms of disadvantage, and therefore may not be appropriate for the diversity of need produced for each individual. They may consequently be subject to multiple, service interventions, each with their own systems of assessment, intervention and surveillance. Notions of 'complexity' and 'multiplicity' may therefore describe the services as much as the citizen accessing services, and professionals may need to reflect on how they deliver services in ways that enable engagement.

PAUSE FOR THOUGHT 18.3

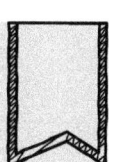

In recent years, the government's Troubled Families Unit have been incentivising local authorities to work with multiply disadvantaged *families* (as opposed to individuals). As you move through this chapter, think about how the concept of intersectionality might be

(Continued)

deployed within a family context. How might it help us to generate anti-oppressive practices within family support services, which challenge the depiction of them as 'troubled' or 'trouble'?

Check the end of the chapter for an answer to this activity.

ECOLOGICAL MODEL

As we have discussed, the individuals that professionals work with in health and social care settings do not live in a vacuum, separate from others. They are interconnected within their families and communities. Social ecology perspectives can therefore be helpful in so far as they emphasise the interdependent and reciprocal relationships between the different levels of individual, family and social environment, and therefore 'remind us that human development is primarily a social affair' (Houston, 2017, p. 58). Originally modelled by Urie Bronfenbrenner (1979) in the context of understanding child development, the social ecology model sees the individual at the heart of a series of nested relationships with others, which all have an impact upon the individual at the centre. His framework has had considerable impact upon social work with children and families in particular (Jack, 2000). In his original formulation, Bronfenbrenner identified four different systems that the individual interacted with.

Microsystem: the most immediate ecosystem around the individual, this reflects their human and interpersonal relationships with others, including family, friends and school teachers.

Mesosystem: the second layer of these nested systems, this reflects direct interactions between those actors within the microsystem, for example between parents and school, which impact upon the individual.

Exosystem: the third layer reflects the actors or services which affect the individual indirectly, through their impact upon the microsystem. This can include health and social care services.

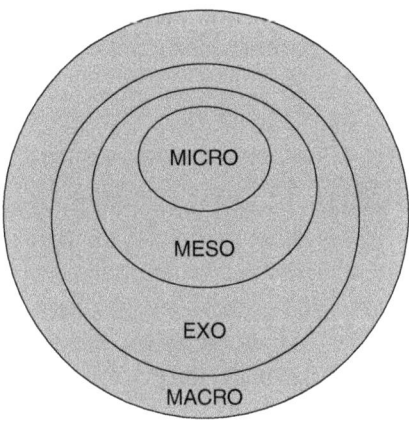

Figure 18.1   Ecological model

Macrosystem: the fourth layer of these nested systems considers the wider social and cultural environment in which the individual lives. It is at this level that historical and cultural constructions of gender, class, race, and so on come into play, impacting upon all of the systems within it.

Bronfenbrenner later added a further layer called the chronosystem, which considers the passing of time and includes all of the events and transitions that an individual experiences in their lifetime, to reflect the impact of these events upon the development of the individual. This demonstrates that the social ecology approach is not limited to our understanding of health and social care work with children. Adults continue to experience these nested systems, which are characterised by specific power relations, although as individuals move from infancy to adulthood, it becomes more important to explore how their interactions with these systems may be complex and multi-directional. In other words, individuals may actively *resist* the influence of the people, services and culture around them, and indeed may *influence* each of them in return. We therefore need to consider questions of agency, power and structure within these nested social relations (Houston, 2017).

The social ecology model is therefore useful in that by seeing the individual in the context of their social ecology, we are encouraged to shift the focus from the individual to the social/structural, such that anti-oppressive practice must take place across the social ecology. The provision of informal social support to families living in impoverished circumstances has therefore been identified as a key task for welfare professionals within an ecological framework (Jack, 2000). However, this will be of limited impact if we do not also consider how to support and empower the wider social groups, communities and economies that surround the individual and their family, and if we do not advocate for policy change at the macro level. Generating supportive social ecologies can build assets for the individual at the centre of the ecological system that can bolster anti-oppressive practice.

ACTIVITY 18.1

Think about an individual that you have worked with in a professional capacity, and reflect upon the range of different challenges they face, as well as their strengths. Draw a series of concentric circles and map the origins of these challenges and strengths within the different levels of the ecological model: What relationships matter? Where is change needed?

Check the end of the chapter for an answer to this activity.

THEME 3: EMBEDDING ANTI-OPPRESSIVE PRACTICE

TWO KEY PRINCIPLES: EMPOWERMENT AND AUTONOMY

We introduced in Theme 1 Zimmerman's empowerment theory, and its emphasis on autonomy in order to promote the individual as expert in their own life. Empowerment and autonomy are thus key principles for anti-oppressive practice, but these terms are not entirely unproblematic. Given that intersectional theory emphasises the need to understand oppression in terms of a complex web of social relations, then anti-oppressive practices within health and social care should be underpinned by relational understandings. This section therefore reflects upon the value of relational interpretations of empowerment and autonomy for the pursuit of equity and social justice.

Empowerment has traditionally been conceptualised either at the *macro* level, in which oppressed communities are supported to develop collective strategies of resistance and liberation (Freire, 1986), or at the *micro* level, in which 'therapeutic' practice promotes the psychological development of an individual's self-belief, attitudes and motivations (Kuokkanen and Leino-Kilpi, 2000). More recent feminist perspectives on empowerment have however rejected these traditional dichotomies between micro (clinical) and macro (community) practice, emphasising how psychological feelings of inadequacy and helplessness are rooted in political and economic structures (Turner and Maschi, 2015), and how control of material resources is essential for the exercise of power (Rowlands, 1997). Furthermore, not all relationships of power need be oppressive. This complexity is addressed within Tew's (2006) typology of power relations in which he distinguishes between *power over* (by which the allocation of resources in society enable certain groups to maintain power whilst others are simultaneously oppressed) and *power together* (whereby individuals benefit from co-operative action to generate greater opportunities for power). Health and social care workers may still retain a position of power, but by working collaboratively with individuals and communities can generate power together. Thompson (2000) thus includes empowerment amongst his list of seven emancipatory social work values, which highlights its importance as a 'golden thread' to health and social care practice.

Zimmerman argued that empowerment and anti-oppressive practices must incorporate an emphasis on autonomy in promoting the oppressed individual to exercise control of their own life and respecting their right to decide on a particular course of action. In advanced liberal democracies, autonomy has tended to be interpreted through the caricature of the autonomous man: a rational, self-sufficient, independent agent, living his life the way he chooses to (Mackenzie and Stoljar, 2000). However, this caricature fails to take into account the interconnectedness between human beings, and the social and embodied contexts within which 'choice' is exercised, creating what has been described as an 'autonomy myth' (Fineman, 2004). Relational theories, by contrast, account for the impairment of autonomy within conditions of oppressive social relations, by moving from *procedural* to *substantive* understandings of autonomy. *Procedural* accounts of autonomy focus solely upon the processes of decision-making in order to identify whether choices appear to have been made without undue influence or coercion. *Substantive* accounts, by contrast, consider the limited range of choices available to the individual in the context of interpersonal and structural inequalities, which restrict the capacity for 'imagining oneself otherwise' (Mackenzie, 2000, p. 124). Moreover, Mackenzie and Stoljar (2000) distinguish between *decisional* and *executional* autonomy, since an individual may be capable of making decisions about their desired course of action, but may not have the capacity or resources to carry out their decisions in the context of oppressive social relationships. Professionals may therefore empower others through collaborative action and the provision of resources which supports executional autonomy, and allows the individual to realise their decisions through action.

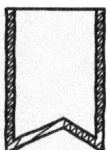

PAUSE FOR THOUGHT 18.4

List what you regard as the main themes of empowering practice when working with a specific group of citizens, for example people with a learning disability or young people who are young carers.

Check the end of the chapter for an answer to this activity.

'WORKING WITH' RATHER THAN 'DOING TO'

The concept of empowerment discussed above is fundamental to all aspects of working with citizens to promote their voice, choice and control. In this section, we will consider the key principles of working in partnership with citizens who access health and social care services. It is good to be mindful from the start that the definitions, meanings and models of 'working with' citizens to gather their views and fully involve them in matters that impact on their life often overlap. For example, there is often an overlap in the idea of 'participation' and 'involvement' (Braye, 2000; Adams, 2008). Thompson's (2012) PCS model provides a valuable mechanism for understanding oppression which draws together some of these discussions around power, inequalities and social ecology. It advocates analysing discrimination in relation to its location at the personal, cultural and structural levels, and can therefore assist us to consider options for tackling barriers to participation which move beyond a stigmatising and responsibilising focus on the individual as 'hard to reach' (Kalathil, 2015).

Citizens who access services can be empowered to have 'active agency', to balance their powers with health and social care professionals, supporting the development of *power together* (Tew, 2006). Arnstein (1969) and later Hart (1992) illustrated participation on a 'ladder' with eight rungs, with each rung representing a model of participation ranging from manipulation/tokenism on the bottom rungs to empowerment/person led on the higher rungs. Therefore, several levels of participation are categorised from the tokenistic perception of citizens as passive recipients of services to the conceptualisation of citizens as 'active agents' working in partnership or directing service delivery. This notion of 'active agency' shifts the landscape towards a model of empowerment. The reality of engaging citizens as 'active agents' in service delivery is complex and should be grounded in their wishes, feelings, experiences and diverse needs. Taking account of citizens' views is important to develop an understanding of the common domains across their narratives and their subjective 'lived' experiences. Also, a range of intersectional needs shape individual reality, which is central to all standpoints. Focusing on enhancing the participation of citizens in the development of services includes their active knowledge and experience from their objective and subjective standpoints to influence service delivery from multiple positions.

Language use can be a barrier to effective engagement and co-production with citizens. Language barriers and the lack of an 'active offer' of language choice can result in ineffective service delivery. Making an 'active offer' of language choice means creating a change in culture that takes the responsibility from the citizen accessing services to ask for a service through the medium of their language choice. Effectively, the model of 'active offer' creates a space that empowers citizens through the provision of a citizen-centred model. For citizens who are vulnerable or who wish to discuss sensitive matters, the use of language and the lack of an active offer of language choice can exacerbate their vulnerability.

The Mental Capacity Act 2005 (MCA 2005) outlines that people have the right to make their own decisions if they have the mental capacity to do so. This includes decisions that others may consider as appropriate or 'unwise'. The assessment of capacity should be based on the individual's understanding of information relevant to particular decisions, the ability to retain and weigh this information to inform his/her decision, and communicating his/her decision through their mode of communication (e.g. verbal, sign language, written/easy read format). For a person who does not have capacity due to his/her learning needs, then decisions must be made for them in their 'best interest'. The law details what factors need to be taken into account to reach a 'best interests' decision. It is only when an individual lacks mental capacity (not able to make their own decisions) that another person (often a relative, friend, advocate) can be authorised to make decisions on behalf of that person and in their 'best interest'. Acting in someone's best interests means considering their past and present wishes, beliefs and values. If a citizen accessing services does not have the mental capacity to provide their views, wishes and feelings, then their 'best interest' should be protected and promoted to ensure that their needs are central throughout. Therefore, the MCA 2005 ensures that a lack of mental capacity should not be a barrier to considering an individual's best interest. However, different power dynamics and the potential for a conflict of interest should be considered, in particular when you have a family member appointed to undertake this role.

CASE STUDY 18.1

Adrian is 55 years old and is resident within a supported living project for adults with a learning disability. He has complex physical, emotional and learning needs. His family visit him each week and have noticed that he is becoming increasingly lethargic and withdrawn. When they checked his personal file log they noticed that the information with regards to his outings in the community is unclear. There was a note in the file log stating that the staff at the local pub have complained that he makes other customers feel uncomfortable when they are eating.

Think:

- In your professional capacity, what would you do next if Adrian's family told you this information?
- What information would you gather to inform your professional decision?
- How would you ensure that Adrian's views were gathered and included as part of this process?

Check the end of the chapter for an answer to this activity.

CONCLUSION

Within this chapter, we have encouraged students of health and social care to reflect upon a range of conceptual ideas relating to equality, equity and anti-oppressive practice. At the heart of our approach is intersectional theory, which highlights the prevalence of interlocking and mutually constitutive forms of discrimination. Importantly, this intersectional interpretation focuses upon the power relations that generate oppressive and harmful inequalities, rather than simply the identity characteristics of the individual who is subject to oppression. We have considered the ways that disadvantage, discrimination and oppression must be considered across different levels of social structure, from the individual, through community and culture to the broader political and economic contexts. For individuals and families facing multiple forms of social and economic exclusion across these different levels of the social ecology, these will intersect in complex ways, leading to greater diversity of experience. This provides additional challenges for professionals in delivering services that can effectively meet their needs.

The legislative framework of the Equality Act 2010 prohibits discrimination on the grounds of nine protected characteristics, but does not consider the complex ways in which these intersect, or the broader forms of disadvantage that lead to inequalities and oppression. For health and social care professionals, anti-oppressive practice involves much more than equal treatment. Rather, it demands that the professional reflect upon their own role within oppressive power structures, through their capacity for exercising control over citizens accessing services or contributing to harm. We have therefore argued that anti-oppressive practice is grounded in respect for diversity, and an emphasis on key principles of empowerment and autonomy. Services must generate space for the individual to exercise voice, choice and control, and develop collaborative approaches that promote active agency.

This chapter has provided you with a number of critical and conceptual tools that can support anti-oppressive practice in a range of health and social care settings, but has been unable to provide a detailed account of the literature and theory around each of these. As you move between learning and practice, consider the value of this toolkit and reflect on the questions below:

- How will you develop your professional understanding of these principles and practices?
- How will you use these principles to help you to work with others in more equitable ways, in pursuit of social justice?
- What are the potential barriers that you may face?
- How would you address these potential barriers?

GO FURTHER ACTIVITY

To assist you to reflect on your learning and application of the key ideas shared in this chapter, complete the mind map activity below. Mind map 1 outlines the key ideas routed in UK based health and social care legislation. Complete mind map 2 and reflect on how each concept will assist your practice development to focus on assisting those accessing services to develop their strengths, capabilities and achieve their individual well-being outcomes.

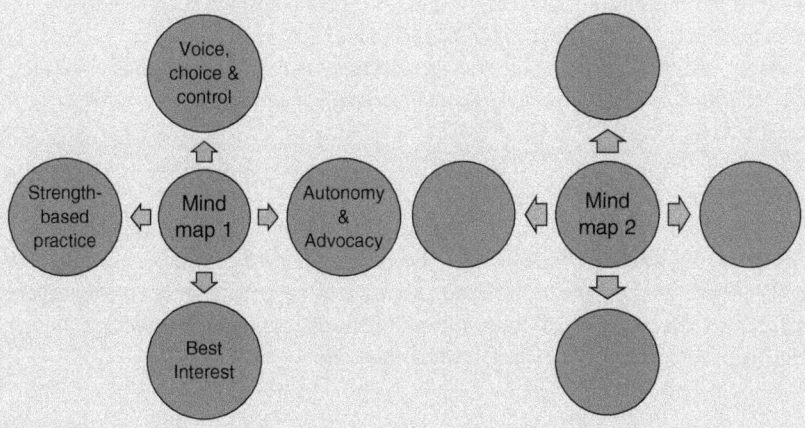

Figure 18.2   Mind map exercise

ANSWERS TO CHAPTER 18 ACTIVITIES

—— Pause for Thought 18.1: Answers

To achieve social justice, equality should be considered in an equitable manner. However, treating individuals equally does not always equate to fairness or social justice. Individuals accessing services should be treated in a manner that promotes their individual needs, and enhances their ability to achieve their individual well-being outcomes by promoting their voice, choice and control. Working in a manner that promotes individual voice and strength will recognise and encourage diversity, social justice and well-being.

—— Pause for Thought 18.2: Answers

- The Social Services and Well-being Act (Wales) 2014 includes children and adults, whilst the Care Act 2014 focuses on adults.
- Greater focus on safeguarding within the Welsh legislation.
- Greater focus on health and social care integration in the Welsh legislation.
- The key principles are similar and have a key focus on promoting well-being:
- The Care Act 2014 key principles: empowerment, prevention, proportionality, protection, partnership and accountability.
- The Social Services and Well-being Act (Wales) 2014 key principles: prevention and early intervention, co-production, voice and control and well-being.

—— Pause for Thought 18.3: Answers

- Multiple intersecting disadvantages can lead to complexity of service responses, which is perceived as costly to the public purse.
- Families tend to be 'responsibilised', i.e. expected to manage their own affairs and overcome the challenges they face. The greater the complexity of support needs within the family, the more difficult families find it to do this.
- Each family member has a unique biography and experience. Together these intersect across the family, with disadvantages compounding, but with the potential for strengths to be shared.
- Working with families must consider how best to meet the needs of family members that are so closely interconnected.
- Work with one family member might impact (positively or negatively) upon another.
- Families may feel overwhelmed by the number of services involved with each family member. They may therefore be 'troubled' as a result of inadequate service co-ordination.
- Support for vulnerable families must also address wider structural inequalities, including poverty and social exclusion within the community.

—— Activity 18.1: Answer

Example: Vicky is experiencing domestic abuse from her husband of ten years.

Micro: In the immediate family, Vicky's husband is coercive, controlling and violent. As a result, she has lost contact with any friends, as well as her mother and sister, with whom she used to have good relationships. Her father passed away when she was a child. Vicky has a son aged ten who is frightened of his father but can also be abusive towards her.

Meso: Vicky's GP referred her to a domestic abuse service and she has been allocated a support worker whom Vicky is starting to trust. A Team Around the Child has been put in place for her son, but Vicky worries that her son will be taken into care if things get worse.

Exo: There are good services within the local community that could support Vicky but she isn't accessing them. These include a local support group for survivors of domestic abuse, a mentoring and friendship scheme for vulnerable women, and a women-only gym that aims to empower through strength and fitness.

Macro: Government cuts to service funding mean that the local domestic abuse refuge recently closed. Changes to the legal framework have broadened the scope of criminal behaviour in the domestic sphere, which might support police responses to Vicky's husband. Wider structural conditions remain underpinned by patriarchal power relations and constructions of masculinity. Public attitudes and media/judicial responses to domestic abuse cases are not always sympathetic to the victim.

——— Pause for Thought 18.4: Answers

- Giving voice, choice and control to citizens accessing services
- Providing citizens with a role to co-produce services
- Promoting an active role for all in service creation and delivery
- The use of effective communication and active listening skills
- A person centred approach to service delivery
- Effective multi-agency working
- Proportionate multi-agency assessment of need that has led to the design of a bespoke well-being outcome focused plan
- Community-based and strength-based practice
- The offer of information, advice and assistance in a preventive manner to work collaboratively with citizens and prevent the need for crisis intervention
- The offer of effective multiple agency services should be specialist and needs led, irrespective of level of needs, age or disability

——— Case Study 18.1: Answers

- **In your professional capacity, what would you do next if Adrian's family told you this information?** Gather all available information from the staff members supporting Adrian. Consider whether Adrian has mental capacity, an ability to share his views, consider also the possible role of family and independent advocacy in promoting Adrian's voice. Review Adrian's needs on a multi-agency basis to see whether his well-being outcomes are being met, address this issue constructively and openly with the local pub to promote Adrian's rights and challenge the view shared.

(Continued)

- **What information would you gather to inform your professional decision?** The views of Adrian and his family members, and the multi-agency team. Undertake a review of the daily log from the supported living project to understand the pattern of Adrian's everyday life and if there's any gap in his support plan in meeting his well-being outcomes, considering whether there have been any key changes to Adrian's life and routine: Is there anyone new living in the supported living project? Have there been any significant staff changes? Has there been a significant change to his health needs? Has there been a significant change to his social needs?
- **How would you ensure that Adrian's views were gathered and included as part of this process?** Consider his ability to share his views, engage with suitable family members who see him frequently, ask the views of staff who support Adrian within the supported living project and if required arrange for an advocate to work with Adrian.

FURTHER READING

Dhamoon, R. K. (2011). Considerations on mainstreaming intersectionality. *Political Research Quarterly* 64(1), 230–243. Dhamoon's article offers a detailed theoretical discussion of different models of intersectionality and considers their relevance and implications for future research and practice.

Houston, S. (2017). Towards a critical ecology of child development in social work: aligning the theories of Bronfenbrenner and Bourdieu. *Families, Relationships and Societies* 6(1), 53–69. This article provides a valuable account of Bronfenbrenner's ecological model, but developed further in light of Bourdieu's critical social theory. More challenging material for those wanting to develop their theoretical understanding.

Maclean, S. (2010). *The Social Work Pocket Guide to...: Reflective Practice*. Lichfield, Staffordshire: Kirwin Maclean Associates. A really accessible book introducing the concept of reflective practice and offering advice for professionals on how to develop this approach in their work.

Ruche, G., Turney, D. and Ward, A. (eds) (2018). *Relationship-Based Social Work: Getting to the Heart of Practice* (2nd edn). London: Jessica Kingsley. An important text for anyone working on the front line in social work and care, including practical and theoretical guidance on why relationships are so important.

Sousa, L. and Rodrigues, S. (2012). The collaborative professional: towards empowering vulnerable families. *Journal of Social Work Practice* 26(4), 411–425. A useful consideration of the role of the professional in empowering vulnerable families, through strategies of collaborative working, building trust and flexibility of approach.

Thompson, N. (2011). *Promoting Equality: Working with Diversity and Difference*. London: Palgrave Macmillan. Highlights the legal and moral imperative for professionals working with vulnerable people to tackle inequality and promote diversity in everything they do.

USEFUL WEBSITES

Crenshaw, K. (2016). The urgency of intersectionality (Ted Talk). Available at: www.ted.com/talks/kimberle_crenshaw_the_urgency_of_intersectionality?language=en

The Equality and Human Rights Commission website contains valuable information about the Equality Act and protected characteristics, as well as their research, publications and other resources: www.equalityhumanrights.com/en

REFERENCES

Adams, R. (2008). *Empowerment, Participation and Social Work* (British Association of Social Workers (BASW) Practical Social Work) (Practical Social Work Series) (4th edn). Basingstoke: Palgrave Macmillan.

Arnstein, S. R. (1969). A ladder of citizen participation. *Journal of American Institute of Planners* 35(4), 216–224.

Braye, S. (2000). Participation and involvement in social care. In H. Kemshall and R. Littlechild (eds), *User Involvement and Participation in Social Care: Research Informing Practice*. London: Jessica Kingsley Publishers.

Bronfenbrenner, U. (1979). *The Ecology of Human Development: Experiments by Nature and Design*. Cambridge, MA: Harvard University Press.

Collins, P. H. (2000). *Black Feminist Thought: Knowledge, Consciousness, and the Politics of Empowerment* (2nd edn). New York: Routledge.

Crenshaw, K. (1989). Demarginalizing the intersection of race and sex: a black feminist critique of anti-discrimination doctrine, feminist theory, and antiracist politics. *University of Chicago Legal Forum*, 139–167.

Fineman, M. A. (2004). *The Autonomy Myth: A Theory of Dependency*. New York: New York Press.

Freire, P. (1986). *Pedagogy of the Oppressed*. Harmondsworth: Penguin.

Hart, R. (1992). *Children's Participation: From Tokenism to Citizenship*. Florence: UNICEF International Child Development Centre.

Houston, S. (2017). Towards a critical ecology of child development in social work: aligning the theories of Bronfenbrenner and Bourdieu. *Families, Relationships and Societies* 6(1), 53–69.

Jack, G. (2000). Ecological influences on parenting and child development. *British Journal of Social Work* 30(6), 703–720.

Kalathil, J. (2015). 'Hard to reach'? Racialised groups and mental health service user involvement. In P. Staddon (ed.), *Mental Health Service Users in Research: Critical Sociological Perspectives*. Bristol: Policy Press.

Kuokkanen, L. and Leino-Kilpi, H. (2000). Power and empowerment in nursing: three theoretical approaches. *Journal of Advanced Nursing* 31(1), 235 –241.

Mackenzie, C. (2000). Imagining oneself otherwise. In C. Mackenzie and N. Stoljar (eds), *Relational Autonomy: Feminist Perspectives on Autonomy, Agency and the Social Self*. New York: Oxford University Press.

Mackenzie, C. and Stoljar, N. (2000). Introduction: autonomy refigured. In C. Mackenzie and N. Stoljar (eds), *Relational Autonomy: Feminist Perspectives on Autonomy, Agency and the Social Self*. New York: Oxford University Press.

Rowlands, J. (1997). *Questioning Empowerment: Working with Women in Honduras*. Oxford: Oxfam.

Tew, J. (2006). Understanding power and powerlessness: towards a framework for emancipatory practice in social work. *Journal of Social Work* 6(1), 33–51.

Thompson, N. (2000). *Understanding Social Work: Preparing for Practice*. Basingstoke: Palgrave.

Thompson, N. (2012). *Anti-Discriminatory Practice: Equality, Diversity and Social Justice* (Practical Social Work Series) (5th edn). Basingstoke: Palgrave Macmillan.

Turner, S. G. and Maschi, T. M. (2015). Feminist and empowerment theory and social work practice. *Journal of Social Work Practice* 29(2), 151–162.

Valentine, K. (2016). Complex needs and wicked problems: how social disadvantage became multiple. *Social Policy and Society* 15(2), 237–249.

Zimmerman, M. A. (2000). Empowerment theory: psychological, organizational and community levels of analysis (pp. 43–63). In J. Rappaport and E. Seidman (eds), *The Handbook of Community Psychology*. New York: Plenum Press.

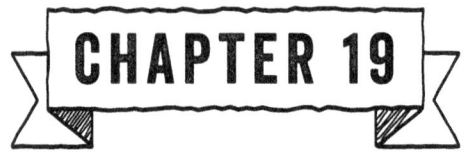

CHAPTER 19

SOCIAL JUSTICE ISSUES IN HEALTH AND SOCIAL CARE

Gideon Calder

OVERVIEW

This chapter is about how health and social care relate to issues of social justice. The first main section sets out three focal points in discussions of social justice: resources, relationships and capabilities. Each is unevenly distributed in any society: some people will have more than others, often in ways which seem harmful or unfair. The next section looks at social justice and health, through the examples of inequalities in children's health and in adult life expectancy. The following section turns to how social care connects up with questions about social justice, and again uses two examples – disability and how we pay for social care. These examples show how the organisation and practice of health and social care are inevitably tied up with questions of social justice – and that a sense of those questions is a vital part of understanding the importance of the field and the challenges faced there.

LEARNING OUTCOMES

By the end of this chapter you will be able to:

- Identify what 'social justice' means in general, and why it is important
- Discuss examples of how social justice issues are related to health
- Discuss examples of how social justice issues are related to social care
- Consider ways in which these issues make a difference to health and social care practice

INTRODUCTION

'Social justice' refers to questions about who should have what, and our rightful relationship to others in society. What should citizens be entitled to? What do they owe each other? How should they expect to be treated? These questions might be connected to anything from taxation (e.g. how much should richer people pay compared to poorer people, and what should that money be spent on?), to education (e.g. should every child have equal access to a good school, and are university tuition fees set the right way?), to our beliefs and lifestyles (e.g. why might people in minority groups be oppressed, and what is the fairest way to manage a multicultural society?). This chapter is about how those questions apply to issues in health and social care. Questions like 'What is a just society?' can seem abstract and vast – and may appear separate from other themes tackled in this book. Yet as we will see, they are right at the heart of why health and social care matter, and closely tied up with various spheres of professional practice. The chapter begins by looking at what 'social justice' means, in general – the kinds of issues we're referring to when we use the term. It then explores some examples of how social justice issues might arise in connection with first health, and then social care. The final section looks further at how all of this matters for how we understand priorities in health and social care in general.

WHAT DO WE MEAN BY 'SOCIAL JUSTICE'?

PAUSE FOR THOUGHT 19.1

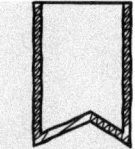

Imagine you have been informed that health and social care are not provided in a fair way in our society. Two questions: (1) What *kinds* of unfairness would spring to mind? (2) Which kinds of *people* do you think would be most likely to be affected by unfairness?

Thinking about unfairness is one way to start to get to grips with what 'social justice' means. (Indeed, one of the most influential theorists of social justice, John Rawls (1999), explicitly presents his approach as based on our shared intuitions about fairness.) Your answers here may partly depend on family experiences, or your knowledge of issues in health and care, or your views on what's wrong with our society as it is. For question (1), typical examples might include: the systems in place favour some kinds of people and discriminate against others; not everyone gets their basic care needs met; access to services is not the same for all of us (e.g. there is a 'postcode lottery'); some people don't get the care they deserve. With (2), you may have thought of those who are financially worse off, those most likely to be vulnerable, or people in a particular age group (perhaps young children or older people), or people with particular medical conditions, or members of minority groups, or people about whom others are likely to have prejudiced views.

Clearly, both of those lists could be much longer. They tell us that social justice issues come in various forms, affecting people in various ways. They are also inherently debatable, or *contested*. While most of us may like the idea of a just society, we are very likely to disagree about what 'justice' actually means, or where our priorities should lie if we are promoting it.

What do we talk *about* when we talk about social justice? Or to put it another way, what kinds of things should people have a right *to*? Here are three common focal points in social justice debates. We can think of each one as ways in which people may be advantaged or disadvantaged, compared to others. When those disadvantages seem unfair or unjust, then we find a social justice issue.

Table 19.1 Social justice issues

Focus	What's involved	Typical questions	Health and social care examples
1 Resources (See, e.g., Rawls, 1999)	Things people can *use*: • income • material goods • opportunities • facilities	• Are resources distributed in a just way? • Are they sufficiently available to those who need them? • Are they available to those who deserve them?	• Should lifelong smokers be entitled to health care paid for at taxpayers' expense? • On what basis (e.g. need or taxes paid) should social care be allocated to older people? • Should we prioritise the worst-off when we are allocating limited care resources, or should we reward the hardest-working?
2 Relationships (See, e.g., Young, 1990)	How people are *perceived and treated*: • laws • attitudes • social norms • power and oppression	• Are all people included in society, in an equal way? • Are some kinds of people viewed as 'inferior' or less important? • Are some unfairly discriminated against?	• Are disabled people treated with equal respect? • Are the particular care needs of people from minority cultures fairly catered for? • Do LGBT people experience barriers in accessing certain services?
3 Capabilities (see, e.g., Nussbaum, 2013; Sen, 1999)	What people can realistically *achieve*: • what people are able to do • what people are able to be • meeting needs • autonomy and flourishing	• Are different people genuinely free to achieve their own particular priorities? • Are people with different needs equally able to flourish? • Are capabilities such as health, emotional attachments, friendship and security against abuse shared fairly?	• Are people with life-limiting conditions able to live as well as possible? • Do people who need extra resources in order to achieve well-being receive what is necessary? • Do we take sufficient steps to enhance the life chances of children in the care system?

It's important to notice that these three categories may overlap with each other. My having good relationships with others may partly depend on my access to resources, for example, and in turn, the quality of my relationships might shape my capabilities to achieve the things most important to me.

While these categories – resources, relationships and capabilities – will generally overlap and affect each other, the ways they do this will differ from person to person. This may make it complex to identify, for example, who are most vulnerable in society, or how best we should respond to individual cases. If a person is poor, isolated and living in circumstances where there are few real opportunities to achieve what they value most, then they seem straightforwardly disadvantaged. But if a person on a similar income has very strong social networks and access to facilities which help them achieve their goals, then their situation may seem more complex. Factors such as age, education, access to housing – all of these may be 'in the mix' when assessing how vulnerable someone is.

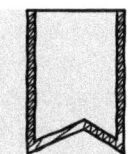

PAUSE FOR THOUGHT 19.2

How has access to resources, relationships and capabilities shaped your own life? How does your position compare to those who seem most disadvantaged in society? Do any differences seem fair? If not, why not?

It is also crucial to recognise that the typical issues in Table 19.1 may differ from one society to another, or between different periods of history. Health needs are partly shaped by social factors – for example, trends in living conditions, jobs and leisure activities. Starvation or lack of adequate shelter may be key threats in some social circumstances, but so rare in others that they would not be recognised as a pressing issue. The public perception of smoking and smokers has changed a good deal in countries like the UK since the mid-twentieth century, in ways which have had a considerable impact on how much of a spending priority the needs of smokers is perceived to be, compared to those of other groups. (For example, they may now be perceived as knowingly responsible for any poor health they suffer as a direct result of smoking.) What counts as a priority case, or a disadvantage to be compensated for, will depend importantly on social context. But we might still say that these three focal points always apply, even if they are interpreted in different ways in different settings. Or to put it another way, my well-being will always be shaped by my access to resources, my relationship to others and to society, and the range of my real capabilities. To some extent, these may be things which I have a choice about. But how much that is so will depend partly on the ways society is organised, or factors – for example, my family background – over which I have no simple control (Calder, 2016), or of what some call 'brute luck' (see Calder, 2018; Dworkin, 2000). And those are key reasons why questions of social justice arise and become pressing.

SOCIAL JUSTICE AND HEALTH

That term 'well-being' provides an important bridge between discussions of health and discussions of social justice. Health itself can be understood in narrow medical terms (focusing on disease, or how well an individual's body is functioning) or in the more general sense that the term 'well-being' suggests. On the one hand, as one contemporary analyst observes, 'perhaps the strongest reason why health is seen as an important element of social justice is the fact that ill health regularly comes with impairments of well-being' (Schramme, 2018, p. 21). So medical health (whether physical or mental) will have an important bearing on well-being.

But it is not the whole picture. Medical health is both a *product* and a *cause* of a life going well. Generally, people who are living better lives are less likely to be ill. My well-being consists not just in the absence of illness, but in the opportunity to live a full and rounded life in the terms which are important to me. While we don't have the scope within this chapter to explore this distinction in full, it is worth stressing that social justice will tend to focus on harms to the person's overall prospects for well-being, rather than simply the eradication of a particular disease. Some diseases, for example, may not necessarily impair an individual's well-being, depending on how that person's life is going in general. And to use another example, someone developing a particular medical condition may not sound like an injustice. But it will sound more like one if this happens because they did not receive treatment which they wanted, were entitled to and was available to others. Similarly, a key aspect of why we care about the distribution of resources, relationships and capabilities in society is the effects that such factors have on individuals' well-being. But how exactly might these two sides link up? When does a bad situation become an *injustice*?

EXAMPLE: CHILDREN'S HEALTH

An example would be the well-being of children. In the early 1800s, 33 per cent of babies born in the UK would die before their fifth birthday – one in three. By 2015, the figure was 0.5 per cent (United Nations, 2017). The first figure now seems horrific. The change has come partly because of advances in medical treatment – and the development of universal health care provision. But it also reflects a sense of urgency about the unfairness of infant mortality, which is much more likely to affect families who are already disadvantaged in other ways. We can certainly call infant mortality a social justice issue – and one which, happily, was well addressed in the twentieth century (although since the 1980s the UK's rates of neonatal mortality have been comparatively worse, in international league tables – and since 2015, it is now the only country in Europe where infant mortality has actually been *rising* – ONS, 2018). But recent figures show that child poverty is rising rapidly – with rates as high as 53 per cent in Tower Hamlets in London – and is projected to rise still further (End Child Poverty, 2018; JRF, 2018). A range of poverty-related health issues not common since the 1800s are now again on the rise – from rickets to scurvy (Savage and Lee, 2017). In 2015/16, the most deprived children infants and pre-school children were 50 per cent more likely to attend A&E than the least deprived. Famously, the Marmot Review (2010) found that babies born to the most disadvantaged households in England were on average 200g lighter, and had a 40 per cent increased risk of dying in the first ten years of life, compared to the least disadvantaged.

Children – especially, younger children – are not typically regarded as being responsible for their circumstances in life, for obvious reasons. They do not choose their parents, or the place they grow up, or the ways they are reared. It is hard to argue from any position that a child of five *deserves* to be in poor health, or that any harms experienced because of this are somehow their own fault. If young children are not responsible for their own diet, and if malnutrition in the early years may have significant impacts on well-being, both for the child and in later life, and if each child is regarded as being equally important, then again it seems that we have not just a twenty-first-century priority. If these are matters of *justice* (rather than, say, just a regrettable feature of a society, or issues which could be left to charities to tackle if they can) then society has a *duty* to address them.

EXAMPLE: HEALTH INEQUALITIES

In early 2019 a series of reports were published confirming that life expectancy in England and Wales is falling (Institute and Faculty of Actuaries, 2019; ONS, 2019; Pike, 2019). Average life expectancy among women rose from 48 years in 1891, to 83 years in 2011 – while for men in the same period, it rose from 44 to 79 (Dorling and Gietel-Basten, 2017). But in recent years it has stopped rising. And now – for the first time since records began, outside of either wartime or a major epidemic – it has actually begun to fall. Why? Some have attributed the fall to worsening obesity, dementia and diabetes, and others to the effects of austerity – the reduction in government spending on welfare, benefits and social care since 2010 (Collinson, 2019; Dorling, 2019). Whatever the cause, it is clearly a major development – and one expected to be a trend, rather than a blip (Pike, 2019).

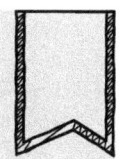

PAUSE FOR THOUGHT 19.3

Women on average live longer than men. Might this be a social justice issue? If so, in what ways?

But that's not the whole story. Behind those headlines lie what for many are more shocking statistics. For while average life expectancy is falling for the poor, it is still rising for the rich. In England, in the period between 2012–14 and 2015–17, it fell by almost 100 days for women living in the most deprived areas – while at the same time *rising* by 84 days for women in the least deprived areas. So the *overall* fall masks a complex, unequal picture. Life expectancy isn't falling for all of us – but it is falling steeply for many, and being a woman, and living in a deprived area, are key predictors. (This may make you reflect again on your response to the 'Pause for Thought' box above. Clearly some women are faring significantly worse than others, in terms of health – even if in general, they still live longer.) To put it another way, if we take life expectancy as an indicator of health, the 'health gap' between the advantaged and disadvantaged is growing.

Again, there are various possible explanations. Deprived areas may themselves be less healthy environments in which to live. Typical jobs done by those who live in those places may carry more health risks. Gender differences may be partly explained by the different likelihood of women and men suffering from acute or chronic illness (see, e.g., Graham et al., 2013). Poorer people may have less healthy diets. They may be less aware of health-related advice, or less well-placed to follow it. They may take less advantage of available services – for example, better-off people make more use of the National Health Service (NHS) over the life-course, and this seems a key reason why the life-course for them lasts longer (Hills, 2017). But it is not simply health care services which determine life expectancy. As one commentator puts it, 'the key to a long and healthy life is not getting sick in the first place' (Barry, 2005, p. 76). And who gets sick and who doesn't seems closely connected to where people live, and how well-off they are. How much people are *responsible* for those features of their lives is difficult to determine. But a large part of the story concerns structural factors which shape life in society – and specifically, aspects of the way society is *stratified*. 'Social stratification' refers to how individuals and groups sit in unequal positions in society – or on 'the social ladder' (see Giddens and Sutton, 2017, ch. 12). Stratification could be based on, for example, economic resources, gender, age, religious affiliation, or geographical location. Having more money, being of a certain gender or age or religion, or living in one place or another – all of these are examples of how people are positioned in ways which have clear implications for how well their lives go. And none of them can be said to be 'up to the individual', in any simple way – something we have choice or control over, in a way that makes related disadvantages our 'own fault'. Again, this is why these are *social justice* issues.

ACTIVITY 19.1   RESEARCH AND EVIDENCE-BASED PRACTICE

Marmot (2016) and Wilkinson and Pickett (2018) have both provided major, widely read studies of factors relating to health inequalities. Looking at either book, and using the index, explore particularly what they say about health inequalities among children. What suggestions are made, to improve children's well-being and reduce the gap between the advantaged and the disadvantaged? In what ways (if any) do you think those suggestions might be relevant to practice in health and social care? How much can practitioners in health and social care tackle these challenges in their everyday work?

SOCIAL JUSTICE AND SOCIAL CARE

Social care is by any definition a social practice. While seeing health as a social justice issue might require some thinking 'outside the box', links between social care and our three categories may already seem obvious. Social care happens in and through relationships – and is a kind of relationship itself. One of its purposes is to enhance our capabilities. And it is clearly connected to resources which may be unevenly distributed: some people receive better standards of care than others. And the fact that social care recipients are typically vulnerable (though often in complex ways) places a particular urgency on finding fair ways of organising it. Yet behind these general points lie difficult questions about the nature of care, who should receive it, and on what terms. And those questions are often sharply contentious. During the UK general election of 2017, the Conservative Party found its support dropping sharply when a key policy announcement on social care provision was labelled as a 'dementia tax'. For reasons we will see shortly, there is an urgent need to address the funding of social care – and arguably, politicians of all parties have failed to confront this difficulty head on. But the way in which that policy announcement backfired – and became perceived by many as starkly unjust – tells us that solutions which people find acceptable and fair may be as elusive as they are urgent. We will come back to that example shortly. But first, here is another which shows different dimensions of why and how social justice issues matter in care relationships.

EXAMPLE: DISABILITY

Disability has often been assumed to be a feature of an individual – a lack of physical or mental capacity, sometimes acquired during the life course, but most often inherited at birth. Such a condition may be physical or cognitive. Viewed this way, it seems to be *inherently* disadvantageous – a piece of brute bad luck, or a kind of personal tragedy. In social justice terms, we might be talking about compensating such individuals for the disadvantages which stem from it – and if possible, by providing a medical solution. For example, deafness can now be 'corrected' by the use of cochlear implants. Perhaps, in a fair society, those who are deaf will be compensated for this disadvantage by the provision of appropriate medical responses. From another point of view, this 'medical model' of disability is looking at things back to front and upside down. For the 'social model' of disability, the disadvantage is understood as the product of social forces. Crucial for this alternative model is the distinction between an impairment – a feature of an individual – and disability, which refers to the process by which that impairment becomes a *disadvantage*. Viewed this way, an impairment is not automatically disadvantageous. What makes it so are social circumstances. These create barriers and inequalities which could be challenged and removed, and so take the disadvantage 'out' of an impairment (Oliver, 1990; UPIAS, 1976). So disability becomes a social and political matter, rather than an individual or medical one.

Again, deafness might be used as an example. On the social model, the disabilities associated with the impairment of deafness will be to do with factors such as a 'communication barrier'. A deaf person may find it harder to follow what others are saying, and those others may be unsure about how to communicate with a deaf person. These are social processes, which can be changed through (for example) the learning of sign language, or the provision of an induction loop, or improved lip-reading skills. If we say that the solution lies in 'fixing' the impairment, we are assuming both that the disability lies in the individual, and that it is inherently disadvantageous or degrading. We are assuming that the deaf would prefer not to be deaf. But whether, or how much, deafness feels like a disability to the individual is not so simple. Many in the deaf community see the condition as a positive asset, for example because of the ways in which it opens up forms of communication and culture which are not available to those who do not know sign language (Scully, 2008). And treating the hearing-impaired as if their condition is inherently disadvantageous may itself be oppressive.

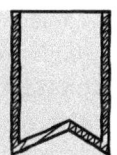

PAUSE FOR THOUGHT 19.4

Often, members of the disability rights movement have objected to policies which seem to treat having an impairment as a reason for pity or compassion. Why do you think this is?

There is a good deal of debate about the relative implications of the medical and social models, with the latter itself attracting criticism from many in the disability rights movement (see, e.g., Shakespeare, 2006; Terzi, 2009). Proponents of 'independent living' have argued that the appropriate response to disability is to find arrangements and support mechanisms which enable disabled people to live life on their own terms, as far as possible – to achieve the kinds of autonomy in their everyday lives which others may take for granted (see Morris, 2015). Meanwhile some have questioned whether independence is a realistic or desirable goal for any human being, given our dependency on each other for most of what is vital and valuable in life (see, e.g., Smith, 2001). Yet at any rate, disability is strongly associated with stark inequalities in each of our three categories. Disabled people are considerably more likely to live in poverty – with very nearly one in three in that situation in 2018 (JRF, 2018). They face barriers in terms of education, employment and general negative stereotyping which together represent a particularly vicious mix of resource-, relationship- and capability-related factors. Disabled people are capable of contributing far more to society than is typically the case, and (whatever the finer points at stake in competing models of disability) this is clearly a social justice deficit, and one which those working in the care sector will confront in the most mundane aspects of working with disabled people.

EXAMPLE: PAYING FOR SOCIAL CARE

In the UK, as in many countries, the population is getting older. In 2018 there were a little over 12 million people of state pension age; by 2040, there are projected to be 16.16 million (Pensions Policy Institute, 2019). That would put 37 per cent of the population in that category. (In 1949, there were 4 million – less than 8 per cent.) These demographic changes will affect various aspects of social policy – most obviously, the increasing proportion of the welfare budget which goes to pensioners, already over 55 per cent (DWP, 2018). They will also shake up social norms and perceptions of age – what it means to be 'old', what is expected of older people, and so on. In countries such as Japan, there has already been a considerable shift in the direction of schemes designed to facilitate retired people getting back into work, and carrying out socially vital tasks which once might have perceived as inappropriately demanding for them (see, e.g., Otake, 2018). All countries with ageing populations will need to rethink their systems and assumptions.

Social care arrangements are among the most fundamental aspects of this. Arrangements for the care of older people will be put under strain as their number grows. The practical challenges here come tied up with social justice issues, in various ways. On the one hand, there is the question of how social care is funded. Should we simply raise general levels of taxation, to raise the revenue for steadily increasing social care budgets? Should there be a specific levy, paid steadily during our working lives, through which individuals effectively invest in the covering of their future care needs? Should families be left to their own devices or encouraged to 'opt out' of local authority care provision, as has become more likely as spending on social care has been depleted under the period of 'austerity' since 2010 (Fyans, 2018; NAO, 2018)?

In terms of our three categories, the resources issues here are very prominent: we will expect there to be quite drastic inequalities among older people when it comes to their (or their family's) ability to pay for their care needs. We will find arguments about whether this is fair at all – whether (as with the NHS) those needs should be met regardless of people's financial means. The 'relationships' aspect of social justice is also integral here. Society's views of older people may be more or less positive. There may be a sense in which how much one is valued or respected as an older person may depend on one's social class, for example – and there are widespread examples of 'ageism', where people are discriminated against on the basis of stereotypes of what older people are like, or capable of. This may be true in general, but may also be a feature of how services geared towards older people function. In 2018, the head of Care England claimed that 'the health and social care system is constantly discriminating against older people' (Hill, 2018). Added to this, care is tied up with family relationships in a way which makes access to it fundamentally uneven. Some of us have more relatives than others – and those relatives may be more or less willing or able to help fund our care needs as we age. Caring is a kind of work, even if it is done by family members on an unpaid basis – and even when those members are below the usual working age (Calder, 2019). That work is not itself fairly distributed: some (especially women) will carry a greater burden. And there is also clear inequality of capabilities between older people, partly in ways which mirror the distribution of resources and relationships. The capacity of older people to achieve their priorities will depend on factors shaping their fortunes across the life course, from the care they received in their early years, to their attainment at school, to what they did for a living, to whether they had children, and a whole range of factors which may inhibit or facilitate the pursuit of goals in later life. In many cases, unfairness experienced in earlier life can accentuate unfairness among older people, as disadvantages are consolidated.

ACTIVITY 19.2

Apart from the funding and provision of social care, what other kinds of social justice issues might be related to an ageing population? List as many examples as you can. How many of those examples are specific to older people, as opposed to being issues which might affect us at all stages of the life course?

CONCLUSION

We have been looking at examples of how social justice matters, and how it is connected to people and factors dealt with by health and social care systems and workers. Those systems and individuals cannot simply solve these problems, however effective they are, and however anti-oppressive and non-discriminatory their practice is. Social justice issues are too large scale, and related to too many complex features and effects of a stratified society, to be fixed by any profession as a whole, let alone any team or individual within it. That requires joined-up responses, over the long term. But this does not mean that social justice issues should be off the radar of people engaged in health and social care. Really it's the other way around. The fact that the real world around us is in many respects an unequal and unfair place is part and parcel of everyday practice in health and social care. We confront the implications of that inequality and unfairness in every case of a girl whose illnesses are poverty related, a man who is expected to die younger because of where he lives and works, a disabled woman denied the resources she needs to live on her own, or a widowed and childless pensioner who has found that he is unable to provide for his own care needs. Those are not fictional examples; they are there, all around us, in the world which health and social care is grappling with. If we aspire to fairness in how those services are organised and delivered, then we should focus precisely on those individuals, and the nuances of their situation, as well as the categories of social justice we have been looking at here.

GO FURTHER ACTIVITY

Having read this chapter, what differences does thinking about social justice make
to how you see policy and practice in health and social care? Do you think the way
we provide health and social care can help make society a fairer place? Can you give a
good example, and describe the positive difference it is making in terms of resources,
relationships or capabilities? Do you think that sometimes, health and social care
practitioners might risk reinforcing unfairness? What kinds of cases might that
happen in? And finally, can you see how some of these questions link up with
themes covered in other chapters of this book?

ANSWERS TO CHAPTER 19 ACTIVITIES

The questions posed in this chapter are interpretive and reflective: each one invites you
to connect up themes raised in the chapter with your own knowledge of society, and of
practice in health and social care. Possible ways of answering them are provided in the
text which follows each box. Yet it's important to stress that there are no simple, generic
answers to them – and the answers you yourself provide will change as your knowledge
expands, of relevant issues and challenges faced in work in these fields. The chapter
itself, however, provides you with a set of tools, and suggestions of how to use them.
Returning to those questions, and applying those tools, should give you a framework for
developing your own critical understanding of how social justice issues matter in health
and social care.

FURTHER READING

Barnes, E. (2009). Disability, minority and difference. *Journal of Applied Philosophy* 26(4), 337–355.
    An illuminating discussion of disability and disadvantage which argues that disability is something
    which makes people different, but can be experienced in different ways, and does not necessarily
    make people worse off.

Barry, B. (2005). *Why Social Justice Matters*. Cambridge: Polity Press. An impassioned, always
    thought-provoking discussion of how social justice issues arise in various contemporary contexts
    and key ideas about how to tackle them, including a (particularly angry) chapter on health.

Bartley, M. (2017). *Health Inequality: An Introduction to Concepts, Theories and Methods* (2nd edn).
    Cambridge: Polity Press. A clear overview of the main ideas, approaches and debates connected
    to current explanations of health inequalities, covering gender and ethnicity as well as class, and
    addressing the whole life course.

Calder, G. (2018). Capabilities, well-being and universalism. In K. T. Galvin (ed.), *The Routledge
    Handbook of Well-being*. London: Routledge. Offers a discussion of issues arising from a focus on
    capabilities in social justice debates, using childhood and disability as examples.

Wolff, J. (2015). Equality and social justice. In C. McKinnon (ed.), *Issues in Political Theory* (3rd edn). Oxford: Oxford University Press. A concise introduction to key concepts and themes in recent theories of social justice – really about as concise as they come, and with a case study on disability which echoes and builds on some of the issues raised here.

The journal *Disability and Society* (Taylor & Francis) comes out ten times a year, and is an excellent place to go for current insights and debates around disability in all its forms – many of these directly related to social justice issues.

USEFUL WEBSITES

Professor Danny Dorling's life expectancy calculator: www.bbc.co.uk/programmes/p00ftllp. A fascinating three-minute run-down of factors which, on average, make our lives more or less long.

www.youtube.com/watch?v=KvwIW2dlUj8

Talks to help you understand social justice: www.ted.com/playlists/445/talks_to_help_you_understand_s. An evolving list of TED Talks on aspects of social justice, right across the spectrum from gun crime to class inequality.

4 Ted Talks on social justice everyone should watch: www.inc.com/peter-economy/4-ted-talks-about-social-justice-every-millennial-should-watch.html. Another batch of TED Talks, this time on gender equality, women's rights, transgender equality, and growing up black.

Social Model of Disability Animation: www.youtube.com/watch?v=9s3NZaLhcc4. A quirky, short cartoon setting out the social model of disability in a very effective way.

Poor kids: forced to grown up poor: www.youtube.com/watch?v=i9aSp9bFmMg. An hour-long documentary looking at the lives of four children living in poverty, from their own perspective.

REFERENCES

Barry, B. (2005). *Why Social Justice Matters*. Cambridge: Polity Press.

Calder, G. (2016). *How Inequality Runs in Families: Unfair Advantage and the Limits of Social Mobility*. Bristol: Policy Press.

Calder, G. (2018). Social justice, single parents and their children. In R. Nieuwenhuis and L. C. Maldonado (eds), *The Triple Bind of Single-Parent Families: Resources, Employment, and Policies to Improve Well-Being*. Bristol: Policy Press.

Calder, G. (2019). Young carers. In H. Lindemann, J. McLaughlin and M. A. Verkerk (eds), *What About the Family? Practices of Responsibility in Care*. Oxford: Oxford University Press.

Collinson, P. (2019). Life expectancy falls by six months in biggest drop in UK forecasts. *Guardian*, 7 March. Available at: www.theguardian.com/society/2019/mar/07/life-expectancy-slumps-by-five-months

Dorling, D. (2019). Austerity bites – falling life expectancy in the UK. *BMJ*, 19 March. Available at: https://blogs.bmj.com/bmj/2019/03/19/danny-dorling/

Dorling, D. and Gietel-Basten, S. (2017). Life expectancy in Britain has fallen so much that a million years of life could disappear by 2058 – why? *The Conversation*, 29 November. Available at: http://theconversation.com/life-expectancy-in-britain-has-fallen-so-much-that-a-million-years-of-life-could-disappear-by-2058-why-88063

Dworkin, R. (2000). *Sovereign Virtue: The Theory and Practice of Equality*. Cambridge, MA: Harvard University Press.

DWP (Department for Work and Pensions) (2018). *Guidance: Government Expenditure and Caseload Tables*, 21 November. Available at: www.gov.uk/government/publications/benefit-expenditure-and-caseload-tables-information-and-guidance/benefit-expenditure-and-caseload-tables-infor mation-and-guidance

End Child Poverty (2018). Figures on level of child poverty in each constituency. Available at: www. endchildpoverty.org.uk/poverty-in-your-area-2018/

Fyans, J. (2018). *On the Ropes: Social Care Provision Under Austerity*. Localis. Available at: www.localis. org.uk/wp-content/uploads/2018/08/022_OntheRopes_PRF1.pdf

Giddens, A. and Sutton, P. (2017). *Sociology* (8th edn). Cambridge: Polity Press.

Graham, R. with Payne, J., Payne, G. and Bond, M. (2013). Health. In G. Payne (ed.), *Social Divisions*. Basingstoke: Palgrave Macmillan.

Hill, A. (2018). UK is 'completely and institutionally ageist'. *Guardian*, 26 December. Available at: www. theguardian.com/science/2018/dec/26/uk-is-completely-and-institutionally-ageist

Hills, J. (2017) *The Welfare Myth of Them and Us* (2nd edn). Bristol: Policy Press.

Institute and Faculty of Actuaries (2019). Longer term influences driving lower life expectancy projections. 7 March. Available at: www.actuaries.org.uk/news-and-insights/media-centre/ media-releases-and-statements/longer-term-influences-driving-lower-life-expectancy-projections

JRF (Joseph Rowntree Foundation) (2018). UK Poverty 2018. Available at: www.jrf.org.uk/report/uk-poverty-2018

Marmot, M. (2016). *The Health Gap: The Challenge of an Unequal World*. London: Bloomsbury.

Marmot, M. et al. (2010). *Fair Society, Healthy Lives: Strategic Review of Health Inequalities in England post-2010*. Available at: www.ucl.ac.uk/marmotreview

Morris, J. (2015). Independent living and disabled people. In L. Foster, A. Brunton, C. Deeming and T. Haux (eds), *In Defence of Welfare 2*. Bristol: Policy Press.

NAO (National Audit Office) (2018). *Adult Social Care at a Glance*. Available at: www.nao.org.uk/ wp-content/uploads/2018/07/Adult-social-care-at-a-glance.pdf

Nussbaum, M. C. (2013). *Creating Capabilities: The Human Development Approach*. Cambridge, MA: Harvard University Press.

Oliver, M. (1990). *The Politics of Disablement*. London: Macmillan.

ONS (Office for National Statistics) (2018). *Deaths Registered in England and Wales*. 23 October. Available at: www.ons.gov.uk/peoplepopulationandcommunity/birthsdeathsandmarriages/deaths/ datasets/deathsregisteredinenglandandwalesseriesdrreferencetables

ONS (Office for National Statistics) (2019). Life expectancy at birth and selected older ages. 22 March. Available at: www.ons.gov.uk/peoplepopulationandcommunity/birthsdeathsandmarriages/deaths/ datasets/lifeexpectancyatbirthandselectedolderages

Otake, T. (2018). 'Turning Ageing Society on its Head', University of Tokyo, 14 September. Available at: www.u-tokyo.ac.jp/focus/en/features/z0508_00007.html

Pensions Policy Institute (2019). Demographics. Available at: www.pensionspolicyinstitute.org.uk/ research/pension-facts/table-1/

Pike, H. (2019). Life expectancy in England and Wales has fallen by six months. *BMJ*, 11 March. Available at: www.bmj.com/content/364/bmj.l1123

Rawls, J. (1999). *A Theory of Justice* (rev. edn). Cambridge, MA: Harvard University Press.

Savage, M. and Lee, D. (2017). I regularly see rickets: diseases of Victorian-era poverty return to the UK. *Guardian*, 23 December. Available at: www.theguardian.com/society/2017/dec/23/poor-er-children-disproportionately-need-hospital-treatment

Schramme, T. (2018). *Theories of Health Justice*. London: Rowman & Littlefield International.

Scully, J. L. (2008). *Disability Bioethics*. Lanham, MD: Rowman & Littlefield.

Sen, A. (1999). *Development as Freedom*. Oxford: Oxford University Press.

Shakespeare, T. (2006). *Disability Rights and Wrongs*. London: Routledge.

Smith, S. R. (2001). Distorted ideals: The 'problem of dependency' and the mythology of independent living. *Social Theory and Practice* 27(4), 579–598.

Terzi, L. (2009). Vagaries of the natural lottery? Human diversity, disability, and justice: a capability perspective. In K. Brownless and A. Cureton (eds), *Disability and Disadvantage*. Oxford: Oxford University Press.

United Nations (2017). World population prospects 2017. Available at: esa.un.org/unpd/wpp/Download/Standard/Interpolated/

UPIAS (1976). *Fundamental Principles of Disability*. London: Union of the Physically Impaired Against Segregation.

Wilkinson, R. and Pickett, K. (2018). *The Inner Level: How More Equal Societies Reduce Stress, Restore Sanity and Improve Everyone's Well-Being*. London: Allen Lane.

Young, I. M. (1990). *Justice and the Politics of Difference*. Princeton, NJ: Princeton University Press.

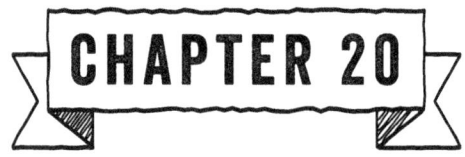

CHAPTER 20

DISABILITY POLICY AND PROVISION IN HEALTH AND SOCIAL CARE

Andrew Dunning

OVERVIEW

This chapter explores key concepts, policy and provision in health and social care with regard to disabled people in the United Kingdom (UK). It begins by scoping disability, followed by a discussion of historical responses of the state towards people with impairments and a brief outline of the policy across the four nations of the UK. The chapter discusses the medical and social models of disability and the profound influence of the disability movement in recasting the meaning of disability and the nature of health and social care policy and provision itself. Finally, there is a consideration of issues for health and social care professionals seeking to work in an ethical and empowering way with disabled people.

LEARNING OUTCOMES

By the end of this chapter you will be able to:

- An awareness of key issues facing disabled people in society
- An understanding of the historical development of state responses to disabled people
- An understanding of the medical model of disability and the social model of disability
- An awareness of the influence of the disability movement
- An awareness of the role of health and social care professionals in supporting the voice, choice and control of disabled people

INTRODUCTION

Disability is a central issue in health and social care. It is also a dynamic and contested one. Health and social care professionals can play a crucial role in the lives of disabled people – but can also be part of the problem or process which disables people in the first place. It is vital that health and social care professionals possess a critical understanding of the historical, political and sociological context of disability. This chapter begins by scoping some of the main issues affecting disabled people in the UK today. There will then be an outline of state responses to disability from the nineteenth century to the present day. This will be followed by an exploration of the two main models in understanding disability – the medical model and the social model. The role and impact of the disability movement in the development of the social model will be explored. Finally, there will be a consideration of the role of health and social care professionals working with disabled people and supporting voice, choice and control.

SCOPING DISABILITY

According to the Equality Act 2010 a person is disabled if that person has a physical or mental impairment that has a substantial and long-term adverse effect on the ability to carry out normal day-to-day activities (www.gov.uk, 2010). Just over one in five (21 per cent) of the UK population has some form of life-limiting long-term illness, impairment or 'disability' (DWP, 2014). That equates to some 13.3 million people, including those of us with physical impairments, sensory impairments, cognitive and learning difficulties, and mental health issues. The prevalence of such impairments increases with age, but it is important to recognise that does not mean impairment in old age is inevitable. Thus, about 8 per cent of children; 18 per cent of adults of working age; and 44 per cent of people of state pension age (67 plus) have some form of long-term life-limiting condition or impairment (DWP, 2019).

According to Swain et al. (2003):

> Disabled people want the same chances and opportunities in life as non-disabled people: to gain an education, and employment, to live in affordable accessible housing, to have relationships, to be able to make their own decisions about the issues that affect their lives.

However, whilst the experience of disability may vary between individuals, there is much evidence to demonstrate that there are many areas in life in which unfair discrimination and disadvantage prevail. These include income, employment, social security, education, housing and the built environment, and criminal justice as well as social, cultural and civic participation.

INCOME

The annual report on poverty in the UK 2018 published by the Joseph Rowntree Foundation shows that whilst 22 per cent of the population is in poverty, 31 per cent of disabled people are in poverty. Moreover, whilst 19 per cent of families without a disabled adult or child are in poverty, 30 per cent of families with a disabled adult or child are in poverty (www.jrf.org.uk). According to the charity Scope, disabled people pay on average £583 per month on extra costs related to their impairment or condition, including diet, heating, equipment, transport and insurance. Furthermore, disabled people are twice as likely to have unsecured debt totalling more than half of their household income, three times more likely to use doorstep loans and have fewer savings and assets than non-disabled persons, including private pensions (www. scope.org.uk).

EMPLOYMENT

Official figures show that although disabled people in the UK are more likely to be employed today than they were at the beginning of the twenty-first century, they are still more than twice as likely to be unemployed than non-disabled people (ONS, 2019a).

Given the rise of in-work poverty and the tendency for disabled people to be stuck in lower-paid work, employment does not necessarily bring a change in material circumstances. Within work, disabled people are significantly more likely to experience unfair treatment by their employers than non-disabled people with regards to job security, pay and conditions as well as promotion (Coleman et al., 2013).

SOCIAL SECURITY

Given the income and employment situation outlined above, social security can be an essential means of support. However, since 2010 the reconfiguration of the social security system and the advent of austerity measures and cuts to public expenditure have disproportionately affected disabled people. The Hardest Hit Coalition of over 90 disabled people's organisations and charities highlighted the fear, stress and ill health experienced by disabled people, as well as the concerns of welfare rights advisors, as the changes began to take effect (Kaye et al., 2012). The Work Capacity Assessment (WCA) for Employment and Support Allowance claims has been one such change. In 2015 following a request from the Information Commissioner, the Department for Work and Pensions officially reported that 2,380 people had died within weeks after being found fit for work and losing their benefit entitlement (BBC, 2015). Furthermore, Barr et al. (2016) found that 600 additional suicides could be related to the WCA process, numbers which continue to rise.

EDUCATION

Disabled people are around three times as likely not to hold any qualifications compared to non-disabled people, and about half as likely to hold a degree-level qualification (DWP, 2014). Approximately 30 per cent of young people aged 16–24 with a limiting long-term illness or disability are not in education, employment or training, compared with 8 per cent of young people without limiting long-term illness or disability (ONS, 2019b). The nature of educational provision has also been subject to change (Haines and Ruebain, 2011). Having largely been subject to segregation since the nineteenth century, during the 1980s there began a significant movement towards the inclusion of disabled children and young people with special educational needs within mainstream education (Barton, 1988; Thomas and Vaughan, 2004). However, for over a decade this development has been under pressure for a range of reasons, including funding and resources as well as calls for greater parental choice and a return to the provision of special education schools under the coalition and Conservative UK governments (Slee, 2011; Warnock and Norwich, 2010).

HOUSING AND THE BUILT ENVIRONMENT

Imrie (1996) noted the denial of space afforded to disabled people, resulting in a 'design apartheid'. Barnes and Mercer (2010) similarly highlight housing and the built environment as being key aspects in the creation of social exclusion and disabling barriers. Disabled people are twice as likely as non-disabled people to live in social housing, more reliant upon the private rental market and less likely to be home owners (DWP, 2014). About a third of households with a disabled person live in poor quality accommodation (Provan et al., 2016). Across tenures, the Equality and Human Rights Commission (2018) found that one in three disabled people lived in unsuitable accommodation in the private rental sector, one in five in social housing and one in seven of disabled people living in their own home. Policies such as the spare room subsidy (or 'bedroom tax') for people living in social housing and in receipt of housing benefit as part of their universal credit adversely affected disabled people needing extra space for equipment or for people to stay (Shelter, 2013). Furthermore, the *Guardian* newspaper reported that the government's own figures showed that the general rise in homelessness since 2010 has been outstripped by rises in the number of homeless households with a person experiencing mental health problems (53 per cent) and physical impairment (49 per cent) (Sparrow, 2016).

CRIMINAL JUSTICE

A range of issues can be seen to affect disabled people within the criminal justice system, including hate crimes and harassment as well as a lack of access to justice. A study on disability-related harassment published by the Equality and Human Rights Commission (EHRC) estimated some 70,000 incidents of disability hate crime in England and Wales alone (Equality and Human Rights Commission, 2017b). Such hate crimes are perceived by the victim, or any other person, to be motivated by a hostility or prejudice based on a person's disability, or perceived disability (Crown Prosecution Service, 2018). They include verbal and physical abuse, threatening behaviour, damage to property, online abuse, stalking and harassment. Disabled people also experience a number of barriers in gaining access to justice and making a complaint, as well as within the investigation process and court proceedings. This is due to a range of issues including affordability, communication, composition of panels, austerity measures and cuts to legal aid and advice services (Flynn, 2016; Disability Rights UK, 2019).

SOCIAL, CULTURAL AND CIVIC PARTICIPATION

Disabled people remain significantly less likely to participate in social, cultural and leisure activities than non-disabled people (DWP, 2014; Equality and Human Rights Commission, 2017a. Around a third of disabled people also reported having difficulties in accessing public, commercial and leisure facilities and services. In a report on digital access and inclusion, the communications regulator Ofcom found that disabled people were less likely than non-disabled people to live in households with access to computers, games consoles or smartphones and less likely use such devices personally (Ofcom, 2019). In a House of Commons briefing paper, Butcher (2018) summarises a range of research showing the way in which disabled people can be socially excluded due to accessibility and cost of transportation, and are also disproportionately affected by cuts to local transport services.

ACTIVITY 20.1

Search for the official definition of disability within the Equality Act 2010 at the following government website address:

www.gov.uk/definition-of-disability-under-equality-act-2010

Then identify three examples which demonstrate that disabled people are being discriminated against in terms of the legislation.

Check the end of the chapter for an answer to this activity.

THE DEVELOPMENT OF DISABILITY POLICY

It is important to note that there is no single 'disability policy', rather a range of legislative and policy measures encompassing disability. These not only cover health and social care but a variety of other substantive policy areas such as education, housing, social security, transport and communities as well as human rights and equalities. The picture is further fragmented by devolution, so that some pieces of legislation and policy pertain to only one of the four nations – England, Northern Ireland, Scotland and Wales – whilst others apply to the UK as a whole.

Today, relevant UK-wide legislation includes the Human Rights Act (1998), in line with the European Convention on Human Rights (1950). The UK Government also ratified the United Nations Convention on the Rights of Persons with Disabilities (UNCRDP) in 2009. The Equality Act (2010), within which disability is a 'protected characteristic', applies to England, Scotland and Wales, whereas in Northern Ireland the Disability Discrimination Act (1995) and Special Educational Needs and Disability (Northern Ireland) Order 2005 form key pieces of legislation. Social Security is another UK-wide or non-devolved area of policy, with significant recent legislation including the Welfare Reform Act (2012) and the Welfare Reform and Work Act (2016). Devolved areas of legislation and policy-making include education, housing, transport and communities. Health and social care are also a substantive area of devolved policy across the four nations. Key legislation relating to health and social care includes the Care Act (2014) in England, the Health and Social Care (Reform) Act (Northern Ireland) (2009); the Social Care (Self-directed support)(Scotland) Act (2013) and the Public Bodies (Joint Working) (Scotland) Act (2014); and the Social Services and Wellbeing (Wales) Act (2014).

The way in which the government responds to disability plays a significant part in how disability is understood and the ways in which disabled people are treated. Drake (1999, p. 45) suggests that since Victorian times, the state has had four successive policy goals regarding disability. They have broadly been containment, compensation, care and citizenship, each of which are briefly explored in turn below. It is important to note that rather than tracing a linear path of progression, these trends have overlapped and elements of each remain apparent in policy development to the present day.

CONTAINMENT

Throughout the nineteenth century the segregation and containment of disabled people was typified by incarceration in prisons, asylums and workhouses (Borsay, 2005). Some authors argue that the rise of capitalism and the Industrial Revolution brought about standardised norms in production during this period, making it more difficult for people with impairments to contribute than they had in earlier agrarian society (Finkelstein, 1980). Ultimately, this led to the exclusion and placement of disabled people in a range of institutional settings. Disabled people were considered to be 'the impotent poor', subject to the poor laws and often placed in workhouses. The Poor Law Amendment Act (1834) separated the 'deserving poor' and 'undeserving poor'. Those deemed to be deserving included people with impairments, along with children and older people, who were unable to work. The undeserving were those who were believed to be poor due to being idle, lazy, feckless and unwilling to work (Fraser, 2017). Conditions inside the workhouses were deliberately harsh in order to deter anyone but the most desperate and destitute from entering. In the scandal of the Andover workhouse, for example, inmates were found to be eating marrow and gristle from putrid animal bones (Anstruther, 1973).

COMPENSATION

At the turn of the twentieth century the state started to provide redress and compensate disabled people for chronic illnesses and injuries received in war or at work, through the provision of direct services or cash allowances. The Workmen's Compensation Act 1897 made it a duty for employers to compensate their employees for loss of earnings due to accidents arising 'out of and in the course of employment', whilst the Workmen's Compensation Act 1906 extended cover to both accidents and diseases caused by work (Borsay, 2005). The National Insurance Act 1911 introduced the twin ideas of insurance and compensation, but it was the outbreak of the First World War that made compensation a common principle of disability legislation (Anderson, 2011). By the end of the First World War three-quarters of a million soldiers had died, with more than twice that number wounded. More disabled ex-servicemen were being seen in public, including those who had lost limbs. The government not only promised 'homes fit for heroes', but also passed legislation to provide war pensions, regulate disability charities, help to find jobs for the injured and more. However, the focus on injured servicemen was to have a detrimental effect on disabled civilians, from prioritisation for work placement to differentiation in the quality of artificial limbs (Borsay, 2005).

CARE

The Beveridge Report (1942) and creation of the welfare state was to herald a more comprehensive commitment to the care of disabled people by the state. Drake (1999) suggests that such 'care' was to take four broad forms. Firstly, rehabilitation, with the Disabled Persons Employment Act 1944 bringing vocational training and subsequently a register of disabled people and employment quotas. Secondly, financial support and resources through the National Assistance Act 1948 and then further legislation such as the social security Acts of the 1970s which introduced sickness and invalidity benefits as well as mobility and attendance allowances. Thirdly, the growth of local authority social services for disabled people, initially by means of the National Assistance Act 1948, the subsequent unification of social services departments under the Seebohm Report 1968 and development of community care services through the Griffiths Report 1988 and NHS and Community Care Act 1990. Fourthly, ad hoc environmental adjustments with measures from the 1951 circular on access to churches and leisure provision to wider requirements and the introduction of the orange badge scheme within the Chronically Sick and

Disabled Persons legislation of the 1970s. However, as Oliver and Barnes (1998) argue, and will be further explored later in this chapter, despite its provisions, the welfare state failed to ensure the basic human rights of disabled people and indeed in part served to perpetuate discrimination, disadvantage and disempowerment.

CITIZENSHIP

Finally, the late twentieth and early twenty-first centuries can be viewed as being a period in which the citizenship of disabled people has entered the legislative and policy framework. Citizenship can be seen to reflect the relationship between the individual and the state. It concerns our rights or entitlements and our responsibilities or duties. In his classic model of citizenship, T. H. Marshall argued that three sets of rights are bestowed upon citizens in Western democracies (Marshall, 1950): civil rights such as freedom of speech, individual liberty and rights to justice; political rights, such as the right to vote and the right to participate in the democratic process; and social rights which enable all individuals to a life in accordance with the standards of the society in which they live, through rights to welfare, social security and participation. Disabled people can be seen to have encountered a range of barriers to such citizenship status in all aspects of life (Oliver, 1990). It was not until 1995 that the first disability discrimination legislation was passed, and that was not without its challenges and shortcomings (Oliver and Barnes, 1998). Indeed, the struggle by disabled people to be able to secure and exercise their citizenship and human rights continues to the present day. Whilst the health and social care legislation appears to encourage a more citizen-directed, broad and progressive approach to the participation of disabled people, as we have already seen this is undermined by cuts in other policy areas such as social security and transport and the lack of availability of accessible and affordable homes.

ACTIVITY 20.2

Identify examples of containment, compensation, care and citizenship in disability policy and provision in health and social care today.

Check the end of the chapter for an answer to this activity.

MODELS OF DISABILITY

The way in which the state has gradually changed in its response to disability and disabled people so far has not simply come about due to the benevolence of politicians, policy-makers and professionals; rather it has been the result of a still ongoing struggle by disabled people themselves. The rise of the disability movement – organised by and for disabled people – has been instrumental in challenging negative approaches to disability and reframing them from the perspectives of disabled people. A crucial component of that endeavour has been the challenge to the traditional medical model of disability and the development of the social model of disability.

A model can be described as being, 'a framework of ideas used to make sense of phenomena and experience in the social worlds we inhabit' (Cameron, 2014, p. 98). As such, it represents the way in which our knowledge and perception of the world is structured and ordered. In doing so, the nature of the ideas and the assumptions behind them need to be understood and made explicit. The explanations and predications provided by a model can be dynamic and depend upon the particular perspectives of powerful groups in society.

Gramsci (2005) and Lukes (2019) show that society can be shaped by the powerful in such a way that those subordinated believe the status quo to be 'natural', normal, inevitable or beneficial even when it is not in their best interests to do so. A patriarchal model of society, for example, is one in which the interests of men dominate and construct the way in which the world is shaped and experienced by men and women. Similarly, the medical model of society has long dominated the way in which disability is understood and can be seen to have been shaped in the interests of particular social and professional groups over those of disabled people. However, the social model of disability offers a critical alternative. We will now explore the medical model of disability and the social model of disability in turn.

THE MEDICAL MODEL

The medical model casts disability as being an individual condition or limitation, with disabled people themselves being problematised, pathologised, and in need of intervention by medical and allied professionals. Barnes and Mercer (2010) highlight the way in which the World Health Organization (WHO) captures such a conceptualisation in its International Classification of Impairment, Disabilities and Handicaps:

> Impairment: any loss or abnormality of psychological, physiological or anatomical structure or function.

> Disability: any restriction or lack (resulting from impairment) of ability to perform an activity in the manner or within the range considered normal for a human being. (WHO, 2011)

In these terms, disability is simply seen as being the consequence of impairment, and with that characterised as being an individual deficit or personal tragedy to be borne by the disabled person themselves. Oliver (1990, p. 30) observes that to be disabled means that there is 'something wrong with you'. It must therefore be endured or put right through a range of medical and professional responses, screening, diagnosing, treating, rehabilitating and fixing the individual to fit into 'normal' society. The expression of the medical model as an individual deficit or personal tragedy is so strong that it is internalised by most people with as well as without impairments (Oliver and Barnes, 2012).

Now included in keeping with the medical model, functionalist sociologist Talcott Parsons (1951) argued that 'good health' represents the 'normal' state of being in the developed world, thus illness and impairment were seen as being forms of 'deviance'. The social system managed such sickness by individuals having to adopt a 'sick role' and readily conforming to the assessments and treatments administered by medical professionals. As such, medical professionals play a crucial part in the management of 'sickness' and as agents of social control. Thus, Barnes in Swain et al. (2014, p. 18) notes, impairment or disability becomes 'ascribed social deviance'.

This notion is extended with further concepts of control and compliance. Siegler and Osmond (1974) recognised that the 'sick role' might be considered as being a temporary phenomenon whereas the 'impaired role' might be used to describe a situation in which a particular condition is unlikely to improve or return to 'normal' and recovery unrealistic. In such circumstances they argue, the individual must come to terms with the prospect of chronic dependency and attendant loss of status. Safilios-Rothschild (1970) on the other hand advances the 'rehabilitation role' in which individuals are encouraged to find ways to make the best of their situation. There is an expectation that individuals will resume as many previous roles as they can and that they will develop new capabilities. There is also an expectation that individuals will comply with rehabilitation professionals in working back towards 'normality'.

Albrecht (1992) describes such explanations as 'facile' and highlights the potential for the objectification, manipulation and mistreatment of disabled people by professionals working within the medical model. The aforementioned segregation and containment of disabled people has to an extent remained since the days of the workhouse, within care homes and other institutions. The negative consequences of institutional regimes highlighted by Goffman (1961, 1963) have resonated through the decades, as highlighted by Goble (2008) and in the findings of inquiries into abuses in health and social care settings such as Winterbourne View (Flynn and Citarella, 2012) and the BBC *Panorama* exposé of Whorlton Hall in May 2019 (BBC, 2019). Similarly, within state responses regarding both compensation and care as outlined above, health and social care staff continue to hold significant power and play a central role in the assessment and categorisation of disabled people across the life-course, from pregnancy to schooling, work capacity to housing options, retirement to end-of-life issues (Oliver and Barnes, 1998).

A number of reasons can be advanced for the longstanding dominance of the medical model and its emphasis upon individual deficit. The medical model might be seen to serve and be supported by the prevailing political and economic system, with medical and allied professionals acting as gatekeepers to resources and even agents of social control (Finkelstein, 1980; Oliver, 1990). Professionals can also be seen to benefit from the development of hierarchical relationships and practices which devalue, distance and disable (Illich et al., 2005). This is not confined to health and social care within the statutory sector, but also those charities which portray disabled people as tragic victims and highlight individual impairments rather than structural issues as being the problem in their fundraising efforts (Drake, 1999). Indeed, as Albrecht (1992, 1999) has argued, there is a whole 'disability industry' or 'business' which is built upon the basis of the structured dependency and subordination of people with impairments, within the medical model of disability. At its most sinister, the de-humanisation and 'othering' of people with impairments can be seen to have reached its nadir in the eugenics movement which gave rise to the sterilisation and slaughter of disabled people in Nazi Germany, with the collusion of medical professionals (Gallagher, 1989; Kerr and Shakespeare, 2002).

PAUSE FOR THOUGHT 20.1

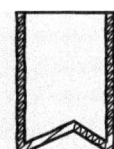

In which areas of health and social care policy and practice does the medical model of disability still prevail? What are its advantages and disadvantages, and to whom?

Check the end of the chapter for an answer to this activity.

THE SOCIAL MODEL

In September 1972 the *Guardian* newspaper published a letter from Paul Hunt, highlighting the segregation of disabled people within institutional settings, and 'subject to authoritarian and often cruel regimes'. Hunt had already written about the stigma, segregation and abuse of disabled people (Hunt, 1966). He invited disabled people to join with him to form a group to devise alternative forms of care and tackle disability issues. Those who responded were to form the Union of Physically Impaired Against Segregation (UPIAS), which can be attributed to the beginning of the disability movement in the UK as we know it today and with it the development of the social model of disability.

The aims adopted by UPIAS in 1974 were stated as follows:

> The Union aims to have all segregated facilities for physically impaired people replaced by arrangements for us to participate fully in society. These arrangements must include the necessary financial, medical, technical, educational and other help required from the State to enable us to gain the maximum possible independence in daily living activities, to achieve mobility, to undertake productive work, and to live where and how we choose with full control over our lives. (UPIAS, 1976)

In its *Fundamental Principles of Disability*, UPIAS went on to radically redefine the meaning of impairment and disability, in clear contrast with the definition used within the medical model,

> We define impairment as lacking all or part of a limb, or having a defective limb, organ or mechanism of the body; and disability as the disadvantage or restriction of activity caused by a contemporary social organisation which takes little or no account of people with physical impairments and thus excludes them from participation in the mainstream of social activities. (UPIAS, 1976, p. 20)

By rejecting the approach of the medical model, disability was reconceptualised from being a personal or individual problem to being seen as a political, cultural and social structural issue, to be challenged (Oliver and Barnes, 2012). In accordance with the social model, a number of barriers must be removed for disabled people to enjoy full citizenship (Swain et al., 2014). They include attitudinal barriers, communication barriers, organisational barriers and environmental barriers (www.inclusionscotland.org). A range of factors can be seen to play a part in the creation of such barriers, from day-to-day language to media stereotypes, segregated schooling to institutional care, the social security system to transport facilities, and assumptions about human value and worth. The proponents of the social model argue that the direct experience and voices of disabled people must be heard at all levels of society. Thus, the social model of disability was, according to Hasler, 'the big idea' of the disability movement (in Hasler, 1993, p. 284).

In 1981, the International Year of Disabled People, the British Council of Organisations of Disabled People was formed and adopted the social model of disability. In the same year, Disabled People's International extended the UPIAS definition to explicitly include people with cognitive, emotional and sensory impairments (Barnes, 1991). The disability movement has grown not only to include people with physical impairments but also people with mental health issues, people with learning difficulties, people with dementia and others (Cameron, 2014). Another key feature of the movement has been the involvement of disabled academics and activists such as Mike Oliver, Colin Barnes, Jenny Morris and others who have developed the thinking as well as campaigning for change.

The disability movement has created a context for solidarity and mutual support between disabled people and to also campaign for a barrier free society, anti-discrimination legislation and independent living (Oliver, 1990). As well as the not inconsiderable feat of forming a social movement, significant achievements of the disability movement include the following.

THE CHANGE IN DISCOURSE

The way in which disability is thought about and discussed in policy, provision and wider society has been questioned by the social model. The language of disability has revised and recast how society sees 'disabled people' regarding social structures rather than 'people with disabilities' in which the attribution is one of individual problems (Barnes and Mercer, 2010). This has found its way into areas of social policy where disabled people are participants rather than passive subjects or service users, and the direct voice of disabled people is heard in politics, policy-making and provision, as exemplified by the slogan: 'Nothing about us, without us!'

THE ADVENT OF DISABILITY DISCRIMINATION LEGISLATION

The disability movement has long battled for rights (Barnes, 1991). Disability discrimination legislation has evolved from the ground-breaking imperfect, Disability Discrimination Act (DDA) (1995) to the broader DDA (2005). As previously mentioned, the UK Government ratified the UNCRDP, granting disabled people a comprehensive set of rights in 2009, whilst the present Equality Act 2010 includes disability amongst its "protected characteristics" and there is an Equality Duty to ensure that disability is considered within relevant policies and provisions (Wadham, 2010). Despite such progress, however, there remains a tendency to adopt a medical model approach towards legal definitions and a need for cultural change in the way in which disabled people are treated (Brown, 2014). Moreover, a damning recent United Nations Inquiry, called for by disabled peoples organisations, into the effects of Government welfare reforms and austerity measures on the human rights of disabled people in the UK, found that, 'there is reliable evidence that the threshold of grave or systematic violations of the rights of persons with disabilities has been crossed by the State party' (United Nations Committee on the Rights of Persons with Disabilities, 2017, p. 18).

THE RISE OF INDEPENDENT LIVING

The concept of independent living arose out of the negative experiences of disabled people segregated in institutions and in receipt of 'care'. Hasler (2003) summarises definitions of independent living as being, 'the emancipatory philosophy and practice which empowers disabled people and enables them to exert influence, choice and control in every aspect of their life'. Independent living is located within the social model of disability, human rights based and enshrined in the UN Convention on the Rights of Persons with Disabilities (2006). It is ostensibly supported by a shift in government policy towards personalisation, direct payments and self/ citizen directed budgets. Centres for Independent Living (CIL) controlled by disabled people have also emerged across the UK, offering a range of support for disabled people to be able to meet their needs for living independently and to be a part of inclusive communities. Spectrum was founded as Southampton CIL in 1984 (http://spectrumcil.co.uk/), whilst others include Dewis CIL in Wales (www.dewiscil.org.uk/), Lothian CIL in Scotland (www.lothiancil.org.uk/) and the Centre for Independent Living Northern Ireland (www.cilni.org/). Such developments are not without threats and challenges, particularly in facing welfare cuts and austerity measures, unequal power relationships and co-option or colonisation by politicians, policy-makers and professionals (Barnes and Mercer, 2006; Morgan, 2014; Woodin, 2014).

FURTHER DEVELOPMENT

The instrumental role of the disability movement in developing the thinking and creation of the social model of disability has already been highlighted. Over the years since its inception the model has been subject to further debate and development. Tregaskis (2002) notes the initial influence of materialist accounts of disability (Finkelstein, 1980; Oliver, 1990), which she demonstrates has been augmented within disability studies by feminist perspectives (Morris, 1991; Thomas, 1999), analyses of cultural representations (Barnes, 1991; Hevey, 1992) and notions of embodiment and the disabled body (Garland-Thomson, 1997; Wendell, 1996).

Shakespeare (2014) argues that the social model has been overly concerned with social structure and does not take full account of the lived experience of disabled people themselves. He suggests that the social model has polarised debate regarding medical and social perspectives, impairment and disability, disabled and non-disabled. He posits that it promotes disability identity politics at the cost of recognising inter-sectionality, diversity and the differential experience of disabled people with regard to age, race, ethnicity, gender, sexuality and other factors. He proposes a more sophisticated analysis beyond the removal of barriers. Nevertheless, Shakespeare (2014) also acknowledges the progress made from the position of disabled people prior to the introduction of the social model.

A crucial issue here is the relationship between disability politics in daily life and disability studies as an academic field (Cameron, 2014). The disability movement has sought to promote an understanding of disability based upon a social model which is inclusive and relevant to lived experiences and relations. The development of critical disability studies over the past two decades might well have provided a number of illuminating insights and new perspectives from a range of disciplines (Goodley, 2011, 2014; Shildrick, 2012). However, as Sheldon (2014) points out, such theorising might not necessarily help to confront the problem of disablism or inform the political action required to combat it. Whilst acknowledging that the social model of disability is 'a simplified representation of a complex social reality', it provides 'a practical guide to action' which attempts to make sense of living with impairment in a disabling society and a much needed alternative to the medical model (Oliver and Barnes, 2012, p. 22).

ACTIVITY 20.3

View Sisters of Frida Website: www.sisofrida.org/

How do the Sisters of Frida challenge the medical model of disability?

What other types of discrimination and exclusion are of concern to the Sisters of Frida?

Check the end of the chapter for an answer to this activity.

THE ROLE OF HEALTH AND SOCIAL CARE PROFESSIONALS

Although the social model of disability and rise of organisations of disabled people stand in opposition to the predominance of medical model, professional power and associated systems, that is not to say that there is no place for health and social care professionals today. Indeed, the initial policy statement of UPIAS, whilst criticising the oppressive nature of the institutions and the practices of medical and other professionals for telling disabled people how to live, withholding information and making decisions on their behalf, also highlighted the need for 'the right kind of help' (UPIAS, 1996).

Finkelstein (1981) called for a new kind of helper/helped relationship 'reformed into one of equality', within which professionals ensure the involvement of the disabled person in the decision-making process, access to all records and participation in planning. More recently Brandon (2014) has stressed that professionals are not 'the enemy', but values, ideology, power and control are key to understanding their relationship with disabled people (p. 121). This is echoed by others, including Oliver et al. (2012), suggesting that it is not a question of 'if' but 'how' health and social care professionals work with disabled people within the prevailing context of policy and practice.

At a fundamental level there is a need to question the term 'care' within health and social care and the work of professionals in the field. Care is a contested and more complex concept than it might first appear, but crucial to consider. Indeed, it is so problematic that there are some calls for different or alternative terms to be used, including help, support or assistance (Harris and Roulstone, 2011; Priestley, 1999; Shakespeare, 2000). There is a danger that care is only approached as being about 'the alleviation of burden' (Roulstone and Prideaux, 2012, p. 7). Jack (1999, p. 22) warned against the 'myopia of therapeutic good intention' in which well-meaning paternalism through care serves to effectively disempower disabled people. Care can also become a means of control or the creation of dependency on the part of powerful institutions, organisations and professionals (Barton, 1989).

Wood (1991), the then chair of the British Council of Organisations of Disabled People, is unequivocal in his assertion that 'WE DON'T WANT CARE!', in terms of disabled people being 'done to' as the objects of intervention by professionals and as passive recipients of health and social care services. Rather, Wood called for greater independence and the autonomy of disabled people. Alternatively, Morris (2001) proposes a new ethics of care drawn from feminist as well as disability studies, which instead emphasises interdependence and reciprocity whilst also recognising difference and our common humanity, concluding:

> We need an ethics of care which recognises that anyone – whatever their level of communication or cognitive impairment – can express preferences. We need an ethics of care which aims to enable people to participate in decisions which affect them and to be involved in the life of their community. Most importantly we need an ethics of care which, while starting from the position that everyone has the same human rights, also recognises the additional requirements that some people have in order to access those human rights.' (p. 15)

Shakespeare (2006, 2014) notes the complexities, dilemmas and variety of care and support that might be needed by disabled people. He argues for a pluralistic approach to care based upon the support needs, aspirations and values of the individual, from those in residential care to independent living. He also calls for the forms of care and support adopted to be based upon mutual respect for both those providing and those receiving care.

It must be said that maintaining a principled ethical and empowering approach in practice can be tough, even when it appears to be going with the grain of seemingly progressive health and social care policy. Beresford et al. (2011), for example, found that despite the rhetoric of person-centred care, personalisation and self/citizen directed budgets, in reality there continue to be a number of obstacles in offering such support. Such obstacles include inadequate funding, workforce limits, institutionalisation, organisational structures, accessibility of services and an 'occupational practice that is still often paternalistic, inflexible and reflects a disempowering one-size-fits-all culture' (p. 346). This consequently calls upon practitioners to undertake more critical refection upon the political and organisational context of health and social care as well as their own personal and professional values, and their individual attitudes and actions.

Given the challenges of developing policy and practice based upon the evolving social model of disability, it is important for health and social care professionals themselves to develop alliances that offer mutual support, shared learning and a common commitment to change. That might involve making links between like-minded health and social care colleagues as well as disabled people at a local level, within teams or across local authorities, boards and other agencies. Developing relationships and meaningful connections with local organisations of disabled people can provide an essential touchstone for practice. There are also national bodies that attempt to support such alliances and action, for example the Social Work Action Network (SWAN) which aims to 'promote a model of social work rooted in social justice, valuing both individual relationship-based practice and collective approaches' (www.socialworkfuture.org).

ACTIVITY 20.4

List what you would consider disempowering practice, followed by a list of what you would consider empowering practice, in health and social care.

Check the end of the chapter for an answer to this activity.

CONCLUSION

This chapter has scoped the issue of disability in the UK today and provided an outline of the historical development of policy responses towards disabled people. It has described the key elements of the medical model of disability and the social model of disability. Finally, there has been a consideration of the role that health and social care professionals can play to support disabled people in more progressive and empowering ways.

GO FURTHER ACTIVITY

Having read this chapter what are the main issues confronting disabled people in the UK today? How might your understanding of disability affect the way in which you practise as a health and social care professional? Moving forward, in what ways might you seek to support the voice, choice and control of disabled people in your work? What might be the challenges in doing so and how might they be overcome?

ANSWERS TO CHAPTER 20 ACTIVITIES

—————— Activity 20.1 Answers

Search for the official definition of disability within the Equality Act 2010 at the following government website address: www.gov.uk/definition-of-disability-under-equality-act-2010

Then identify three examples which demonstrate that disabled people are being discriminated against in terms of the legislation

- You are disabled under the Equality Act 2010 if you have a physical or mental impairment that has a 'substantial' and 'long-term' negative effect on your ability to do normal daily activities.

    o   Losing your job due to disability related absence
    o   Not being offered a job due to your disability
    o   An employer's lack of consideration for provision of suitable other employment (failure to make reasonable adjustments)
    o   Being either harassed or victimised due to your disability

—————— Activity 20.2 Answers

Identify examples of containment, compensation, care and citizenship in disability policy and provision in health and social care today.

- Containment: keeping disabled people in institutions for example in some mental health provision
- Compensation: for example, the Disabled Living Allowance
- Care: for example, social care support for a child with additional needs
- Citizenship: for example, the Disability Rights Movement

—————— Pause for Thought 20.1 Answers

In which areas of health and social care policy and practice does the medical model of disability still prevail? What are its advantages and disadvantages, and to whom?

- The medical model still prevails in many areas of healthcare where the challenges the healthcare professional thinks the person is facing may not be the same as the individual believes are the problem.
- Advantages for the person are that attention is given to the disability
- Disadvantages for the person is they (as an individual) may be neglected and opportunities may be missed

—————— Activity 20.3 Answers

View Sisters of Frida Website: www.sisofrida.org

How do the Sisters of Frida challenge the medical model of disability?

- They are a collective of women seeking to develop a network (or several networks) of disabled women.

What other types of discrimination and exclusion are of concern to the Sisters of Frida?

- For example, sexuality, accessibility, advocacy, violence against women

───── Activity 20.4 Answers

List what you would consider disempowering practice, followed by a list of what you would consider empowering practice, in health and social care.

- Disempowering practice could be considered as care being provided in a paternalistic 'the health or social care practitioner knows best' manner with little time or thought given to the preferences of the individual.
- Not asking the person what care they want, what are their expectations of care and what do they want to do with their lives.

FURTHER READING

Borsay, A. (2005). *Disability and Policy in Britain since 1750: A History of Exclusion*. Basingstoke: Palgrave Macmillan.

Cameron, C. (ed.). (2014). *Disability Studies: A Student's Guide*. London: Sage.

Oliver, M. and Barnes, C. (2012). *The New Politics of Disablement*. Basingstoke: Palgrave Macmillan.

Swain, J., French, S., Barnes, C. and Thomas, C. (eds). (2014). *Disabling Barriers – Enabling Environments* (3rd edn). London: Sage.

USEFUL WEBSITES

Key academic journals in disability studies include:

Disability and Society: www.tandfonline.com/loi/cdso20

Journal of Disability Policy Studies: https://journals.sagepub.com/home/dps

The Leeds University disability studies website provides a rich and unique disability studies archive and repository of material from the disability movement: https://disability-studies.leeds.ac.uk/library/

Disability News Service: www.disabilitynewsservice.com/

Key organisations include:

Disability Wales: www.disabilitywales.org/

Inclusion Scotland: https://inclusionscotland.org/

Disability Action Northern Ireland: www.disabilityaction.org/

The Disability Rights UK: www.disabilityrightsuk.org/

The Independent Living Institute: www.independentliving.org

Shaping Our Lives: www.shapingourlives.org.uk/

www.dewiscil.org.uk/

www.lothiancil.org.uk/

www.cilni.org/

http://spectrumcil.co.uk/

Disabled People Against Cuts (DPAC) https://dpac.uk.net/

REFERENCES

Albrecht, G. (1992). *The Disability Business: Rehabilitation in America*. London: Sage.

Albrecht, G. (1999). *Handbook of Disability Studies*. London: Sage.

Anderson, J. (2011). *War, Disability and Rehabilitation in Britain: Soul of a Nation*. Manchester: Manchester University Press.

Anstruther, I. (1973). *The Scandal of the Andover Workhouse*. London: Geoffrey Bles.

Barnes, C. (1991). *Disabled People in Britain and Discrimination: The Case for Anti-Discrimination Legislation*. London: Hurst and Co. in association with British Council of Organisations of Disabled People.

Barnes, C. and Mercer, G. (2006). *Independent Futures: Creating User-Led Disability Services in a Disabling Society*. Bristol: Policy Press.

Barnes, C. and Mercer, G. (2010). *Exploring Disability* (2nd edn). Cambridge: Polity.

Barr, B. et al. (2016). Fit-for-work or fit-for-unemployment? Does the reassessment of disability benefit claimants using a tougher work capability assessment help people into work? *Journal of Epidemiology and Community Health* May, 70(5), 452–458. DOI: 10.1136/jech-2015-206333

Barton, L. (1988). *The Politics of Special Educational Needs*. Lewes: Falmer Press.

Barton, L. (1989) (ed.). *Disability and Dependency*. Lewes: Falmer Press.

BBC (2015). More than 2,300 died after fit for work assessment – DWP figures. Available at: www.bbc.co.uk/news/uk-34074557 (accessed 15 May 2019).

BBC (2019). Whorlton Hall: Hospital 'abused' vulnerable adultsAvailable at:. www.bbc.co.uk/news/health-48367071 (accessed 21 July 2019).

Beresford, P. et al. (2011). *Supporting People: Towards a Person-Centred Approach*. Bristol: Policy Press.

Borsay, A. (2005). *Disability and Policy in Britain since 1750: A History of Exclusion*. Basingstoke: Palgrave Macmillan.

Brandon, T. (2014). Professionals. In C. Cameron (ed.), *Disability Studies: A Student's Guide*. London: Sage.

Brown, J. (2014). Rights and legislation. In C. Cameron (ed.), *Disability Studies: A Student's Guide*. Sage: London.

Butcher, L. (2018). Access to transport for disabled people. *House of Commons Briefing Paper Number CBP601*, 30 October. https://researchbriefings.files.parliament.uk/documents/SN00601/SN00601.pdf

Cameron, C. (ed.) (2014). *Disability Studies: A Student's Guide*. London: Sage.

Coleman, N., Sykes, W. and Groom, C. (2013). *Barriers to Employment and Unfair Treatment at Work: A Quantitative Analysis of Disabled People's Experiences*. Research Report 88.

Crown Prosecution Service (2018). Disability Hate Crime and other crimes against Disabled people– prosecution guidance. Available at: www.cps.gov.uk/legal-guidance/disability-hate-crime-and-other-crimes-against-disabled-people-prosecution-guidance

Department of Work and Pensions Office for Disability Issues (2014). Disability facts and figures. Available at: www.gov.uk/government/publications/disability-facts-and-figures/disability-facts-and-figures

Department for Work and Pensions (2019). Family Resources Survey 2017–18. Available at: https://assets.publishing.service.gov.uk/government/uploads/system/uploads/attachment_data/file/790000/family-resources-survey-2017-18.pdf

Disability Rights UK (2019). *DR UK Response to Access to Justice Reforms*. Available at: www.disabilityrightsuk.org/news/2019/march/accesstojusticereformresponse (accessed 11 March 2019).

Drake, R. F. (1999). *Understanding Disability Policies*. Basingstoke: Palgrave Macmillan.

Equality and Human Rights Commission (2017a). *Being Disabled in Britain: A Journey Less Equal*. Available at: www.equalityhumanrights.com/en/publication-download/being-disabled-britain-journey-less-equal (accessed 19 October 2019).

Equality and Human Rights Commission (2017b). *Tackling Disability-Related Harassment: Final Progress Report*. Available at: www.equalityhumanrights.com/sites/default/files/tackling_disablity-related_harassment_final.pdf (accessed 30 April 2019).

Equality and Human Rights Commission (2018). *Housing and Disabled People: Britain's Hidden Crisis*. Available at: www.equalityhumanrights.com/sites/default/files/housing-and-disabled-people-britains-hidden-crisis-main-report_0.pdf (accessed 22 July 2019).

Finkelstein, V. (1980). Disability and the helper/helped relationship: an historical view. In A. Brechin, P. Liddiard and J. Swain (eds), *Handicap in a Social World: A Reader*. Sevenoaks: Hodder & Stoughton/Open University Press.

Flynn, M. and Citarella, V. (2012). *Winterbourne View Hospital: A Serious Case Review*. South Gloucestershire Safeguarding Adults Board. Available at:https://hosted.southglos.gov.uk/wv/report.pdf (accessed 10 May 2019).

Flynn, E. (2016). *Disabled Justice? Access to Justice and the UN Convention on the Rights of Persons with Disabilities*. Abingdon: Routledge.

Fraser, D. (2017). *The Evolution of the British Welfare State: A History of Social Policy since the Industrial Revolution* (5th edn). London: Red Globe Press.

Gallagher, H. G. (1989). *By Trust Betrayed: Patients, Physicians and the Licence to Kill in the Third Reich*. New York: Henry Holt & Co.

Garland-Thomson, R. (1997). *Extraordinary Bodies: Figuring Physical Disability in American Culture and Literature*. New York: Columbia University Press.

Goble, C. (2008). Institutional abuse. In J. Swain and S. French (eds), *Disability on Equal Terms*. London: Sage.

Goffman, E. (1961). *Asylums: Essays on the Social Situation of Mental Patients and Other Inmates*. London: Penguin.

Goffman, E. (1963). *Stigma: Notes on the Management of Spoiled Identity*. London: Penguin.

Goodley, D. (2011). *Disability Studies: An Interdisciplinary Introduction*. London: Sage.

Goodley, D. (2014). *Dis/ability Studies: Theorising Disablism and Ableism*. London: Routledge.

Gov.uk (2010). Definition of Disability under the Equality Act 2010. Available at: www.gov.uk/defini tion-of-disability-under-equality-act-2010

Gramsci, A. (2005). *Selections from the Prison Notebooks*. London: Lawrence & Wishart.

Haines, S. and Reubain, D. (eds) (2011). *Education, Disability and Social Policy*. Bristol: Policy Press.

Harris, J. and Roulstone, A. (2011). *Disability Policy and Professional Practice*. London: Sage.

Hasler, F. (2003). Philosophy of independent living. Independent Living Institute. Available at: www. independentliving.org/docs6/hasler2003.html (accessed 20th October 2019).

Hevey, D. (1992). *The Creatures that Time Forgot: Photography and Disability Imagery*. London: Routledge.

Hunt, P. (ed.) (1966). *Stigma: The Experience of Disability*. London. Geoffrey Chapman.

Illich, I. et al. (2005). *Disabling Professions*. London: Marion Boyars.

Imrie, R. (1996). *Disability and the City*. London: Sage.

Inclusion Scotland (2017) *The Social Model of Disability*. Available at: http://inclusionscotland.org/ socialmodelofdisability/ (accessed 20 October 2019).

Jack, R. (ed.) (1999). *Empowerment in Community Care*. London: Chapman & Hall.

Kaye, A., Jordan, H. and Baker, M. (2012). *The Tipping Point: The Human and Economic Costs of Cutting Disabled People's Support. The Hardest Hit Coalition*. Available at: https://thehardesthit.files.word press.com/2012/10/the_tipping_point_oct_2012.pdf.

Kerr, A. and Shakespeare, T. (2002). *Genetic Politics: From Eugenics to Genome*. Cheltenham: New Clarion Press.

Lukes, S. (2019). *Power: A Radical View* (2nd edn). London: Red Globe Press.

Marshall, T. H. (1950). *Citizenship and Social Class*. Cambridge: Cambridge University Press.

Morgan, H. (2014). User-led organisations: facilitating independent living? In J. Swain et al. (eds), *Disabling Barriers – Enabling Environments* (3rd edn). London: Sage.

Morris, J. (1991). *Pride Against Prejudice: Transforming Attitudes to Disability*. London: The Women's Press.

Morris, J. (2001). Impairment and disability: constructing an ethics of care that promotes human rights. *Hypatia* 16(4), 1–16.

Ofcom (2019). *Disabled Users Access to and Use of Communication Devices and Services*. Available at: www.ofcom.org.uk/__data/assets/pdf_file/0023/132962/Research-summary-all-disabilities.pdf (accessed 22 July 2019).

Oliver, M. (1990). *The Politics of Disablement*. London: Macmillan.

Oliver, M. and Barnes, C. (1998). *Disabled People and Social Policy: From Exclusion to Inclusion*. London: Addison Wesley Longman.

Oliver, M. and Barnes, C. (2012). *The New Politics of Disablement*. Basingstoke: Palgrave Macmillan.

Oliver, M., Sapey, B. and Thomas, P. (2012). *Social Work with Disabled People* (4th edn). Basingstoke: Palgrave Macmillan.

ONS (2019a). Dataset A08: Labour market status of disabled people. Available at: www.ons.gov.uk/ employmentandlabourmarket/peopleinwork/employmentandemployeetypes/datasets/labour marketstatusofdisabledpeoplea08 (accessed 20 October 2019).

ONS (2019b). Proportion of young people aged 16 to 24 years that are not in education, employment or training (NEET) by disability status, UK, 2014 to 2017. Available at: www.ons.gov.uk/employ mentandlabourmarket/peoplenotinwork/unemployment/adhocs/009631proportionofyoung peopleaged16to24yearsthatarenotineducationemploymentortrainingneetbydisabilitystatusuk- 2014to2017

Parsons, T. (1951) *The Social System*. Glencoe, IL: The Free Press.

Priestley, M. (1999). *Disability Politics and Community Care*. London: Jessica Kingsley Publishers.

Provan, B., Burchardt, T. and Suh, E. (2016). *No Place Like an Accessible Home: Quality of Life and Opportunity for Disabled People with Accessible Housing Needs*. London School of Economics, CASE Report 109. Available at: www.lse.ac.uk/business-and-consultancy/consulting/assets/documents/No-Place-Like-an-Accessible-Home.pdf (accessed 20 May 2019).

Roulstone, A. and Prideaux, S. (2012). *Understanding Disability Policy*. Bristol: Policy Press.

Safilios-Rothschild, C. (1970). *The Sociology and Social Psychology of Disability and Rehabilitation*. London: Random House.

Scope (2016). John, E., Thomas, G. and Touchet, A. (2019). *The Disability Price Tag 2019: Policy Report*. Scope. Available at: www.scope.org.uk/campaigns/extra-costs/disability-price-tag

Shakespeare, T. (2000). *Help: Imagining Welfare*. Birmingham: Venture Press.

Shakespeare, T. (2006). *Disability Rights and Wrongs*. London: Routledge.

Shakespeare, T. (2014). *Disability Rights and Wrongs Revisited*. London: Routledge.

Sheldon, A. (2014). The future of Disability Studies. In J. Swain, S. French, C. Barnes and C. Thomas (eds), *Disabling Barriers – Enabling Environments* (3rd edn) (pp. 326–331). London: Sage.

Shelter (2013). *What's Wrong with the Bedroom Tax? Briefing*. Available at: https://england.shelter.org.uk/__data/assets/pdf_file/0020/650630/Bedroom_tax_-_Shelter_briefing_March_2013.pdf (accessed 30 March 2019)

Shildrick, M. (2012). Critical Disability Studies: rethinking the conventions for the age of postmodernity. In N. Watson, A. Roulstone and C. Thomas (eds), *Routledge Handbook of Disability Studies* (pp. 30–41). London: Routledge.

Siegler, M. and Osmond, H. (1974). *Models of Madness: Models of Medicine*. New York: Macmillan.

Slee, R. (2011). How do we make inclusive education happen when exclusion is a political predisposition? *International Journal of Inclusive Education* 17(8), 895–907. https://doi.org/10.1080/1360311 16.2011.602534

Social Work Action Network (SWAN) (2009). The SWAN Constitution. Available at: https://socialwork future.org (accessed 28 April 2019)

Sparrow, A. (2016). Families and disabled people 'hit worse by rising homelessness', *The Guardian*. Available at: www.theguardian.com/society/2016/dec/23/families-and-disabled-people-hit-worse-by-rising-homelessness (accessed 2 April 2019).

Swain, J., French, S. and Cameron, C. (2003). *Controversial Issues in a Disabling Society*. Buckingham: Open University Press.

Swain, J., French, S., Barnes, C. and Thomas, C. (eds) (2014). *Disabling Barriers – Enabling Environments* (3rd edn). London: Sage.

Thomas, C. (1999). *Female Forms: Experiencing and Understanding Disability*. Buckingham: Open University Press.

Thomas, G. and Vaughan, M. (2004). *Inclusive Education: Readings and Reflections*. Maidenhead: Open University Press.

Tregaskis, C. (2002). Social Model Theory: the story so far... *Disability & Society* 17(4), 457–470. https://disability-studies.leeds.ac.uk/wp-content/uploads/sites/40/library/UPIAS-UPIAS.pdf

United Nations Committee on the Rights of Persons with Disabilities (2017). *Inquiry Concerning the United Kingdom of Great Britain and Northern Ireland Carried out by The Committee under Article 6 of the Optional Protocol to the Convention: Report of The Committee*. Available at: https://docu ments-dds-ny.un.org/doc/UNDOC/GEN/G17/326/14/PDF/G1732614.pdf?OpenElement (accessed 20 October 2019).

UPIAS (1976). Fundamental Principles of Disability. London: Union of the Physically Impaired.

Wadham, J. (2010). *Blackstone's Guide to the Equality Act 2010*. London: Blackstone Press Limited.

Warnock, M. and Norwich, B. (2010). *Special Education Needs: A New Look*. London: Continuum.

Wendell, S. (1996). *The Rejected Body: Feminist Philosophical Reflections on Disability*. Routledge: London.

Wood, R. (1991). Care of disabled people. In G. Dalley (ed.), *Disability and Social Policy*. London: Policy Studies Institute. Available at: www.psi.org.uk/publications/archivepdfs/Disability%20and%20 social/WOOD.pdf (accessed April 2019)

Woodin, S. (2014). Care: controlling and personalising budgets. In J. Swain et al. (eds), *Disabling Barriers – Enabling Environments* (3rd edn). London: Sage.

World Health Organization (2011) *World Report on Disability*. Available at: www.who.int/disabilities/ world_report/2011/report.pdf

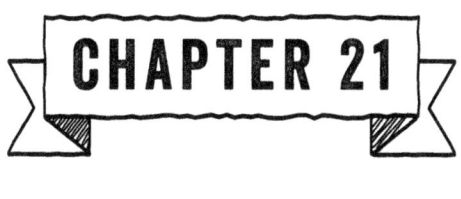

CHAPTER 21

HEALTH INEQUALITIES

Benny Goodman

OVERVIEW

It is clear to anyone who cares to look that we live in very unequal societies. There is inequality in the distribution of wealth and of income, of access to health services, of access to education, food, water and sanitation. These social inequalities are linked to unequal health outcomes, one of the most striking of which is the difference in mortality rates within and between countries. These are the 'wider determinants of health', which impact on life expectancy and the number of years of good health enjoyed by different groups in society. This chapter aims to introduce the reader to the concept of health inequalities, outlining some of the causes, providing an overview of explanations and addressing a theory of human action towards health.

LEARNING OUTCOMES

By the end of this chapter you will be able to:

- Identify key indicators that outline health inequalities
- Describe the theory of structured agency and how that contributes to undertaking inequalities in health
- Discuss the options for taking action on the wider determinants of health

INTRODUCTION

Rudolph Virchow in 1848 argued that: 'medicine is a social science and politics is nothing more than medicine on a grand scale'. Friedrich Engels wrote in 1848:

When society places hundreds of proletarians in such a position that they inevitably meet a too early and an unnatural death, one which is quite as much a death by violence as that by the sword or bullet, its deed is murder just as surely as the deed of the single individual.

These two quotes imply that health inequalities and their social causes have been of concern for a very long time. In 1980 the Black Report also drew attention to material conditions and health outcomes, followed by both the Acheson Report (1998) and the World Health Organization's Commission on the Social Determinants of Health (2005). In 2010, 'Fair Society, Healthy Lives' (The Marmot Review) was published. Nearly ten years later its message remains relevant, only the detail has changed. We know enough already about what determines health and we have a mass of data describing inequalities in both access to health services and of health outcomes. Universal health care is still a global goal not yet achieved.

What we do not have is an agreed explanation of, or theory about, why we continue to see health inequalities. However, there are global outcomes agreed at international level such as the globalgoals.org which sets out 17 sustainability development goals to address the continuing misery experienced daily by the global 'bottom billion' in the poorest level 1 income level of under $2 per day (Rosling et al., 2018).

ROSLING'S INCOME LEVELS

Hans Rosling, professor of public health, argues that the labels 'developed and developing or rich/poor' countries are outdated and unhelpful. Describing the United States as 'rich or developed' obscures the income levels experienced within it. He uses four income levels instead to better describe how people's lives can change gradually with money:

Income per person in dollars per day adjusted for price differences:

> Level 1. Under $2
>
> Level 2. $2–$8
>
> Level 3. $8–$32
>
> Level 4. Above $32

Note that these levels completely obscure the 0.01 per cent of billionaires and their activities.

Note that this is especially relevant for those who link material conditions of life with health outcomes.

In the United Kingdom life expectancy (LE) in the poorest areas are on average ten years less than in the most affluent (2016 ONS figures). Male LE in Kensington was 83.4 while in Glasgow it was 73.4. The Office for National Statistics publishes annual 'Health State Life Expectancies' where these figures can be found. The World Health Organization reports that the risk of a child dying before getting to five is highest in the African region (74 per 1000 live births), which is eight times higher than the European region (9 per 1000 live births). Figures can be found in the Global Health Observatory (GHO) data published by the WHO.

This chapter briefly points to some of the data on health inequalities, but then addresses the 'why' question, by illuminating contested explanations for inequality before finally providing a theory of human action towards health that more adequately addresses causal mechanisms.

ACTIVITY 21.1

Go to YouTube and watch Michael Marmot on 'Close the Health Gap' discussing the social determinants of health.

WHAT DO WE MEAN BY HEALTH INEQUALITIES?

Health inequalities are the *unjust* and *avoidable* differences in people's health across the population and between specific population groups, such as ethnicity, gender and class. Health inequalities are also about unequal access to health services.

Because they are avoidable, and not a result of chance, they become an issue of social justice and hence become political. The concept of 'social justice' is dealt with in Chapter 19. Health and health inequalities are largely socially and politically determined as well as partly arising out of differences in biology. The facts of the wider (social, political, economic and environmental) determinants of health makes this field of enquiry contested and political with a very basic division arising over explanations for inequalities and thus for policy options. The division is around what is seen as the proper role of the state and transnational bodies such as the World Health Organization on the one hand and of individual responsibility for health on the other. Should people be left free to eat sugar or should governments tax it?

The very idea of 'social justice' itself is highly charged and value laden in which those who now advocate for local, national and international policy interventions are at times labelled 'social justice warriors' in a pejorative sense (Ohlheiser, 2015).

ACTIVITY 21.2

'**Marmot Indicators**' are indicators of the social determinants of health, health outcomes and social inequality. You can find them here: https://fingertips.phe.org.uk/profile/wider-determinants and include well-known indicators such as 'life expectancy at birth'.

'Health inequality' can refer to differences between social groups in specific and measurable empirical outcomes such as 'life expectancy' or 'disability free life years', or to epidemiological data on specific diseases such as diabetes. It can also refer to unequal access and use of health

Table 21.1 GPs per patient in 2018 per deprivation area

Least Deprived	Most Deprived
53 GPs per 100,000	47 GPs per 100.000
1 GP per 1869	1 GP per 2125
1 in 10 unable to get GP appointment	1 in 7 unable to get GP appointment

Source: Nuffield Trust (2018).

services such as GP practices where, for example, some of the most deprived socio-economic areas of the country also have the least amount of GPs per patient.

As for life expectancy in the UK, the Office for National Statistics (ONS) reported (2018):

- In England, the least deprived males at birth in 2014 to 2016 could expect to live almost a decade longer than the most deprived (9.3 years), while for females the gap was 7.4 years.
- In 2014 to 2016, the least deprived males and females at birth in Wales could expect to live 8.9 years and 7.3 years more than the most deprived, respectively.
- Large gaps in longevity by level of deprivation exposure persisted at age 65 years in England and Wales; the gap for men exceeded 4.7 years and the gap for women exceeded 4.6 years.
- The gap in healthy life expectancy at birth exceeded 18 years for both males and females in England whereas in Wales, it surpassed 17 years for both males and females.
- There were increases in the socio-economic inequality in male and female life expectancy at birth and at age 65 years between 2011 to 2013 and 2014 to 2016 in both England and Wales; however, the increases were only statistically significant in England.

NHS Scotland (2019) report:

- In the most affluent areas of Scotland, men experience 23.8 more years of good health and women experience 22.6 more years compared to the most deprived areas.
- The life expectancy of people with learning disabilities is substantially shorter than the Scottish average.
- Gender-based violence is experienced unequally, with 17 per cent of women and 7 per cent of men having experienced the use of force from a partner or ex-partner at some point in their lives.

ACTIVITY 21.3

- Access Scotland's 'Inequality Briefing' for a more detailed discussion: www. healthscotland.scot/publications/health-inequalities-what-are-they-and-how-do-we-reduce-them
- Go to the BBC News site and watch 'Dying Young in Stockton – England's Most Unequal Town': www.bbc.co.uk/news/health-44985650. Note what explanation is made for the ill health discussed.
- See also BBC *Panorama* 'Get Rich or Die Young': www.bbc.co.uk/programmes/b0bdm7zm

---

The differences hold not only in the UK of course but globally. There is a wealth of data describing the differences (Dorling, 2013, Wilkinson and Pickett, 2010) such as the Global Health Observatory, and so it is sufficient in this chapter to point to the myriad resources you can access to understand the detail.

DATA ON HEALTH INEQUALITIES

1   The World Bank: Health: www.worldbank.org/en/topic/health/overview
2   World Health Organization: ten facts about health inequities and their causes: www.who.int/features/factfiles/health_inequities/en/
3   World Health Organization. Tracking universal health coverage: 2017 Global Monitoring report: www.who.int/healthinfo/universal_health_coverage/report/2017/en/
4   *The Lancet*. The health inequalities and ill health of children in the UK. February 2017: www.thelancet.com/journals/lancet/article/PIIS0140-6736(17)30264-7/fulltext
5   The King's Fund. Health Inequalities: www.kingsfund.org.uk/topics/health-inequalities
6   Gapminder.org: www.gapminder.org
7   Public Health England. Health Profile for England (2018): www.gov.uk/government/publications/health-profile-for-england-2018. Data exists of course for other UK countries – see their Public Health Observatories.

*The data changes each year and so you will need to keep accessing the above organisations.

To understand why there are these differences, there is a need to consider what population and individual health is based upon: a) biology; b) the provision of health services; c) individual behaviour; d) the wider determinants of health. The latter is the next focus of attention. This is clearly outlined by Public Health England in the 'Health Profile for England 2018', Chapter 6 'Wider Determinants of Health. Note especially the work of Dahlgrend and Whitehead's model of the main determinants of health in that chapter. One's biology is of course a determinant of health and for the individual can be the most pertinent; however, the data suggests the wider determinants play a larger part in unequal health outcomes than does biology or even health services (WHO, 2008).

ACTIVITY 21.4   RESEARCH AND EVIDENCE-BASED PRACTICE

What are the key health inequalities indicators for your local area as published by Public Health England's 'Local Authority Health Profiles'?

1   Go to https://fingertips.phe.org.uk/profile/health-profiles
2   Enter 'Blackpool' and then 'Kensington and Chelsea' in the search box
3   Download the two reports

Comparing the two local authorities, what is the difference between:

a   Male life expectancy;
b   Female life expectancy; and
c   The under-75 all-cause mortality rate?

Check the end of the chapter for an answer to this activity.

THE WIDER DETERMINANTS OF HEALTH

The World Health Organization, noting 'social gradients' in health (WHO, 2008) and persistent inequities, set up a Commission on Social Determinants of Health (CSDH) in 2005.

The Commission argued:

> The social determinants of health are the conditions in which people are born, grow, live, work and age, including the health system. *These circumstances are shaped by the distribution of money, power and resources at global, national and local levels*, which are themselves influenced by policy choices. The social determinants of health are mostly responsible for health inequities – the unfair and avoidable differences in health status seen within and between countries. (My emphasis).

> *Source*: www.who.int/social_determinants/en/

The CSDH takes a *holistic* view of the determinants of health. It argues that the unequal distribution of power, resources, wealth, income and services across the globe have a direct effect on the health of the poor and result in a social gradient in health within countries and between countries. In addition, inequities in health are not natural or inevitable; they are a result of economic, political and policy failures.

The CSDH also argues that the global community can put this right but it will take urgent and sustained action, globally, nationally and locally.

Traditionally, society has looked to the health sector to deal with its concerns about health and disease. Unequal access to health services is one of the determinants of health. However, the high burden of illness responsible for premature loss of life arises because of the conditions in which people are born, grow, live, work and age.

Therefore, action on the social determinants of health must involve the whole of government, civil society and local communities, business, global forums and international agencies. The ministers of health and national departments of health are also critical to global change.

The social determinants of health approach thus challenges the notion that health is the sole domain of the NHS and brings it squarely into the arena of local government and other agencies. For example, the *Foresight Report* (Butland et al., 2007) argues that obesity cannot be addressed by the NHS alone. The report makes clear that the overwhelming scientific consensus is that 'modern life' is a major driver of obesity. Obesity is an indicator of socio-economic inequality (Bambra et al., 2013).

Barton and Grant's (2006) health map and Horton et al.'s (2014) 'Planetary Health' paradigm point to climate change, biodiversity and global ecosystems as the ultimate determinants of health and even these factors impact unequally across the globe (Dupar, 2018; Islam and Winkel, 2017).

Buck (2018) argues that health services such as the NHS have a crucial role in reducing health inequalities even though it is third after the wider determinants and behaviour in affecting health. He suggests that 10–20 per cent of health outcomes are directly determined by the NHS. He then lists eight action points for the NHS to address health inequalities. At the end of this chapter there is an activity for you to undertake to understand and take forward his arguments.

Note that it is the role of government that is often contentious. Governments are criticised for doing too much as well as doing too little. The reasons why are outlined below.

EXPLANATIONS

Explanations given for inequalities in health can be grouped as follows:

- **Hereditarian** explanations: everyone has a biologically determined natural capacity, thus little can be done (an individualist explanation).
- **Behavioural** explanations: the lifestyle choices of individuals are the cause; the answer is education (or 'nudges' or punishment).
- **Environmental** explanations: the cause is a person's social position and material deprivation, so the answer is structural.

The wider determinants of health approach accepts all three as causally efficacious for health but emphasises the social, political and environmental. This is a live issue, because the solutions to inequalities in health depend on why you think they exist in the first place. If you believe in the primacy of individual behaviour, you will seek policies that focus on individual behaviour change and education, such as 'Change4Life'.

Underlying the explanations are what are known as 'discourses'. These are mental conceptions about the nature of human action and existence, and involves often unexamined or taken for granted personal theories, epistemologies, ontologies, values and philosophies.

Three competing discourses (Table 21.2) for explaining inequalities (Carlisle, 2001) can be remembered using the mnemonics RED, SID and MUD:

- **Red**istribution
- **S**ocial **I**ntegrationist
- **M**oral **U**nderclass

Table 21.2 Competing discourses to explain health inequalities

Discourse	Source of problem is	Explanatory level	Causal mechanism	Solution level	Action level
RED	The concentration of resources in higher socio-economic (SE) groups	Social structure (SS), of class primarily	Inequitable social distribution of resources	Redistribute resources downwards	Socio-economic policy by international and national governance
SID	Social polarisation of SE groups	Interaction between the individual and their SS – 'status anxiety'	Relative inequality and social stress in disadvantaged groups	Reduce gap and increase social integration	Community
MUD	The culture and behaviour of the lower SE groups themselves	Individual experiences and their chosen actions, e.g. to smoke	Narrow resource margins, individual 'bad' behaviour	Help poor people develop their coping strategies – to take responsibility	Individual – must change attitudes and behaviour via education

Wilkinson and Pickett's 'The Spirit Level' (2010) focused on 'Inequality' itself as a causal mechanism to explain inequalities in health outcomes. They argue that countries that are equal almost always do better than unequal countries on a range of indicators such as life expectancy and even rates of incarceration. According to the Equality Trust:

The most plausible explanation for *income inequality's* apparent effect on health and social problems is 'status anxiety'. Income inequality is harmful because it places people in a steep hierarchy that increases status competition and causes stress, which in turn leads to poor health and other negative outcomes. There is little consensus on how these mechanisms, particularly 'status anxiety,' work in practice, given different people's different reference groups, their knowledge (or lack of knowledge) about social stratification and the complex nature of 'status' and self-esteem. Other possible mechanisms put forward include stress in the womb and early life and the socioeconomic status of your parents.

* This explanation draws from the social integrationist discourse (SID):

Thus there is ongoing debate about the exact causes of health inequalities and the mechanisms involved. Some of these debates are ideologically driven, such as the political ideology of right-wing libertarianism that views government interference as force, ineffective or dangerous. Some debates neglect the evidence, or are based in limited understanding of social and psychological theory/research. Some exclude considering that there might be such a thing as society (social ontology) that provides the context for individual behaviour (Scambler, 2018), preferring instead to think that there are only individuals making choices out of free will. 'Positivism' is prone to leading health practitioners, and others, to perhaps confuse 'cause and correlation' so that one variable in the epidemiological data, such as life expectancy, correlates with another variable such as socio economic status as measured by the NS SEC, but could be seen as causal, but without examining the *underlying mechanisms that might be at play* for this link. The above is covered in detail in Scambler (2018) which is highly recommended for a more detailed discussion of theory.

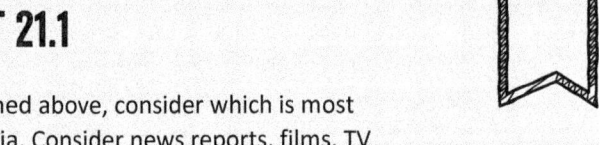

PAUSE FOR THOUGHT 21.1

Of the three 'discourses' outlined above, consider which is most commonly invoked in the media. Consider news reports, films, TV and radio programmes, especially 'phone in' shows. Think about the headlines printed by the UK's newspapers especially since 2010.

THEORY

Humans, I have contended elsewhere, are simultaneously the products of biological, psychological and social mechanisms whilst retaining their agency. Acknowledgement must be made also of the sometimes mundane and sometimes dramatic interruptions of contingency. Thus, humans can be said to be biologically, psychologically and socially 'structured' without being structurally determined. (Scambler, 2013).

This is a theory of 'structured' human agency which tries to explain *why* we do *what* we do: smoke, drink alcohol, eat too much, be sedentary or even drive recklessly. We need a theory of human agency to assist in understanding the differentials in health outcomes and to help with deciding which discourse has the most explanatory power. It draws heavily from the 'Redistribution and Social Integrationist discourses' while avoiding the moralising, the victim blaming, the shaming and stigmatising that often explicitly arises from the 'moral underclass discourse' which focuses mostly on individualistic/behaviourist explanations manifest in the oft repeated phrase 'take responsibility for health'.

By 'contingency', I think Scambler refers to the existence of random, unpredictable events and developments that impact upon our exercise of agency. An example is the explosion of social media into our lives, the effects of which on our choices to act we are yet to fully understand. Current developments such as mapping the human genome or the development of artificial intelligence may well introduce contingency and could have enormous effects on human health and well-being.

STRUCTURED AGENCY

The theory of structured agency rests upon three propositions:

1 **Ontological realism**: There exists both a *natural* world and a *social* world *independent* of our knowledge of them. There *is* such a thing as society in which powerful global actors take decisions that affect the health of billions. Society pre-dates us and 'exists' whether we believe it does or not.
2 **Epistemological relativism**: what we can know is unavoidably a function of time and place. This knowledge is also fallible and is 'socially constructed' by us in our everyday lives. For example, many of those who believe that the moral underclass is responsible for the ills they experience, do so based in a knowledge that has been created within the time and place(s) of their lives. Health secretaries who urge the 'skivers' to take responsibility for health understand the determinants of health very differently from public health academics.
3 **Judgemental rationality**: Despite knowledge being socially constructed by our position in time and place, we can decide between alternative theories and discourses, for example about poverty and health, on rationally compelling grounds, if we so wish to do so. It remains possible for health care professionals to move beyond individualistic biomedical frames of reference or overly simplistic positivist epidemiology which describes patterns but does not explain them.

In Archer's 'trilogy' (2000, 2003, 2012), we are asked to think about human agency in the context of social *structure* and *culture* and how reflexivity (our inner conversations) mediates the relationship between objective social conditions and human agency. Archer here rejects completely the notion that there is no such thing as society existing 'outside' of individual human actors, and thus Archer is rooted in 'ontological realism'.

However, it is arguable that a dominant discourse around health outcomes does just that, in focusing on the individual and expecting behaviour change as the main thrust for policy, it downplays the role of powerful social actors and the 'behind our backs' social and political mechanisms at play. The Grenfell Tower fire is an extreme example of how 'behind our backs' decisions result in death, and underpins arguments that socio-economic, e.g. austerity, policies can kill (Stuckler and Basu, 2013) through mechanisms of institutional and structural violence (Cooper and Whyte, 2017). Try exercising agency for better health while living in a fire trap.

A 'behind our backs' (unseen or unacknowledged) mechanism is our social class position as it affects our daily decisions whether we acknowledge it or not. For example, we smoke because we like it, because our friends do, because we can't stop, we have a fatalistic attitude to life, because we underestimate the risk, because relatives smoked and died at an old age. We see these factors and we acknowledge them. We don't see class, we don't invoke 'social class' as a reason, despite the evidence that smoking is more common if we earn less than £10,000 or are looking for work. Note that around one in four in routine and manual occupations smoke compared to one in ten in managerial and professional occupations according to the ONS's adult smoking in the UK 2018 data.

The 'moral underclass discourse' is rooted in a view of human agency that separates out the individual from structures and cultures and expects rational action – the weighing up of the pros and cons of action. This is the Enlightenment's 'man of modernity' – the utility maximising rational actor – and while it may seem a very crude outline of the theory of human action that perhaps no one today adheres to, I would argue it implicitly underpins many a policy decision and media exhortation to people to 'take responsibility'.

Health professionals will hear echoes of this 'man's' voice when they hear such statements as 'only the individual should and can take responsibility for health', 'there is no such thing as society, just individuals and families' and rational injunctions to 'Just say No', 'I stopped smoking, so can you'. The uncritical acceptance of the 'sovereign individual' lays the foundation for victim blaming and shaming, for if there is no social structure or culture what else is there to blame for their poverty and health inequalities except the behaviour of the 'moral underclass' themselves? This view argues that we stand alone, making foolish choices about smoking, food, exercise and alcohol. This is just 'common sense'. The actions of powerful global actors who have a vested interest in making profits rather than in public health (Freudenberg, 2014) are ignored or dismissed.

As for the role of personal agency in the adoption of unhealthy behaviours, I do not erase the primacy of human action and decision-making. However, we must refer to the context, the culture and structures in which people live their lives. I contend that social structures, for example of class, ethnicity, gender and cultures, *do* have 'causal' mechanisms (ontological realism) but we engage reflexivity, and perhaps some judgemental rationality, to choose a course of action.

We retain our agency but not in the circumstances of our own choosing.

Some will exercise their agency to resist the drift towards adopting sedentary lifestyles, others will be not able to do so quite so easily. Biological, psychological and social mechanisms impact on our decision-making but we might still be able to exercise our 'judgemental rationality'. I suggest, however, that people who are poorly paid, stressed, demoralised, devalued, stigmatised, shamed and ill-educated might find it harder to do so as the knowledge they draw upon (epistemic relativism) may be inadequate and the social, economic and political pressures they face (their 'ontological realism') may be too high. Too many people may be what Archer refers to as 'fractured reflexives' who find it difficult to make sense of their experiences or think about healthy routes out of poverty and distress.

PAUSE FOR THOUGHT 21.2

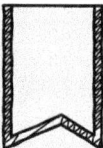

If our agency is highly structured, but not of course 'determined', think about how your life and your choices would differ if you had experienced a different culture and social structure from the one in which you were brought up. You did not choose your time and place of birth, neither did you choose who your parents would be, how healthy they were, where you lived, whether you were blessed to be born without any biological impediments, whether you experienced childhood trauma or abuse. You only need to compare yourself with your parents or grandparents, let alone a different ethnicity or class, to begin to see how the decision to smoke, drink alcohol or undertake cosmetic surgery might have been very different. What seems like decisions taken out of free will, rationally, are actually highly structured and mediated by culture as well as your reflexivity (your inner deliberations).

SCAMBLER'S 'GREEDY BASTARDS HYPOTHESIS'

'This asserted that health inequalities in Britain were first and foremost an unintended consequence of the "strategic" behaviours at the core of the country's capitalist-executive and power elite' (Scambler, 2012). These strategic behaviours may also be *behind our backs mechanisms* causing ill health.

Ill health and death result in part, and both directly and indirectly, from decision-making that takes place in boardrooms, council chambers, cabinet meetings and at country clubs. The evidence for this assertion derives from examining the results of Austerity policies on public health outcomes especially since 2010 (Stuckler and Basu, 2013). Examples such as the Volkswagen emissions scandal and the continuing issue of respiratory disease and death linked to air pollution from diesel particulates also provide support for the hypothesis.

Scambler here points to the everyday business of 'business' and 'politics' that results in flammable cladding on buildings; reduction in services for children; social care issues for older people and lack of provision for those with mental health problems; poor and expensive housing; climate change; plastic pollution in the oceans; inaccessible and expensive health care; deforestation; ocean acidification; biodiversity loss; species extinctions; oil spills and other pollutant externalities – that is the 'wider determinants of health'. These together are injurious to health and in many cases injure the poorer members of society disproportionally.

Scambler implies that 'business as usual' is primarily aimed at capital accumulation rather than sustainable development and poverty reduction, despite the protestations of enlightened business leaders at places such as the World Economic Forum. It is of course easy to see how some businesses are taking up these challenges and that in 2019 some politicians are making overt speeches about such issues as climate change. However, counter-examples do not necessarily negate the overall hypothesis as it has operated over the past 50 years.

If taken seriously, this hypothesis would direct the attention of public health workers onto the activities of certain powerful groups, the 0.01 per cent, as both the CSDH and Ottersen et al. (2014) imply. The CSDH argue: 'The social determinants of health are the conditions in which people are born, grow, live, work and age. These circumstances are shaped by the distribution of money, power and resources at global, national and local levels', and who else is largely responsible for that 'global distribution of money, power and resources', if it is not Scambler's GBs? Ottersen et al. argue for the need for 'Global Governance for Health'. They accept that the health sector has a crucial role in addressing health inequalities, yet efforts often come into conflict with 'powerful global actors in pursuit of other interests such as protection of national security, safeguarding of sovereignty, or economic goals' (such as capital accumulation).

When Scambler talks about 'social mechanisms', as well as the biological and psychological, that are partly causal for human action, this is an example of what is meant. Agency is structured by much wider socio-economic and political forces at work.

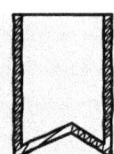

PAUSE FOR THOUGHT 21.3

Dawn Foster wrote in the *Guardian* on 14 May 2019: 'We're deluged with images of "beauty", no wonder many of us feel so bad … one company has bombarded me with adverts offering interest free credit for several procedures.' See: www.theguardian.com/commentisfree/2019/may/13/images-beauty-feel-bad-adverts-social-media. Read this article and consider her points about social media, e.g. Instagram.

A young woman's decision to have botox, dermal fillers or other cosmetic procedures is an example of structured agency. What are the social structures in place, what is the cultural milieu and who profits from her actions? To what degree do you think this is a fully thought through rational action aimed at 'maximising utility'? What does the data say about eating disorders, body dysmorphia and poor body image?

Is this an example of an inequality in health based on age/gender?

CONCLUSION

The facts of health inequalities are well known and published. The facts of social inequalities are also very well documented and are of contemporary concern for many. The links between the two are known to those who study the field and is the focus of global governance initiatives to address them. Journals such as *The Lancet*, organisations such as the WHO and academics such as Kate Pickett and Richard Wilkinson, Danny Dorling and Michael Marmot have produced a mass of data and have provided tentative explanations rooted in epidemiological data. Graham Scambler provides a hypothesis based on his argument that we need a theory of causal mechanisms to explain the relationship between the variables of socio-economic position and unequal health outcomes described by Marmot et al. His theory links an understanding of wider determinants of health with the actions of a core cabal of powerful social and political actors who take decisions with often unintended consequences injurious to the health of millions. Using the work of Margaret Archer, Scambler provides a theory of human agency that accounts for the interplay of social structures, cultures and human agency. This perspective renders totally inadequate the theorising of those who adhere to the 'moral underclass' discourse; that is those who can only see education and individual behaviour change policy as efficacious for addressing the lifestyles of people. This ignores the fact that some people are without strong positive material, psychological, social, spatial, cultural, symbolic or biological health assets that assist in lifestyle changes and responses to education.

Yet, the issue remains a contentious one. The facts speak for themselves but what the proper course of action should be is quite another. If the arguments over smoking, diet, drug and alcohol use (and even climate change) are unpicked, you may see that there are those who wish to root the cause of the behaviour firmly within the individual and thus they seek solutions from within those individuals. Many in this camp abhor state intervention, using terms like 'nanny state' or fears about liberty and personal choice being curtailed. They adhere to an inadequate theory of humanity, discounting society, culture or power. On the other hand there are many who ask us to examine the role of powerful individuals, groups and corporate actors whose ordinary daily business results in death, lower life expectancy and increased morbidity for certain groups of people. Exhorting young women not to be affected by body image issues arising in association with social media, telling poorly paid and overworked people in precarious employment to save more for their futures or to give up smoking, or expecting the population to avoid en masse high calorie, sweet, enjoyable and readily available food is pie in the sky. The odds are stacked against many of us. It is in the interests of others that we continue to buy products and services that are unhealthy if taken in quantity. Exercising agency for better health in the social and cultural circumstances in which we find ourselves is a full-time job that millions of us fail at daily in the UK as illustrated in indicators such as obesity rates and the differentials in life expectancy. Conclusively, unequal social conditions make unequal health outcomes inevitable.

ACTIVITY 21.5   TEST YOURSELF

1   Define the 'social determinants of health'.
2   How can Scambler's theory of structured agency be applied to actions on obesity?
3   What inequalities in health can you identify that are based on a) social class, b) ethnicity, c) gender, d) sexual orientation, e) mental health?

GO FURTHER ACTIVITY

Buck (2018) outlines an eight-point plan for the NHS to address inequalities in health.

Discuss these with colleagues and consider what your actions could be in your clinical area.

Go to the King's Fund site: search for 'Health Inequalities: the NHS plan needs to take more responsibility': www.kingsfund.org.uk/blog/2018/09/health-inequalities-nhs-plan-needs-take-more-responsibility

ANSWERS TO CHAPTER 21 ACTIVITIES

———— Activity 21.4: Answers

What are some health inequalities indicators for your local area as published by Public Health England's 'Local Authority Health Profiles'?

1   Go to https://fingertips.phe.org.uk/profile/health-profiles
2   Enter 'Blackpool' and then 'Kensington and Chelsea' in the search box.
3   Download the two reports.

What is the difference in a) male life expectancy b) female life expectancy and c) the under 75 all-cause mortality rate for both Local Authorities?

———— Blackpool	Kensington and Chelsea
a Male: 74.2	Male: 83.7
b Female: 79.5	Female: 86.4
c Under 75: 545.7	Under 75: 241.2

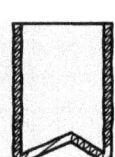

PAUSE FOR THOUGHT 21.1

There is no definitive answer to this, but consider the difference in approach in films such as Ken Loach's 'I Daniel Blake' (2016) and 'Sorry We Missed You' (2019) to the Front page headlines of Tabloid newspapers regarding poverty and responsibility for health.

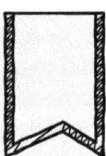

PAUSE FOR THOUGHT 21.2

There is no definitive answers to this as it requires you to think about your own personal circumstances and the decisions you could and could not make.

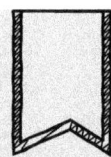

PAUSE FOR THOUGHT 21.3

Social structures and culture: Just one aspect of social structure is the gendered nature and positioning of women in society for certain functions and roles. Although women enjoy access to occupations and roles which once were the preserve of men, there is a continued emphasis on beauty and attractiveness for young women.

Both the fashion industry and social media platforms such as Instagram support and encourage young women to engage in displays of their bodies and promote certain ideals of beauty. The reach of media portrayal of beauty and attractiveness is pervasive in many cultures putting pressure on even schoolgirls to conform to new ideals of feminine attractiveness. The resultant pressure to conform, to be part of the 'in group', can lead to any number of adaptive and maladaptive coping mechanisms. However, the phenomenon cannot simply be reduced to media pressure alone. See the following further reading:

Brown, Z. and Tiggemann, M. (2016). Attractive celebrity and peer images on Instagram: effect on women's mood and body image. *Body Image* 19, 37–43.

Maltby, J., Giles, D., Barber, L. and McCutcheon, L. (2005). Intense-personal celebrity worship and body image: evidence of a link among female adolescents. *British Journal of Health Psychology* 10, 17–32.

Mental Health Foundation (2019). Body Image – Executive Summary. Available at: www.mentalhealth.org.uk/publications/body-image-report/exec-summary (accessed 15 May 2019)

Orbach, S. (1978). *Fat is a Feminist Issue.* London: Arrow Books.

Polivy, J. and Herman, P. (2004). Sociocultural idealisation of thin female body shapes: an introduction to the special issue on body image and eating disorders. *Journal of Clinical Psychology* 23(1), 1–6.

Tiggemann, M. and Slater, A. (2013). NetGirls: the internet, Facebook, and body image concern in adolescent girls. *International Journal of Eating Disorders* 46(6), 630–633.

Wolf, N. (1990). *The Beauty Myth. How Images of Beauty Are Used Against Women.* London: Chatto & Windus.

FURTHER READING

BOOKS

Bartley, M. (2017). *Health Inequality: An Introduction to Theories, Concepts and Methods* (2nd edn). Cambridge: Polity Press. By examining influences of social class, income, culture and wealth as well as gender, ethnicity and other factors in identity, this accessible book provides a key to understanding the major theories and explanations of what lies behind inequality in health.

Scambler, G. (2018). *Sociology, Health and the Fractured Society*. London: Routledge. An important text outlining the philosophical and theoretical basis analysing health inequalities.

Goodman, B. (2019). Chapter 4: Inequalities, health outcomes and nursing practice. In *Psychology and Sociology in Nursing* (3rd edn). London: Sage. Discusses in more detail some of the theory underpinning human action and the notion of discourses. Although aimed at undergraduate nurses, it is applicable for all health care professionals.

JOURNALS

Carlisle, S. (2001). Inequalities in health: contested explanations, shifting discourses and ambiguous policies. *Critical Public Health* 11(3), 267–281.

Scambler, G. (2019). Dimensions of vulnerability salient for health: a sociological approach. *Society, Health and Vulnerability* 10.

Scambler, G. (2019). Sociology, social class, health inequalities, and the avoidance of 'classism'. *Frontiers in Sociology*, 5 July: https://doi.org/10.3389/fsoc.2019.00056

WEBSITES

Public Health England (2018). Health Profile for England 2018. Chapter 5: Inequalities in health. www.gov.uk/government/publications/health-profile-for-england-2018/chapter-5-inequalities-in-health. Although using data for England, this resource provides a wealth of information explaining the concept while illustrating the scale of the issue.

The Equality Trust. For a wealth of information in social inequality and indicators: www.equalitytrust.org.uk.

WHO: World Health Organization Social Determinants of Health: www.who.int/social_determinants/en. A comprehensive resource packed with data and explaining the concept.

REFERENCES

Archer, M. (2000). *Being Human: The Problem of Agency*. Cambridge: Cambridge University Press.

Archer, M. (2003). *Structure, Agency and the Inner Conversation*. Cambridge: Cambridge University Press.

Archer, M. (2012). *The Reflexive Imperative in Late Modernity*. Cambridge: Cambridge University Press.

Bambra, C., Hiller, F., Moore et al. (2013). Tackling inequalities in obesity: a protocol for a systematic review of the effectiveness of public health interventions at reducing socioeconomic inequalities in obesity on adults. *Systematic Reviews* 2(27).

Barton, H. and Grant, M. (2006) A health map for the local human habitat. *Journal of the Royal Society for the Promotion of Public Health* 126(6), 252–261.

Buck, D. (2018). *Health Inequalities: The NHS Plan Needs to Take More Responsibility*. The King's Fund, 27 September. Available at: www.kingsfund.org (accessed 14 May 2019)

Butland, B., Jebb, S., Kopelman, P et al. (2007) Foresight. Tackling Obesities Future Choices. Available at: www.gov.uk/government/publications/reducing-obesity-future-choices (accessed 20 October 2019)

Carlisle, S. (2001). Inequalities in health: contested explanations, shifting discourses and ambiguous policies. *Critical Public Health* 11(3), 267–281.

Cooper, V. and Whyte, D. (2017). *The Violence of Austerity*. London: Pluto Books.

Dorling, D. (2013). *Unequal Health: The Scandal of Our Times*. Bristol: Bristol University Press.

Dupar, M. (2018). Opinion: IPCC Special report on 1.5.C highlights challenge to achieve climate stability and end poverty. 8 October. Available at: www.cdkn.org (accessed 14 May 2019)

Freudenberg, N. (2014). *Lethal But Legal: Corporations, Consumption and Protecting Public Health*. New York: Oxford University Press.

Horton, R., Beaglehole, R., Bonita, R. et al. (2014). From public to planetary health: a manifesto. *The Lancet* 383(9920). https://doi.org/10.1016/S0140-6736(14)60409-8

Islam, S. and Winkel, J. (2017). *Climate Change and Social Inequality*. United Nations. DESA working paper No. 152. ST/ESA/2017/DWP/152 October.

Marmot, M. (2016). *The Health Gap: The Challenge of an Unequal World*. London: Bloomsbury.

NHS Scotland (2019). What are health inequalities? Available at: www.healthscotland.scot/health-inequalities/what-are-health-inequalities (accessed 14 May 2019)

Nuffield Trust (2018). Poor areas left behind on standards of GP care, research reveals. Available at: www.nuffieldtrust.org.uk/news-item/poor-areas-left-behind-on-standards-of-gp-care-research-reveals (accessed 15 May 2019)

Office for National Statistics (2018). Health state life expectancies by national deprivation deciles, England and Wales: 2014 to 2016. 1 March. Available at: www.ons.gov.uk/ (accessed 14 May 2019)

Ohlheiser, A. (2015). Why 'social justice warrior,' a Gamergate insult, is now a dictionary entry. *The Washington Post*, 7 October.

Ottersen, O., Dasgupta, J. and Blouin, C. (2014). The political origins of health inequity: prospects for change. *The Lancet* 383(9917), 630–637.

Rosling, H, Rosling, O. and Rosling, A. (2018). *Factfulness: 10 Reasons Why Were Wrong about the World*. London: Hodder & Stoughton.

Scambler, G. (2012). GBH: greedy bastards and health inequalities. 4 November. Available at: www.grahamscambler.wordpress.com (accessed 14 May 2019)

Scambler, G. (2013). Resistance in Unjust Times: Archer, Structured Agency and the Sociology of Health Inequalities, *Sociology*. 47(1):142–156.

Scambler, G. (2018). *Sociology, Health and the Fractured Society*. London: Routledge.

Stuckler, D. and Basu, S. (2013) *The Body Economic – Why Austerity Kills: Recessions, Budget Battles and the Politics of Life and Death*. New York: Basic Books.

Wilkinson, R. and Pickett, K. (2010). *The Spirit Level*. London: Penguin.

World Health Organization (2008). 'Closing the gap in a generation' taking action on the social determinants of health. Commission on Social Determinants of Health Final Report. Key Concepts. Available at: www.who.int/social_determinants/final_report/key_concepts_en.pdf?ua=1 (accessed 14 May 2019)

CONCLUSION

Darren J. Edwards and Stephanie Best

This textbook has discussed the main topic areas covered in a health and social care BSc degree. There were three main sections: (1) 'Underpinning Knowledge', including psychological and sociological principles, academic skills, introduction to research, the law relating to social care, reflective practice and normal physiological effects; (2) 'Health and Social Care in Action' exploring safeguarding children and adults, childcare provision, health promotion and health psychology, working with young people, working with people in mental illnesses, and adopting child's rights and participatory approaches to health and social care; and (3) 'Contemporary Topics' such as evidence-based practice, management and leadership, legal and ethical issues, equity, care and social justice, and disability and inequalities.

Reading this textbook provides you with a consolidated background in health and social care which will allow you to consider the impact of some of the current contemporary political issues such as Brexit on health and social care or the growing discussion around the privatisation of the NHS. Even though the health and social care systems differ in each of the home nations there are many common challenges such as the ageing population and concomitant pressures on services or sustainability of health and social care systems. One of the main political focuses in the UK across the four nations recently has been on how health and social care will be funded in the future (Thorlby et al., 2018).

Brexit (if the UK actually leaves the EU) will also impact on the health and social care provision both directly and indirectly. For example, a King's Fund report (Baird and McKenna, 2019) suggested that the recruitment and retention of EU nationals will exacerbate pre-existing staff shortages. This may mean that the UK will need to find new innovative ways to recruit and retain staff in the future.

One area of reform to health and social care may come from the way in which care is delivered. The NHS was established to provide universal health care, free at the point of delivery (which is in contrast to the provision of social care services). However, there has recently been a move towards more person-centered care. The NHS in England (NHS, 2019) has developed a long-term plan to deliver more personalised care which is planned to be rolled out to 2.5 million people by 2023/24 and with the aim of doubling this within a decade. Personalised care means that people will have more choice and control over the planning and delivery of their care representing a shift in power away from the system and into the hands of the patients. Moving the care provision in this direction will fundamentally change the relationship between the patient and health and social care provision, placing increased responsibility on patients and communities, whilst contributing to significant changes in practice for health professionals. Personalised care raises the significance of growing an evidence base in what has worked in shared decision-making; personalised care and support planning; enabling choice; and social prescribing involving community support and personalised health budgets.

Of course, many of these issues will likely lead to some fundamental shifts in the health and social care system for the future. However, for many of these, such as Brexit and personalised care, it is simply too early to understand the full impact of these on the health and social care system. A second edition of this textbook in a few years will, however, be able to explore some of these socio-political issues in more detail. For now though, we hope this textbook will allow you to think more broadly about these contemporary issues in the health and social care provision of the UK, providing you with concrete academic support in your health and social care BSc degree.

REFERENCES

Baird, B. and McKenna, H. (2019). Brexit: the implications for health and social care. Available at: www. kingsfund.org.uk/publications/articles/brexit-implications-health-social-care

NHS England (2019). What is personalised care. Available at: www.england.nhs.uk/personalisedcare/ what-is-personalised-care/

Thorlby, R., Starling, A., Broadbent, C. and Watt, A. (2018). The NHS at 70: What's the problem with social care, and why do we need to do better? Available at: www.kingsfund.org.uk/publications/ nhs-70-whats-the-problem-with-social-care

INDEX

Page numbers in *italics* refer to Figures and page numbers in **bold** refer to Tables and Boxes.